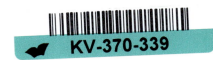

Contents

Perspectives in Coeliac Disease

Perspectives in Coeliac Disease

Edited by B. McNicholl, C. F. McCarthy and P. F. Fottrell

Departments of Paediatrics, Medicine and Biochemistry, University College and the Regional Hospital, Galway, Ireland

Proceedings of the Third Symposium on Coeliac Disease, held at University College, Galway, September 19–21, 1977

MTP PRESS LIMITED *International Medical Publishers*

Published by
MTP Press Limited
St Leonard's House
Lancaster, England

ISBN: 0 85200 224–6

Printed in Great Britain by Blackburn Times Press,
Northgate, Blackburn, Lancs. BB2 1AB

CONTENTS

CONTENTS

List of Chairmen and Co-ordinators

Chairmen
P. F. Fottrell
J. S. Trier
C. F. McCarthy
A. Ferguson
B. McNicholl
C. C. Booth
A. H. Ch. Haex
A. E. Read
W. Th. J. M. Hekkens
C. M. Anderson
T. Cooke

Co-ordinators
E. Wauters
T. J. Peters
J. Houghton
J. Flynn
J. Fielding
G. Connolly
A. P. Douglas
G. Love
H. Grimes
B. Egan-Mitchell
R. Comerford

List of Participants

L. AKSNES
The Children's Hospital, Bergen, Norway

E. ALBERT
Universitäts-Kinderklinik, D-800
Munich 2, West Germany

B. S. ANAND
Nuffield Department of Clinical
Medicine, The Radcliffe Infirmary,
Oxford OX2 6HE

A. ANDREAS
The Children's Hospital, Bergen,
Norway

P. ASQUITH
The Alastair Frazer and John Squire
Metabolic and Clinical Investigation
Unit, East Birmingham Hospital,
Birmingham B9 5ST

A. BAER
The Johns Hopkins Hospital, Baltimore,
Maryland 21205, USA

B. G. BAKER
Department of Medicine, University of
Bristol Medical School, Bristol

S. H. BAKER
Department of Medicine, Regional
Hospital, Galway, Ireland

K. BAKLIEN
Institute of Immunology and
Rheumatology, Oslo 1, Norway

R. E. BARRY
Department of Medicine, University of
Bristol Medical School, Bristol

M. K. BASU
The Alastair Frazer and John Squire
Metabolic and Clinical Investigation
Unit, East Birmingham Hospital,
Birmingham B9 5ST

T. M. BAYLESS
The Johns Hopkins Hospital, Baltimore,
Maryland 21205, USA

J. J. BERNIER
Hôpital St Lazare, F-75010 Paris, France

R. BERTELE
Universitâts-Kinderklinik, D-8000
Munich 2, West Germany

H. S. BESTERMAN
Department of Medicine and
Histochemistry, Royal Postgraduate
Medical School, Hammersmith Hospital,
London W12 0HS

S. R. BLOOM
Royal Postgraduate Medical School,
Hammersmith Hospital, London
W12 0HS

MARY A. BOURKE
Department of Medicine, Regional
Hospital, Galway, Ireland

C. BOZIC
Clinique Universitaire de Pediatrie,
CH-1211 Geneva, Switzerland

xiii

P. BRANDTZAEG
Institute of Immunology and
Rheumatology, Oslo 1, Norway

K. D. BUCHANAN
The Queen's University of Belfast,
Institute of Clinical Science, Belfast
BT12 6BJ, Northern Ireland

A. BUGE
Clinique Neurologique, Hôpital de la
Salpetriere, F-75634 Paris cedex 13,
France

D. N. CHALLACOMBE
The Children's Research Unit, Musgrove
Park Hospital, Taunton, Somerset
TA1 5DA

H. M. CHAPEL
The Alistair Frazer and John Squire
Metabolic and Clinical Investigation
Unit, East Birmingham Hospital,
Birmingham B9 5ST

L. CHARBONNIER
Unité de Recherches de Génétique
Médicale, U 12 (INSERM), Hôpital des
Enfants-Malades, F-75730 Paris cedex 15,
France

H. F. CHIU
Department of Pathology, The University
of Western Ontario, London, Ontario,
W6A 4G5, Canada

W. F. CLEERE
Department of Medicine, University
College, Galway, Ireland

O. J. J. CLUYSENAER
Division of Gastroenterology,
Department of Medicine, St Radboud
Ziekenhuis, Nijmegen, The Netherlands

F. R. COMERFORD
Department of Medicine, University
College, Galway, Ireland

W. T. COOKE
Postgraduate Medical Centre, Selly Oak
Hospital, Birmingham B29 6JD

B. T. COOPER
Gastroenterology Unit, Royal
Postgraduate Medical School,
Hammersmith Hospital, London
W12 0HS

J. COX
Clinique Universitaire de Pediatrie,
CH-1211 Geneva, Switzerland

P. D. DAWKINS
The Children's Research Unit, Musgrove
Park Hospital, Taunton, Somerset
TA1 5DA

G. DELÉZE
Clinique Universitaire de Pediatrie,
CH-1211 Geneva, Switzerland

D. DENVIL
Clinique Neurologique, Hôpital de la
Salpetriere, F-75634 Paris cedex 13,
France

A. P. DOUGLAS
Division of Gastroenterology, University
of Southern California, Los Angeles,
California 90033, USA

B. EGAN-MITCHELL
Department of Medicine, Regional
Hospital, Galway, Ireland

R. EIFE
Universitäts-Kinderklinik, D-8000
Munich 2, West Germany

M. ELMES
Department of Medicine, The Queen's
University of Belfast, Belfast BT12 6BJ,
Northern Ireland

A. ENDERS
Universitäts-Kinderklinik, D-8000
Munich 2, West Germany

K. P. ETERMAN
Department of Auto-immune Diseases,
Central Laboratory of the Netherlands
Red Cross Blood Transfusion Service,
Amsterdam, The Netherlands

Z. M. FALCHUK
Peter Bent Brigham Hospital, Boston,
Massachusetts 02115, USA

O. FAUSA
Institute of Immunology and
Rheumatology, Oslo 1, Norway

T. E. W. FELTKAMP
Laboratory of Experimental and Clinical
Immunology, University of Amsterdam,
Amsterdam, The Netherlands

R. FÈTE
Clinique Universitaire de Pediatrie,
CH-1211 Geneva, Switzerland

K. FISCHER
Universitäts-Kinderklinik, D-2000
Hamburg 20, West Germany

G. FLUGE
The Children's Hospital, Bergen,
Norway

P. F. FOTTRELL
Department of Biochemistry, University
College, Galway, Ireland

N. E. FRANCE
The Queen Elizabeth Hospital for
Children, London E2 8PS

H. GAZE
Laboratory of Gastroenterology,
University Hospital, Leiden, The
Netherlands

M. K. GOLDEN
Department of Medicine, The Queen's
University of Belfast, Belfast BT12 6BJ,
Northern Ireland

D. M. GOODENBERGER
National Institutes of Health, Bethesda,
Maryland 20014, USA

R. GRÜTTNER
Universitäts-Kinderklinik, D-2000
Hamburg 20, West Germany

B. HADORN
Laboratory of Gastroenterology,
University Hospital, Leiden, The
Netherlands

M. R. HAENEY
Regional Immunology Laboratory,
East Birmingham Hospital, Birmingham
B9 5ST

A. J. Ch. HAEX
Department of Gastroenterology,
University Hospital, Leiden, The
Netherlands

K. HAFFEN
U 61 (INSERM),
Strasbourg, France

M. R. HAENEY
Department of Experimental Pathology,
University of Birmingham, East
Birmingham Hospital, Birmingham
B9 5ST

H. K. HARMS
Universitäts-Kinderklinik, D-8000
Munich 2, West Germany

J. T. HARRIES
Institute of Child Health, London
WC1N 1EH

H. P. HAURI
Universitäts-Kinderklinik, CH-3010
Bern, Switzerland

J. J. HAUW
Laboratoire de Neuropathologie Ch.
Foix (Pr. Escourolle), Hôpital de la
Salpetriere, F-75634 Paris cedex 13,
France

J. A. HECK
Department of Gastroenterology,
University Hospital, Leiden, The
Netherlands

W. Th. J. M. HEKKENS
Laboratory of Gastroenterology,
University Hospital, Leiden, The
Netherlands

T. R. HENDRIX
The Johns Hopkins Hospital, Baltimore,
Maryland 21205, USA

C. HENRY
Department of Medicine, University of
Bristol Medical School, Bristol

C. l'HIRONDEL
Hôpital Saint Lazare, F-75010 Paris,
France

G. K. T. HOLMES
Postgraduate Medical Centre, Selly Oak
Hospital, Birmingham B29 6JD

G. HÜBNER
Universitäts-Kinderklinik, D-8000
Munich 2, West Germany

W. J. JENKINS
Department of Medicine, Royal
Postgraduate Medical School,
Hammersmith Hospital, London
W12 0HS

P. E. JONES
Department of Medicine, Royal
Postgraduate Medical School,
Hammersmith Hospital, London
W12 0HS

J. JOS
Unité de Recherches de Génétique
Médicale, U 12 (INSERM), Hôpital des
Enfants-Malades, F-75730 Paris cedex 15,
France

J. H. van de KAMER
Centraal Instituut voor
Voedingsonderzoek TNO, Zeist, The
Netherlands

D. D. KASARDA
Western Regional Research Laboratory,
US Department of Agriculture, Berkeley,
California 94710, USA

A. J. KATZ
The Children's Hospital Medical Center,
Boston, Massachusetts 02115, USA

M. KEDINGER
Laboratory of Gastroenterology,
University Hospital, Leiden, The
Netherlands

ANNE KILBY
The Queen Elizabeth Hospital for
Children, London E2 8PS

P. J. KUMAR
Department of Gastroenterology,
St Bartholomew's Hospital, London EC1

B. KUNTZ
Universitäts-Kinderklinik, D-8000
Munich 2, West Germany

A. van LEEUWEN
Laboratory of Gastroenterology,
University Hospital, Leiden, The
Netherlands

P. H. LEMS-VAN KAN
Laboratory of Gastroenterology,
University Hospital, Leiden, The
Netherlands

U. LÖHRS
Universitäts-Kinderklinik, D-8000
Munich 2, West Germany

M. S. LOSWOSKY
Department of Medicine, University of
Leeds, St James's Hospital, Leeds
LS9 7TF

A. H. G. LOVE
Department of Medicine, The Queen's
University of Belfast, Belfast BT12 6BJ,
Northern Ireland

C. F. McCARTHY
Department of Medicine, Regional
Hospital, Galway, Ireland

D. McMASTER
Department of Medicine, The Queen's
University of Belfast, Belfast BT12 6BJ,
Northern Ireland

A. McNICHOLAS
Universitäts-Kinderklinik, D-8000
Munich 2, West Germany

B. McNICHOLL
Department of Paediatrics, Regional
Hospital, Galway, Ireland

D. L. MANN
Immunophysiology Section, Metabolism
Branch, National Cancer Institute,
National Institutes of Health, Bethesda,
Maryland 20014, USA

J. A. MANNING
Institute of Child Health, London
WC1N 1EH

D. K. MECHAM
Western Regional Research Laboratory,
US Department of Agriculture
Agricuture, Berkeley, California 94710,
USA

A. MÉGEVAND
Clinique Universitaire de Pediatrie,
CH-1211 Geneva, Switzerland

R. D. MONTGOMERY
The Metabolic Research Unit, East
Birmingham Hospital, Birmingham
B9 5ST

J. MOSSÉ
Unité de Recherches de Génétique
Médicale, U 12 (INSERM), Hôpital des
Enfants-Malades, F-75730 Paris cedex
15, France

J.-F. MOUGENOT
Unité de Recherches de Génétique
Médicale, U 12 (INSERM), Hôpital des
Enfants-Malades, F-75730 Paris cedex
15, France

D. P. R. MULLER
Institute of Child Health, London
WC1N 1EH

J. A. NICHOLSON
Department of Medicine, Royal
Postgraduate Medical School,
Hammersmith Hospital, London
W12 0HS

D. NUSSLÉ
Clinique Universitaire de Pediatrie,
CH-1211 Geneva, Switzerland

F. A. O'CONNOR
Department of Medicine, The Queen's
University of Belfast, Belfast BT12 6BJ,
Northern Ireland

D. P. O'DONOGHUE
Department of Gastroenterology,
St Bartholomew's Hospital, London
EC1

R. E. OFFORD
Laboratory of Molecular Biophysics,
University of Oxford, Oxford

A. S. PEÑA
Laboratory of Gastroenterology,
University Hospital, Leiden, The
Netherlands

T. J. PETERS
Department of Medicine, Royal
Postgraduate Medical School,
Hammersmith Hospital, London
W12 0HS

J. J. PHELAN
Department of Biochemistry, University
College Galway, Ireland

J. PIRIS
Gibson Laboratories, The Radcliffe
Infirmary, Oxford OX2 6HE

J. M. POLAK
Department of Medicine, Royal
Postgraduate Medical School,
Hammersmith Hospital, London
W12 0HS

C. O. QUALSET
Department of Agronomy and Range
Science, University of California, Davis,
California 95616, USA

J. C. RAMBAUD
Hôpital Saint Lazare, F-75010 Paris,
France

G. RANCUREL
Clinique Neurologie, Hôpital de la
Salpetriere, F-75634 Paris cedex 13,
France

P. M. RAWCLIFFE
Nuffield Department of Medicine, The
Radcliffe Infirmary, Oxford OX2 6HE

A. E. READ
Department of Medicine, University of
Bristol Medical School, Bristol

P. REISSINGER
Universitäts-Kinderklinik, D-8000
Munich 2, West Germany

J. REY
Unité de Recherches de Génétique
Médicale, U 12 (INSERM), Hôpital des
Enfants-Malades, F-75730 Paris cedex 15,
France

K. ROBERTSON
The Children's Research Unit, Musgrove
Park Hospital, Taunton, Somerset

J. J. van ROOD
Laboratory of Gastroenterology,
University Hospital, Leiden, The
Netherlands

F. W. M. de ROOIJ
Laboratory of Gastroenterology,
University Hospital, Leiden, The
Netherlands

P. C. M. ROSEKRANS
Department of Gastroenterology,
University Hospital, Leiden, The
Netherlands

I. N. ROSS
The Metabolic Research Unit, East
Birmingham Hospital, Birmingham
B9 5ST

E. ROSSIPAL
Universitäts-Kinderklinik, A-8036 Graz,
Austria

M. ROULET
Clinique Universitaire de Pediatrie,
CH-1211 Geneva, Switzerland

B. SCHIESSEL
Universitäts-Kinderklinik, D-8000
Munich 2, West Germany

P. H. M. SCHILLINGS
Department of Morbid Anatomy, St
Radboud Ziekenhuis, Nijmegen, The
Netherlands

J. SCHMITZ
Unité de Recherches de Génétique
Médicale, U 12 (INSERM), F-75730 Paris
cedex 15, France

S. SCHOLZ
Universitäts-Kinderklinik, D-8000
Munich 2, West Germany

B. B. SCOTT
Lincoln County Hospital, Lincoln
LN2 5QY

D. G. SCOTT
Department of Medicine, University of
Leeds, St James's Hospital, Leeds
LS9 7TF

D. H. SHMERLING
Department of Paediatrics, University of
Zurich, The Children's Hospital,
CH-8032 Zurich, Switzerland

M. SINAASPPEL
University of Amsterdam,
Binnengasthuis, Amsterdam, The
Netherlands

E. E. STERCHI
Biochemistry Research Laboratory,
Department of Biological Sciences,
University of Keele, Keele, Staffs,
ST5 5BG

M. STERN
Universitäts-Kinderklinik, D-2000
Hamburg 20, West Germany

FIONA M. STEVENS
Department of Gastroenterology,
Regional Hospital, Galway, Ireland

W. STROBER
Immunophysiology Section, Metabolism
Branch, National Cancer Institute,
National Institutes of Health, Bethesda,
Maryland 20014, USA

LIST OF PARTICIPANTS

R. A. THOMPSON
The Regional Immunology Laboratory,
East Birmingham Hospital,
Birmingham B9 5ST

J. H. M. van TONGEREN
Division of Gastroenterology,
Department of Medicine, St Radboud
Ziekenhuis, Nijmegen, The Netherlands

J. H. TRIPP
Institute of Child Health, London
WC1N 1EH

S. C. TRUELOVE
Nuffield Department of Medicine, The
Radcliffe Infirmary, Oxford OX2 6HE

R. R. P. de VRIES
Department of Gastroenterology,
University Hospital, Leiden, The
Netherlands

J. A. WALKER-SMITH
The Queen Elizabeth Hospital for
Children, London E2 8PS

W. C. WATSON
Department of Medicine, University of
Western Ontario, London, Ontario,
W6A 4G5, Canada

D. W. WATT
Department of Medicine, Regional
Hospital, Galway, Ireland

E. A. K. WAUTERS
Wilhelmina Kinderziekenhuis,
Universitetskinderkliniek, Utrecht, The
Netherlands

Ch. WEESER-KRELL
Universitäts-Kinderklinik, D-8000
Munich 2, West Germany

M. M. WEISER
Gastrointestinal Unit, Massachusetts
General Hospital, Boston, Massachusetts
02114, USA

H. WETZMÜLLER
Universitäts-Kinderklinik, D-8000
Munich 2, West Germany

J. F. WOODLEY
Biochemistry Research Laboratory,
Department of Biological Sciences,
University of Keele, Keele, Staffs,
ST5 5BG

J. H. YARDLEY
The Johns Hopkins Hospital, Baltimore,
Maryland 21205, USA

Preface

The Third International Coeliac Symposium was held in University College, Galway, Ireland, from September 18 to 21, 1977. The decision to hold the meeting in Galway resulted from the very high incidence of the disease in the West of Ireland and the presence there of a group with strong and continuing interests in studying the disease. It is unlikely that the meeting would have taken place without the enthusiastic involvement and financial support of Mr Jerry Milner, of Milner Scientific and Medical Research, who also played a prominent part in the previous meetings in London and Leiden. We also owe much to the other members of the Organizing Committee, particularly in the selection of the papers. The 150 invited participants represented varied scientific and medical disciplines and came from those parts of the world where an awareness of the disease and its problems has been highlighted. If groups elsewhere have contributions to make these would be welcomed by the organizers of the next symposium. Approximately 60 came from the United Kingdom, 60 from Continental Europe, 15 from North America and 15 from the Republic of Ireland. Since Galway is a little off the beaten track, those who participated deserve a special commendation.

The 51 papers that were presented at the meeting are printed in this book, each being followed by a slightly edited version of the ensuing discussion. Listed also are the titles and authors of the posters that were exhibited. There has been no attempt to edit the papers, except in as much as the phrasing of some of the papers has been slightly altered in the interests of conformity. The editors would like to record with gratitude the help they have received over a number of years from the Medical Research Council of Ireland, the Wellcome Trust, the Western Health Board, the National Science Council, University College, Galway and our colleagues at the Regional Hospitals and University College, Galway. Finally, we are much indebted for secretarial work to Maura Greaney, Una Cradock, Maureen Hansberry and Lily Johnston, and to Stewart Baker for help with illustrations and photography.

B. McNicholl
C. F. McCarthy
P. F. Fottrell

Section I
Protein chemistry and toxicity

1

The toxicity of gliadin, a review

W. Th. J. M. HEKKENS

Protein toxicity in coeliac disease (CD) must describe the interaction between one or perhaps more than one molecule from the mixture that we define as gliadin and the cells from the intestinal wall. We need a test system to determine this interaction. These three elements will be considered in this review.

GLIADIN PROTEINS

Gliadin can be defined in different ways. The definition is not strict but depends on the separation method used. About 40% of the total protein from wheat is gliadin, though the composition differs in each variety of wheat[1]. In electrophoresis, even in a simple system, a great number of bands can be seen (Figure 1.1). When we look at the individual molecules, we can see that the main part of a protein is formed by its backbone, the strain of amino acids linked together by amide bonds. The first thing we can ask is if there is something special in that main structure of gliadin molecules. From the amino acid analysis follows a high content of proline (16%).

This proline interferes with the proteolytic activity of some enzymes and this could, at least to some extent, explain why gliadin is hydrolysed more slowly *in vitro* as well as *in vivo* than for instance casein or albumin[2]. We know on the other hand that 'gliadin' can be hydrolysed *in vitro* by pepsin and pancreatic enzymes without loss of toxicity. Although we do not know about the resistance to hydrolysis of each molecule in the gliadin mixture, we know from different authors[3,4] that degraded molecules are toxic, when the molecular weight is greater than 2000 and smaller than 10 000.

The next level to look at in the molecule concerns the side-chain. Different amino acids give these different chains. In gliadin the high content of glutamine is of special interest. About one in every three

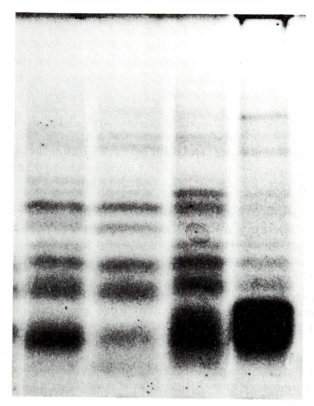

Figure 1.1 Polyacrylamide gel electrophoresis of gliadins. A, B and C, three batches of gliadin; D, a crude α-gliadin preparation

amino acids is glutamine. The consequence for the toxicity has already been demonstrated by van de Kamer[5]. Deamidation abolishes the toxicity if the 15% of hydrolysis of the peptide bonds that occurs at the same time did not have any influence on the toxicity. There is no experimental evidence to rule out this last possibility.

The third structural element that can contribute to the toxicity is the conjugates. They consist of molecules covalently bound to the side-chains of the amino acids. Phelan[6] claimed that carbohydrates are not only bound to proteins in gliadin but also that enzymatic elimination of that carbohydrate from the protein abolishes the toxicity. Bernardin[7] could not demonstrate the presence of glycoproteins in his A-gliadin that proved to be toxic in an *in vitro* system.

Apart from these chemically bound conjugates there is a possibility that those molecules in gliadin that are mainly low-charged due to the high content of aliphatic amino acids and the glutamine, bind other molecules by hydrogen bridges or by absorption. Lipids and glycolipids[8] for instance are known to be bound to the surface and could possibly contribute to the toxicity. De Rooy[9] has studied this possibility and will report on it later. As far as the protein is concerned we come to the following conclusions:

a. Information about the composition of the protein mixture is incomplete.

b. Although backbone and side-chains are different from other proteins, there is no direct indication for a toxic action. Indirectly the low charge of the molecules could interact with the cell membranes.

c. Conjugates or molecules otherwise bound to the proteins of gliadin could play a role in toxicity, but information is not yet sufficient to draw this conclusion.

d. A better definition of the material used in the different studies would contribute very much to the definition of the common part in the mixtures of proteins in all these studies.

THE TARGET ORGAN

How can a structural element in one or more of the molecules from gliadin interact with some component from the intestinal wall? We can look at that from a morphologic or from a functional point of view.

Rubin[10] was the first who tried to localize gliadin after instillation of wheat by an immunofluorescent technique. He found gliadin mainly localized near the brush border. We tried to demonstrate gliadin after instillation with rabbit antigliadin serum and a peroxidase labelled goat antirabbit gammaglobulin, but we were unable to demonstrate any binding in this way. No other publication that has localized gliadin in intestinal epithelium has come to my attention.

Functional disturbances of gliadin are studied with more success. We will review part of these functions.

Enzymes

Apart from the missing enzyme hypothesis—the first hypothesis in the pathogenesis of CD that still has support and cannot yet be rejected on experimental evidence—a number of enzymatic reactions can be influenced by gliadin. A direct effect can be expected on those enzymes that come in contact with gliadin in the intestinal tract. Pancreatic enzymes are responsible for the first degradation steps of gliadin in normal conditions. We therefore measured the action of gliadin, and for comparison, of casein on the activity of α-amylase and trypsin with synthetic substrates (Table 1.1). Amylase is inhibited specifically

Table 1.1 The action of gliadin, casein and a gliadin degradation product (fraction III) on the activity of serum amylase and crystalline trypsin with synthetic substrates

Enzyme	Substrate	Addition	Activity in % of no addition
Amylase	blue α-amylosepolymer (Pharmacia)	—	100
,,	,,	casein 4 mg	93
,,	,,	α-gliadin 4.3 mg	2
,,	,,	fraction III 4 mg	80
,,	,,	20 mg	12
Trypsin	tosyl-L-arginine methylester	—	100
,,	,,	casein 4 mg	94
,,	,,	gliadin 4 mg	95
,,	,,	fraction III 4 mg	110

whereas trypsin is not.

The decrease in activity of the brush border enzymes of the enterocytes can, according to Wright and Watson[11] be explained by the enteroblastic hyperplasia of the intestinal mucosa in CD.

These changes as well as the changes in lysosomal activity[12] are the consequence of the presence of gliadin. Their content and activity return to normal on a gluten-free diet, so we either have to accept the hypothesis that all these enzymes in patients with CD are different from those of normal people or to accept the hypothesis that these effects are secondary and a consequence of structural changes in the enterocyte.

Immunity

Humoral immunity has in my opinion two important points to show in relation to CD. The first point of interest is that in CD not only antibodies to gliadin are raised but also antibodies to all kinds of food[13]. That means that not only gliadin passes the intestinal wall but all kinds of protein do. Baklien and Fausa[14] concluded therefore that 'the local immunocyte pattern seen in bowel diseases is probably determined by the extent of the antigen and mitogen penetration and may thus reflect the degree of mucosal damage'. Also in normal people antibodies to food components including gliadin are present, so penetration of proteins always happens and an explanation must be found for the increased antigen level in CD. The second phenomenon is the formation of immune complexes[15,16], giving rise to tissue damage and possibly to association with other diseases when deposition occurs in other organs. It seems logical to me that immune complexes are formed but nobody to my knowledge has looked if these immune complexes are only related to gliadin or also to other food proteins.

If this complex formation occurs only in coeliacs and only with antibodies to gliadin, then this phenomenon could be primary in CD.

In cell-mediated immunity the recognition of gliadin by immune-competent cells in the gastrointestinal tract of coeliacs is the central event.

As a result of the normal protein passage an immune reaction occurs. This reaction is inherited by an immune response gene. There should be no reaction to other proteins that cross the intestinal wall. An alternative hypothesis is also possible. A change in permeability of the cell membrane could give rise to an increased transport with as a consequence an immune response. In this hypothesis the membrane structure is the genetically determined factor. Specificity of the reaction again is a crucial point. The question of specificity however is difficult to answer as there is heterogeneity in even a pure α-gliadin preparation is demonstrated by means of humoral antibody formation by de Rooy[9]. This stresses again the importance of the utilization of pure proteins to prove that the toxic action and the immune response are identical.

Hormones

The regulation of intestinal function is under hormonal control. Therefore it seems logical to investigate how hormones are influenced by gliadin in CD. The gut hormones and especially secretin have been investigated.

Polak[17] found that in CD there is hyperplasia of endocrine cells, especially of S-cells. According to O'Connor[18] this hyperplasia is caused by a failure of release rather than an excessive synthesis. Infusion of acid causes a flat curve in secretin response in coeliac patients. In response to food, CCK also shows a flat curve but the unchallenged CCK level is significantly increased above normal[19]. On the other hand, gallbladder response to CCK–PZ is normal[20], but pancreas response to secretin–CCK is increased.

Hormonal changes on the level beyond the intestine are also described.

Eggermont[22] found lower levels of plasma growth hormone following insulin administration. Green[23] measured a rise in total plasma testosterone and other androgens. These values returned to normal on a gluten-free diet.

The question if gliadin acts directly beyond the intestine or if the changes in hormonal levels are secondary to changes in the intestinal wall is still unanswered.

The same is true for the mediator 5-hydroxytryptamine. According to Challacombe[24] the level in intestinal biopsies is increased in untreated coeliacs and this could contribute to the morphological changes[25].

Related diseases

Some other questions about the action of gliadin are not yet answered. Why is CD more frequently found in infertile women as claimed by Wilson and Wright[26]? Why is CD more frequently found in schizophrenic patients and why is, according to Dohan[27], the incidence of schizophrenia in coeliacs greater than normal? In my opinion immune complexes alone cannot explain these phenomena as suggested by Scott and Losowski[15].

Only in some diseases a common locus in the HLA typing has been found. Inheritance of CD can be explained by postulating two different genes[28]. A related disease could be caused by a combination of one of these loci with a minor change in the second locus.

Membranes

One of the genetic factors is most probably related to the cellular immune response. In my opinion the other one is related to membranes. Weiser and Douglas[29] propose a membrane receptor and have isolated a glycoprotein from gluten with a lectine-like activity. Differences in permeability giving rise to increased food antibody titres and disturbances of membrane-bound and lysosomal enzymes like the disaccharidases all point in the direction of changes in permeability of the enterocyte.

Conclusions

Gliadin toxicity in relation to the target organ allows for the following conclusions:

a. Enzymes are involved in toxicity but are as far as known are not a primary cause of the disease.

b. Membrane permeability and binding are altered in CD and could be part of the primary cause.

c. Alterations in the secretion of hormones and mediators exist and are mainly unexplained.

d. Humoral antibody synthesis is changed secondary to the disease.

e. Cell-mediated immunity is changed, is genetically determined and may be primarily related to CD.

TEST SYSTEMS

Establishing toxicity means that we have to perform a test. Until recently these tests were done only with human material. The only test system that is non-human is based on the fragility of rat liver lysosomes. Cornell and Townley[30] claim that fractions from gliadin digests increase the acidphosphatase release when lysosomes are incubated with these fractions. We repeated this test with gliadin and with a peptic–tryptic digest similar to Frazer's fraction III. We did the same tests with casein. As shown in Figure 1.2 no different reaction was obtained with gliadin, so in our opinion the test lacks specificity and therefore does not discriminate between gliadin toxicity to coeliacs and a general cytotoxic effect of some proteins and peptides.

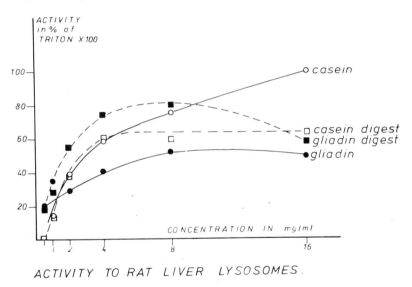

Figure 1.2 Influence of gliadin, casein and their peptic–tryptic digests on the stability of rat liver lysosomes

From the tests with human material the *in vitro* tests are the most preferable ones, being non-offending and utilizing small amounts of material. Serum tests are used only in the demonstration of antibodies to gliadin. With a quantitative technique it is possible to screen patients and to compare results over a longer period of time. We have used the ELISA technique in screening and in family studies as Rosekrans[31] will report. Blood lymphocytes are used by Peña[32] in his test for B-cell alloantigens. Leucocyte adherence is inhibited in CD according to Allardyce[33]. The surfaces of these cells recognize gliadin not only in the intestinal wall but also *in vitro*. The tests are specific and in this way promising in relation to toxicity. Other cell types have also been considered as targets for gliadin. Cordone[34] utilized fibroblasts from skin or intestine of gluten-sensitive patients. He claims *in vitro* degeneration of fibroblasts after addition of peptide fractions to the medium. In our hands the test was not very reproducible and not specific to gliadin only.

From *in vitro* tests with biopsies only Jos[35] claims results that are comparable with *in vivo* studies, so the overall results are rather poor, thus leaving us with *in vivo* tests as the most definitive. With *in vivo* tests we can choose between absorption tests (xylose, fat), skin tests or intestinal tests.

Absorption tests were discussed in the previous symposium; they are

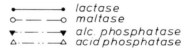

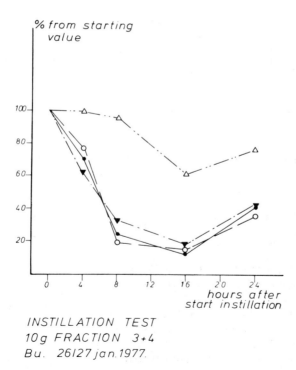

INSTILLATION TEST
10 g FRACTION 3+4
Bu. 26/27 jan.1977.

Figure 1.3 Instillation test of 5 g peptic–tryptic digest of gliadin in a biopsy-proven coeliac patient in remission

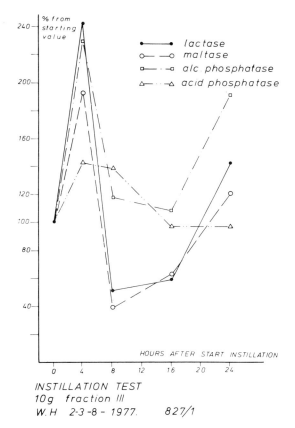

Figure 1.4A Instillation test of 5 g peptic–tryptic digest of gliadin in a normal person

of value but not decisive. Skin tests[36] measure the amount of infiltration and their specificity remains to be proven by utilizing digests
from other proteins in the same system.

We have proposed some years ago[37] an instillation test, being not
harmful to the patient, of short duration and requiring moderate
amounts of protein in comparison to long-term challenge. We have
utilized this test for determination of toxicity for several fractions.
When we express the results as a relative change in brush border
enzyme activity we obtain a definite depression when performed in
patients in complete remission (Figure 1.3).

Correlation with xylose absorption and mucosal damage on histological grounds is also found. It turned out, however, that in normal
individuals the curves are not as regular as one would expect (Figure
1.4). An increase in activity within a few hours after instillation of

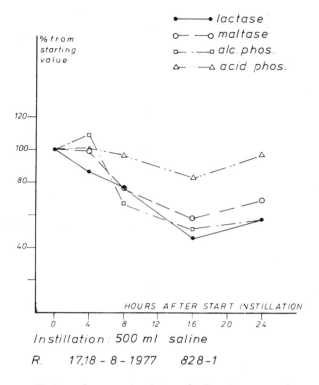

Figure 1.4B Instillation of an equal volume of saline in a normal person

fraction III is often found whereas instillation of saline in one case caused a slow and moderate decrease in enzyme activity. In all cases, however, the values remained within the limits of normal[38].

In the end we are left with the problem of having no single unequivocal test to prove the toxicity of an ill-defined protein to cause an effect that lacks uniform interpretation. I think it one task of this symposium to come to a more open exchange of materials and methods in order to be able to compare the results obtained by the different groups. Only in this way can a more rapid progress in the solution of the gliadin toxicity be expected.

References

1. Kasarda, D.D. (1976). Wheat Proteins. In: Y. Pomeranz (ed.). *Advances in Cereal Science,* **1.** pp. 158–236. (St. Paul, Minn: Am. Ass. of Cereal Chemists)
2. Zimmerman-Nielsen, C. and Schønheyder, F. (1962). On the rate of disappearance of protein from the small intestine in vivo. *Biochim. Biophys. Acta,* **63,** 201

3. Jos, J. and Rey, J. (1975). L'apport de la culture organotypique a l'étude pathogenique de la maladie coeliaque. *Archs. Fr. Mal. App. Dig.*, **64**, 461
4. Dissanayake, A. S., Jerrome, D. W., Offord, R. E., Truelove, S. C. and Whitehead, R. (1974). Identifying toxic fractions of wheat gluten and their effect on the jejunal mucosa in coeliac disease. *Gut*, **15**, 931
5. Van de Kamer, J. H. and Weyers, H. A. (1955). Some experiments on the cause of the harmful effect of wheat gliadin. *Acta Ped.*, **44**, 465
6. Phelan, J. J., McCarthy, C. F., Stevens, F. M., McNicholl, B. and Fottrell, P. F. (1974). The nature of gliadin toxicity in coeliac disease: A new concept. In: W. Th. J. M. Hekkens and A. S. Peña (eds.) *Coeliac Disease*, pp. 60–70 (Leiden: Stenfert Kroese)
7. Bernardin, J. E., Saunders, R. M. and Kasarda, D. D. (1976). Absence of carbohydrate in celiac-toxic A-gliadin. *Cereal Chem.*, **53**, 612
8. Greene, F. C. (1975). On mechanisms of surfactant dough conditioner functionality. *Bakers's Digest*, **49**, 16
9. De Rooy, F. W. M., van Duyn, W., Lems-van Kan, P. H. and Hekkens, W. Th. J. M. (1977). Heterogeneity of α-gliadin. Ibid
10. Rubin, W., Fauci, A. S., Sleisinger, M. H. and Jeffries, G. H. (1965). Immuno-fluorescent studies in adult celiac disease. *J. Clin. Invest.*, **44**, 477
11. Wright, N. A. and Watson, A. J. (1974). The morphogenesis of the flat avillous mucosa of coeliac disease. In: W. Th. J. M. Hekkens and A. S. Peña (eds.) *Coeliac Disease*, pp. 141–150 (Leiden: Stenfert Kroese)
12. Peters, T. J., Heath, J. R., Wansbrough-Jones, M. H. and Doe, W. F. (1975). Enzyme activities and properties of lysosomes and brush borders in jejunal biopsies from control subjects and patients with coeliac disease. *Clin. Sci. Mol. Med.*, **48**, 259
13. Kumar, P. J., Ferguson, A., Lancaster-Smith, M. and Clark, M. (1976). Food antibodies in patients with dermatitis herpetiformis and adult coeliac disease—relationship to jejunal morphology. *Scand. J. Gastroenterol.*, **11**, 5
14. Baklien, K., Fausa, O., Thune, P. O. and Gjone, E. (1977). Immunoglobulins in jejunal mucosa and serum from patients with dermatitis herpetiformis. *Scand. J. Gastroenterol.*, **12**, 161
15. Scott, B. C. and Losowsky, M. S. (1975). Coeliac disease: A cause of various associated diseases? *Lancet*, **ii**, 956
16. Mohammed, I., Holborow, E. J., Fry, L., Thompson, B. R., Hoffbrand, A. V. and Stewart, J. S. (1976). Multiple immune complexes and hypocomplementaemia in dermatitis herpetiformis and coeliac disease. *Lancet*, **ii**, 487
17. Polak, J. M., Pearse, A. G.E., van Noorden, S., Bloom, S. R. and Rossiter, M. A. (1973). Secretin cells in coeliac disease. *Gut*, **14**, 870
18. O'Connor, F. A., McLoughlin, J. C. and Buchanan, K. D. (1977). Impaired immunoreactive secretin release in coeliac disease. *Br. Med. J.*, **294**, 811
19. Low-Beer, T. S., Harvey, R. F., Rhys Davies, E. and Read, A. L. (1975). Abnormalities of serum cholecystokinin and gallbladder emptying in celiac desease. *N. Engl. J. Med.*, **18**, 961
20. Colombato, L. O., Parodi, H. and Cantor, D. (1977). Biliary studies in patients with celiac sprue. *Dig. Dis.*, **22**, 96
21. Rolny, P. and Gillberg, R. (1976). Pancreatic exocrine secretion in patients with coeliac disease. *Scand. J. Gastroenterol.*, **11**, (suppl.), 31
22. Vanderschueren-Lodeweyckx, M., Wolter, R., Molla, A. Eggermont, E. and Eeckels, R. (1973). Plasma growth hormone in coeliac disease. *Helv. Paediat. Acta*, **28**, 349
23. Green, J. R. B., Edwards, C. R. W., Goble, H. L. and Dawson, A. M. (1977). Reversible insensitivity to androgens in men with untreated gluten enteropathy.

Lancet, **i,** 280

24. Challacombe, D. N., Dawkins, P. D. and Baker, P. (1976). Duodenal tissue concentrations of 5-hydroxytryptamine in coeliac disease. *Lancet,* **ii,** 522

25. Challacombe, D. N., Dawkins, P. D., Baker, P. and Robertson, K. (1977). 5-Hydroxytryptamine metabolism in patients with coeliac disease. Presented at the *10th Annual Meeting ESPGAN,* May 13–14, Utrecht

26. Wilson, C., Eade, O. E., Elstein, M. and Wright, R. (1976). Subclinical coeliac disease and infertility. *Brit. Med. J.,* **III,** 215

27. Dohan, F. C. (1970). Coeliac disease and schizophrenia. *Lancet,* **i,** 897

28. Meehra-Khan, P. *et al.* (1978). Genetics of coeliac disease. Presented at this symposium.

29. Weiser, M. M. and Douglas, A. P. (1976). An alternative mechanism for gluten toxicity in coeliac disease. *Lancet,* **i,** 567

30. Cornell, H. J. and Townley, R. R. W. (1973). The effect of gliadin peptides on rat-liver lysosomes in relation to pathogenesis of coeliac disease. *Clin. Chim. Acta,* **49,** 181

31 Rosekrans, P. C. M., Peña, A. S., Hekkens, W. Th. J. M., de Vries, R. R. P. and Haex, A. J. Ch. (1978). Coeliac disease. A family study in the Netherlands. Presented at this symposium

32. Peña, A. S., Mann, D. L., Hague, N. E., Heck, J. A. and Strober, W. (1978). B-cell alloantigens and the inheritance of coeliac disease. Presented at this symposium.

33. Allardayce, R. A. and Shearman, D. J. C. (1975). Leukocyte reactivity to α-gliadin in dermatitis herpetiformis and adult coeliac disease. *Int. Arch. Allergy Appl. Immunol.,* **48,** 395

34. Cordone, G., Gemme, G., Comelli, A., Vianello, M. G. and Calodoni, S. (1975). Peptidase and coeliac disease. *Lancet,* **i,** 807

35. Jos, J., Lenoir, G., de Ritis, G. and Rey, J. (1975). In vitro pathogenic studies of coeliac disease. *Scand. J. Gastroenterol.,* **10,** 121

36. Anand, B.S. and Truelove, S. C. (1977). Skin test for coeliac disease using a subfraction of gluten. *Lancet,* **i,** 118

37. Hekkens, W. Th. J. M., Haex, A. J. Ch. and Willighagen, R. G. (1970). Some aspects of gliadin fractionation and testing by a histochemical method. In: C. C. Booth and R. H. Dowling (eds.) *Coeliac Diesease* p.11. London: Churchill Livingstone)

38. Sinaasappel, M. and Hekkens, W. Th. J. M. (1978). Alterations of the jejunal mucosa after short-time instillation of gliadin fractions in children with coeliac disease. Presented at this symposium

Discussion of chapter 1

Phelan I would like to pay tribute to the work of Van de Kamer *et al.*, but I wish to point out that following boiling with HCl not only de-amidation occurs, many other reactions will take place when gliadin is incubated with normal HCl at 100°C for several hours.

Hekkens I agree with you and I pointed out that Van de Kamer *et al.* said in their paper that they had at least 15% of hydrolysis together with the deamidation and that is one of the aspects not generally realized. However, hydrolysis of this kind might well have something to do with removal of toxicity also.

2

The heterogeneity of α-gliadin

F. W. M. DE ROOIJ, W. VAN DUYN, P. H. LEMS-VAN KAN
and W. TH. J. M. HEKKENS

INTRODUCTION

The α-gliadin fraction used for instillation experiments by Hekkens[1,2] contains proteins with an electrophoretic mobility that differs from the main part of this fraction. These proteins are classified as albumins using the electrophoretic mobility classification according to Woychik[3] in 1961. The presence of such fast-moving proteins is also described for gluten[3,4]. Gliadin as an extract with alcohol also contains these albumins[5]. In the Second International Coeliac Symposium, Kasarda[6] mentioned these faster-moving proteins in a fraction obtained by an extraction with diluted acid of wheat flour. The toxicity of gliadin defined as an extract with alcohol is proved, but how sure are we about the toxicity of an electrophoretically pure gliadin fraction? We have investigated the presence and the similarity in these electrophoretic non-gliadin proteins in toxic fractions such as gluten and gliadin, and compared them with our α-gliadin fraction. We have developed a preparative method to make an electrophoretically pure gliadin fraction, containing mainly proteins in the α-gliadin region, and tested this fraction for toxicity. Finally we have used preparative isoelectric focussing (IEF) for further fractionation of our α-gliadin fraction, and we have screened our α-gliadin fractions on their reaction with pooled sera from coeliac patients with high antigliadin titre.

Abbreviations used IEF = isoelectric focussing.

MATERIALS

The gluten was a commercial preparation. The gliadin fraction is obtained by extraction of wheat flour (Scout 66) with 60% ethanol. The

α-gliadin fraction, as used in instillation experiments, is obtained using the following isolation procedure, which is, up to the second centrifugation step, a modified procedure of the method according to Bernardin[7] et al.

—extraction of wheat flour (Scout 66) with 0.01 acetic acid (500 g/ 1500 ml)

—centrifugation step: 33 000 g × 20 min

—the supernatant is brought to pH 5.0 with 1 M NaOH

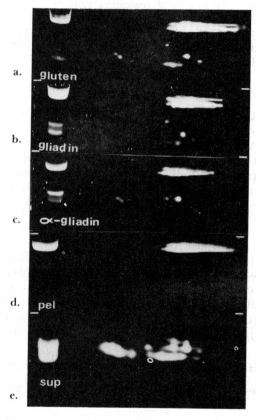

Figure 2.1, a–e Protein maps of gluten (2.1a), gliadin (2.1b) as an alcohol extract with wheat flour (Scout 66), our α-gliadin (2.1c) as used in instillation experiments, the pellet material (pel)(2.1d) and the supernatant material (sup)(2.1e), the last two obtained by precipitation at pH 9.7 The protein maps are obtained by combined isoelectric focussing (IEF) and polyacrylamide (PAA) electrophoresis at pH 2.3. At the left side of each map the normal pattern of the PAA electrophoresis is added. Vertical (PAA): the fastest group of proteins has a mobility equal to wheat albumins and is clearly separated from the gliadin proteins. Horizontal (IEF): from left to right a linear pH gradient from pH 3.5–10

—centrifugation step: $53\,000\,g \times 16\,h$
—the pellet material (crude α-gliadin)
—a Sephadex G-100 column ($14.5 \times 25\,cm$). Fractionation of the crude α-gliadin fraction in $0.01\,M$ acetic acid
—α-gliadin fraction

PROTEIN COMPOSITION

We have investigated the protein compositions of gluten and gliadin, and compared them with our α-gliadin fraction. To do this we used a two-dimensional electrophoresis system, which is in principle the same as the system used by Wrigley and Shepherd[8] studying the proteins in gliadin, and by Aragoncillo[9] studying the non-gliadin proteins in the alcoholic extract.

The two-dimensional electrophoresis system

Isoelectric focussing is used in the first dimension. The proteins move in the electric field to a place in the pH gradient, where their net charge is zero. After this step the gel is layered on top of a poly-acrylamide (PAA) gel. In the second dimension the electrophoretic mobility of the proteins mainly depends on differences in molecular weight and the number of positive charges. The proteins are fixed with trichloroacetic acid solution.

The protein maps

The protein maps (Figure 2.1,a–c) of gluten, gliadin as an extract of wheat flour with alcohol, and our α-gliadin fraction as used in the instillation experiments by Hekkens[1,2] contain proteins which should be classified as albumins according to the electrophoretic definition of Woychik[3]. Most albumin proteins are on the same place in each of the three protein maps, but they differ in concentration.

ORIGIN OF THE CONTAMINATION WITH THE ALBUMINS

During the process of gluten preparation polar lipids and lipoproteins[4] become bound and are no longer extractable with lipid solvents. When the lipids of the wheat flour are extracted before extraction with alcohol, about 8% less protein is extracted. This 8% consists of lipid-bound proteins[5], including albumins. Even glycolipids[10] are mentioned in binding to gliadins. A binding of apolar lipids to α-gliadin[11] is also described. This binding is strong in an acid solution, whereas in an alkaline solution there is almost no binding. The whole isolation procedure of our α-gliadin fraction is performed in an acid solution, therefore a possible reason for the contamination of this α-gliadin fraction can be found in this lipid binding.

ELECTROPHORETICALLY PURE GLIADIN

Our α-gliadin fraction still contains proteins, which are electrophoretically defined as albumins[3]. The binding of lipids[4,5,10] possibly plays a role in the presence of these albumins in the α-gliadin fraction. The binding of these lipids with α-gliadin is negligible in an alkaline solution. Therefore we have chosen these conditions to prepare an electrophoretically pure gliadin fraction.

Preparation

The α-gliadin fraction, obtained after the Sephadex G-100 column is dissolved in 8 M urea, adjusted to pH 9.7 with ammonia at 4 °C, and dialysed against a solution of diluted ammonia with a pH of 9.7. During the dialysis a precipitate is formed, and collected by centrifugation. After a second precipitation step the protein map of the precipitate (Figure 2.1,c–e) only shows proteins in the gliadin region, whereas the supernatant material only has proteins in the albumin region. No deamidation could be measured at pH 9.7.

Toxicity

We have tested these fractions in two coeliac patients, each with one fraction. In an instillation experiment the pellet material, an electrophoretically pure gliadin fraction containing mainly proteins in the α-gliadin region, gives a clinical reaction, histological damage of the mucosa and a decrease of the brush border enzymes, together with a decreased D-xylose excretion. These experiments will be repeated, but from these preliminary results we conclude that our α-gliadin fraction, which is electrophoretically pure, is toxic to coeliac patients.

OTHER ASPECTS OF THE HETEROGENEITY OF THE α-GLIADIN FRACTION

The presence of the faster-moving proteins is the only heterogeneity aspect of the α-gliadin fraction that is mentioned until now. But there are other aspects of heterogeneity in this fraction such as a difference in isoelectric point (pI), in electrophoretic mobility, in aggregation behaviour and also a difference in reaction with antibodies present in sera of coeliac patients with a high antigliadin titre.

Heterogeneity in isoelectric point

The heterogeneity in pI of the proteins in the pellet pH 9.7, as an electrophoretically pure gliadin fraction containing mainly proteins in the α-gliadin region, is visible in a two-dimensional electrophoresis (Figure 2.2). The differences in pI are useful for separating these proteins, because IEF can also be used in a preparative way. We have used a sucrose gradient (5–50%) in a preparative IEF column for further separation of the proteins in the pellet pH 9.7, and Figure 2.3 shows the IEF gel patterns of the fractions of the preparative IEF column.

Heterogeneity in electrophoretic mobility

When electrophoresis in the second dimension (Figure 2.2) is continued for a longer time a better resolution is obtained in the gliadin region of the protein map. For most proteins in the pellet pH 9.7 there are no large differences in mobility in the second dimension. Because the differences in molecular weight of these proteins are negligible, the mobility is mainly determined by the number of positive charges on the molecules. So the difference in the amino acid composition of these proteins, as far as it concerns the charged amino acids, is expected to be

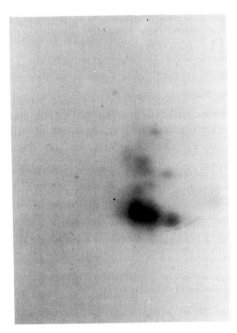

Figure 2.2 The protein map of the pellet material obtained by precipitation at pH 9.7 Vertical: polyacrylamide electrophoresis. Horizontal: from left to right a linear pH gradient from pH 3.5–10. There is a better vertical resolution in the gliadin region, because of a longer time of electrophoresis in the second dimension. The weak spot in the most alkaline region with the α-gliadin mobility does not aggregate. The gel is stained with Coomassie Brilliant Blue G 250

.53 .51 .28 .27 .28 .29 .20 .26

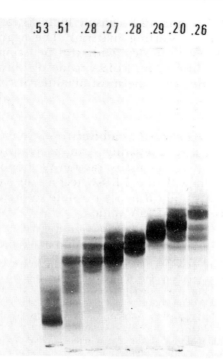

Figure 2.3 The isoelectric focussing (IEF) gel patterns of a preparative IEF column. A linear pH gradient from pH 3.5–10 from top to bottom. The values obtained with the ELISA technique for these fractions are given in arbitrary units above the gels

in the degree of deamidation.

Heterogeneity in aggregation behaviour

If we repeat the aggregation step with the pellet pH 9.7 material in the medium as described by Bernardin *et al.*[7], not all these α-gliadins aggregate. For instance the α-gliadin with the most alkaline pI (Figures 2.2 and 2.3) does not aggregate.

Heterogeneity in antibody reaction

In our laboratory, sera of untreated coeliac patients are screened for antibodies against gliadin by an Enzyme Linked Immunoabsorbent Assay (ELISA) according to Engvall and Perlmann[12]. With the same technique we have investigated the differences in reaction of α-gliadin in fractions with pooled sera from patients with a high antigliadin titre, because of the possibility that differences in reaction might correlate with toxicity. The most alkaline fraction obtained with preparative IEF of the pellet pH 9.7 (Figure 2.3) has a high ELISA value, about 170% of the value of the starting material. The aggregate obtained by repeating the aggregation step with the pellet material termed A-gliadin by Kasarda[6] has a low ELISA value of only 40% and does not contain the α-gliadin with the most alkaline pI.

CONCLUSION

If the toxicity of the pellet pH 9.7 as an electrophoretically pure gliadin fraction containing mainly α-gliadins, can be confirmed in further toxicity tests, it is still a heterogeneous fraction We hope that the type of heterogeneity measured with the ELISA technique has a correlation with toxicity, but at this point it is not possible to predict toxicity of a fraction on the basis of its ELISA value.

References

1. Hekkens, W. Th. J. M., Haex, A. J. Ch. and Willighagen, R. G. J. (1970). Some aspects of gliadin fractionation and testing by a histological method. In: C. C. Booth and R. H. Dowling (eds.) *Coeliac Disease. Proc. Int. Coeliac Symp.*, pp. 11–19 (Edinburgh: Churchill Livingstone)
2. Hekkens, W. Th. J. M., van den Aarsen, C. J., Gilliams, J. P., Lems-van Kan, P. H. and Bouma-Frölich, G. (1974). α -Gliadin structure and degradation. In: W. Th. J. M. Hekkens and A. S. Peña (eds.) *Coeliac Disease Proc. 2nd Int. Coeliac Symp.*, pp. 39–45 (Leiden: Stenfert Kroese)
3. Woychik, J. H., Boundy, J. A. and Dimler, R. J. (1961). Starch gel electrophoresis of wheat gluten proteins with concentrated urea. *Arch. Biochem. Biophys.,* **94**, 477
4. Hoseney, R. C., Pomeranz, Y. and Finney, K. F. (1970). Functional (breadmaking) and biochemical properties of wheat flour components. VII. Petroleum ether-soluble lipoproteins of wheat flour. *Cereal Chem.,* **47**, 153
5. Charbonnier, L. (1973). Etude des protéins alcoolo-solubles de la farine de blé. *Biochimie,* **55**, 1217
6. Kasarda, D. D., Nimmo, C. C. and Bernardin, J. E. (1974). Structural aspects and genetic relationships of gliadins. In: W. Th. J. M. Hekkens and A. S. Peña (eds.) *Coeliac Disease. Proc. 2nd Int. Coeliac Symp.*, pp. 25–36 (Leiden: Stenfert Kroese)
7. Bernardin, J. E., Kasarda, D. D. and Mecham, D. K. (1967). Preparation and characterization of α -gliadin. *J. Biol. Chem.,* **242**, 445
8. Wrigley, C. W. and Shephard, K. W. (1973). Electrofocusing of grain proteins from wheat genotypes. *Ann. N.Y. Acad. Sci.,* **209**, 154
9. Aragoncillo, M. A., Rodriguez, L. M. A., Carbonere, P. and Garcia-Almedo, F. (1975). Chromosomal control of non-gliadin proteins from the 70% ethanol extract of wheat endosperm. *Theor. Appl. Genet.,* **45**, 322
10. Wehrli, H. P. and Pomeranz, Y. (1970). A note on the interaction between glyco-lipids and wheat flour macromolecules. *Cereal Chem.,* **47**, 160
11. Greene, F. C. and Kasarda, D. D. (1971). Apolar interactions of α-gliadin: Binding of 2-p-toluidinylnaphthalene-6-sulphonate. *Cereal Chem.,* **48**, 601
12. Engvall, E. and Perlmann, P. (1972). Enzyme-Linked Immunosorbent Assay, ELISA. III. Quantitation of specific antibodies by enzyme-labelled anti-immuno-globulin in antigen-coated tubes. *J. Immunol.,* **109**, 129

Discussion of chapter 2

Kasarda How many components had Dr de Rooij found in the α-gliadin fractions that he is working with?

de Rooij There are about seven major protein components and four or five minor components.

Kasarda C. Wrigley in Australia analysed our α-gliadin preparation, which we call A-gliadin. There were about 16 protein components in our preparation according to isoelectric focussing by Dr Wrigley; five or six of these were major components and the rest although minor, were clearly visible in the pattern. We therefore find a very high degree of heterogeneity in this A-gliadin.

3

Further subfractionation of digests of gluten

R. E. OFFORD, B. S. ANAND, J. PIRIS and S. C. TRUELOVE

It is of interest to try to prepare the smallest fragments of wheat protein that are toxic to coeliac patients. The advantages of obtaining small fragments are that they are more readily purified to chemical homogeneity, and once this is done, their molecular structures are more easily determined. If a structure is known in detail it is much more easy to modify it in useful or informative ways if the molecule is small. We obtained some time ago a mixture of fairly small peptides derived from gluten that retains enteropathic activity[1]. Our fraction was further separated and, rather unexpectedly, a toxic subfraction was found to show, more clearly than did more crude mixtures of gluten peptides, specific stimulatory activity against maintained lymphocytes of coeliacs[2] and to produce an Arthus-like skin reaction[3].

The purpose of the present paper is to review the protein-chemical aspects of the separation schemes that we use, and to report preliminary results on further purification and characterization of our products.

We decided at the outset to secure the highest probability of our correctly identifying toxic fractions by relying on the results of jejunal biopsy after challenge by our fractions. This led us to begin with gluten rather than a more purified gliadin because we felt that it would be very difficult to obtain, in the large amounts that would be needed for feeding, any gliadin fraction that was purified to a really useful extent.

The need for bulk samples also led us to adopt a separation scheme which under more favourable circumstances would be far from ideal, and which calls for explanation in some detail. The first step was a membrane filtration scheme (Figure 3.1). Membrane separations are based on molecular size: one pays for their ability to handle large quantities by having to accept their very poor resolving power. Of the fractions that retained toxicity, fraction B had the components of smaller molecular weight. The range of molecular weight is not what

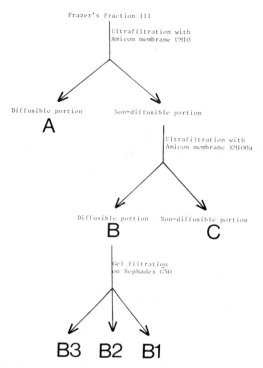

Figure 3.1 The fractionation scheme. Fractions C, B, B2 and B3 are toxic. 100 g of gluten was normally taken at a time and gave approximately 15 g of B. 35 g of B gave about 15 g each of B2 and B3

would be expected on the basis of the manufacturers' specifications for the membranes used, but is not in doubt. There was no visible component above M.W. 8000 and the majority were considerably smaller—intact gluten proteins were not detectable even on grossly overloaded gel electrophoreses.

When proteases are used in structure determination, it is often observed that even under severe conditions leading to extensive digestion, small quantities of protein remain more or less untouched. Our observations gave no grounds for thinking that the toxicity of fraction B is due to some minute contamination by such surviving material, but in view of the largely qualitative nature of the feeding assay it could not be finally excluded at that stage. However, the fractionations reported below settle the point with reasonable finality.

It is normally the practice to follow a separation based on size with one based on some other molecular property. Net charge is normally the property chosen, and differences are usually exploited by means

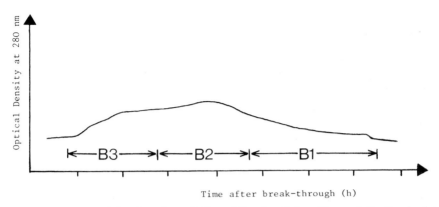

Figure 3.2. The subfractionation of 35 g of fraction B (see Figure 3.1), dissolved in 2 l of 0.5% NH_4CO_3 on a column of Sephadex G-50, fine grade, in 0.5% (w/v) NH_4CO_3 at room temperature. The column consisted of five sections, 37 cm in diameter × 15 cm high, placed in series, and was run at a flow rate of about 250 ml/min. A centrifugal pump was used. the u.v. absorption was measured in Uvicord–II flow monitor (LKB). The high flow rate necessitated the replacement of the standard 3 mm quartz flow cell by one made of Teflon tubing of internal diameter 8 mm. The buffer reservoir was a polythene dustbin (100 l) and the effluent was directed into a series of 15 l plastic buckets which were changed by hand at half-hour intervals

of ion-exchange chromatography. We rejected the use of ion-exchange chromatography, even though it has the required ability to handle large samples, because it can lead to the selective loss of a few components by irreversible adsorption onto the exchanger. That such losses can occur is less of a serious objection than is the fact that they will pass unnoticed. Also, we did not need the high resolving power ion exchange since we are so limited in the number of bioassays that the products of any separation of B would have had to be pooled into no more than three samples. We therefore used gelfiltration, even though it is yet another method based on size. The separation range of Sephadex G-50 most nearly matched the range of sizes that we had observed for fraction B. We were obliged to use an extremely large column (the Pharmacia KS 370) with a total effluent volume of about 100 l. Fraction B2 (Figure 3.2) is the smaller in molecular size of the two enteropathic fractions obtained and shows the immunological activities already mentioned. It is not at present clear if the fact that it seems to show these activities more patently than cruder extracts is due to the removal of inhibitory contaminants or to enrichment in active material.

Paper electrophoresis shows that B2 is still very heterogeneous and the range of mobilities of the components is typical of peptide mixtures with an average molecular weight in the high hundreds, with a considerable dispersion about the mean. This impression is in line with what one would expect for a fraction eluting in the middle of a Sephadex G-50 run.

We have applied the whole of the foregoing scheme (on a smaller scale) to other cereals: barley, rye, maize, and rice. The shapes of the profiles of u.v. absorption of the column effluents do not correlate with the toxicity or non-toxicity of these cereals, but this does not exclude the possibility that toxicity derives from the same or similar sequences, and we are subjecting the column fractions to further separation to investigate the point.

Preparative paper electrophoresis cannot give sufficient material for feeding and further subfractionations for this purpose will certainly require ion-exchange chromatography. But we have used the discovery of the immunological activities of wheat B2 to screen its electrophoretic subfractions. Preparative paper electrophoresis is simple, is rapid if high voltages are used, and there is a fairly low probability of unseen, selective loss of components of the mixture. We have separated wheat B2 at pH 6.5 into ten fractions ranging from strongly acidic to strongly basic (R. E. Offord and M. Perryman, unpublished work). Preliminary experiments suggest that several fractions, especially the basic ones, have immunological activity. We have also examined one peptide fraction called S5γ (mobility at pH 6.5 of -0.36 relative to aspartic acid$= -1.0$) which elutes from the Sephadex column very close to the boundary between fraction B2 and B3. This fraction has been resolved into two components on electrophoresis at pH 1.9 Both of these show lymphocyte stimulatory activity (K. Sikora, private communication). One fraction, S5γ1, has been shown on further electrophoresis (at pH 3.5) to consist of only one major component, together with a small number of faint additional bands. The major peptide has been isolated and its amino acid sequence shown to be Asp–Gln–Gly–Trp (J. D. Priddle, private communication). The molecular weight corresponding to this sequence, 503, is close to the molecular weight calculated from the electrophoretic mobility at pH 6.5 by the method of Offord[4], 600 ± 100, and it seems unlikely that the peptide could carry any large carbohydrate or prosthetic group. We stress that the sequence is simply of the major component of an immunologically active mixture. Even if the immunological activity of S5γ1 is due to this peptide, rather than to some trace component of quite different structure, that activity has yet to be correlated with toxicity to coeliacs. We report the sequence merely to illustrate that, notwithstanding the extreme heterogeneity of the digests, our procedures are proving capable of isolating pure materials of potential interest.

ACKNOWLEDGEMENTS

We thank Dr J. D. Priddle and Dr K. Sikora for permission to use their unpublished results, and the Medical Research Council for a grant. B.S.A. was the holder in succession of a Wellcome Research Training Scholarship and a Coeliac Trust Research Fellowship during the course of this work.

We thank the Central Blood Transfusion Laboratory and M.R.E., Porton, for freeze-drying our materials.

References

1. Dissanayake, A. S., Jerrome, D. W., Offord, R. E., Truelove, S. C. and Whitehead, R. (1974). Identifying toxic fractions of wheat gluten and their effect on the jejunal mucosa in coeliac disease. *Gut*, **15**, 931
2. Sikora, K., Anand, B. S., Truelove, S. C., Ciclitira, P. J. and Offord, R. E. (1976). Stimulation of lymphocytes from patients with coeliac disease by a subfraction of gluten. *Lancet*, **ii**, 389
3. Anand, B. S., Truelove, S. C. and Offord, R. E. (1977). Skin test for coeliac disease employing a subfraction of gluten. *Lancet*, **i**, 118
4. Offord, R. E. (1966). Electrophoretic mobilities on paper and their use in the determination of amide groups. *Nature (Lond.)*, **211**, 591

Discussion of chapter 3

Booth   The evidence you presented suggests that there are three fractions B_1 B_2 and B_3, all of which behave differently in terms of entero-toxicity, skin sensitivity, and stimulatory effect on lymphocytes in culture. For example B_3 is toxic to the intestine but does not stimulate lymphocytes, and yet all fractions produce a positive skin reaction. My question therefore is, what is the effective test system that is being used and what conclusion can you draw from it? Furthermore, when doing skin tests which is of course the area that clinicians and patients are particularly interested in, how does one carry out skin tests, at what time does one read a skin test, how many observers see the test, are the tests done blind, are photographs taken of every test that is done for further storage and analysis by others, how in fact is this achieved because I think on the clinical side it is absolutely vital that sort of data is as tightly controlled as the chemistry.

Offord   Your first question relates to the manner in which different types of assays appear to give different answers for the three fractions. It would not surprise me if this were true. Of course to do an assay properly one has to determine a proper dose response curve and then make sure the assay in use is somewhere near the middle of that curve. It is very difficult as I understand it to do a dose response curve if one is doing a challenge followed by a jejunal biopsy, and the fact that B_3 gave a positive result while the lymphocyte stimulation test seemed negative may simply be because the correct quantities for an optimum assay in two cases were not worked out. This isn't to dispute Professor Booth's point, which rightly emphasizes how much care is needed in the comparison of different types of assay.

Strober   In your lymphocyte stimulation studies the extent of the stimulation was expressed as a stimulation index and something of the order of magnitude of twice background was obtained. I find that somewhat unsatisfactory because in work with other antigens to which individuals are responsive such as *Candida*, a stimulation index of 150 times background is obtained by me. I think therefore that lymphocyte stimulation inducing the order you obtained must be interpreted cautiously.

Offord   You are very correct to point out the low stimulation indices that were observed. However, these stimulatory indices observed were statistically significant and were very useful to us especially in planning subsequent experiments.

Hekkens   You mentioned a molecular weight of a few hundred for fraction

B_2 and you base that on paper electrophoresis and ninhydrin staining as far as I was aware. Do you consider this is the proper technique to monitor molecular size?

Offord I wish to emphasize that I said the average molecular weight of the B_2 components was probably of the order of several hundred. We have used other stains, but all I meant was that the ninhydrin colour on a paper electrophoregram was roughly what one would expect from a given weight of our mixture if it were composed of small peptides. Also the mobilities based on the correlation between electrophoretic mobility, charge and molecular weight that I proposed some years ago suggests that the range of molecular weight peaks at about where I said. But I could not exclude the possibility that materials of very different molecular weight from those have been carried through our separations.

Until we can get really chemically homogeneous preparations which can be characterized chemically, and their structures manipulated and correlated with changes in activity, we can never be sure that there isn't a small contamination of something very much larger which is responsible for all activity. It ties in somewhat with what I said earlier about the need for a dose–response curve. It is all very well to sequence a tetrapeptide, but that tetrapeptide may be lightly contaminated with something very potent and very different in its molecular structure.

4

The detoxification of gliadin by the enzymic cleavage of a side-chain substituent

J. J. PHELAN, FIONA M. STEVENS, W. F. CLEERE, B. McNICHOLL, C. F. McCARTHY and P. F. FOTTRELL

Gluten from wheat and rye was recognized to be the cause of intestinal damage in coeliac disease in the 1950s[1,2] and the toxicity was subsequently shown to be in gliadin, in the 70% ethanolic fraction[3].

Several investigations involving fractionation of gliadin, have demonstrated toxicity in many fractions using patients with coeliac disease in remission, but have not yet identified the precise chemical nature of crude fractions[4-8]. Repeated attempts to abolish toxicity with purified proteolytic enzymes including crystalline papain, have failed[9,10] and from this it was (in our opinion) erroneously deduced that toxicity was due to a small peptide, resistant to proteolytic cleavage. The abolition of toxicity by hog intestinal scrapings[5] then resulted in the hypothesis that coeliacs lacked a specific peptidase.

It seemed more likely to us that the failure of proteolysis to abolish toxicity indicated that the toxicity resided not in particular sequence of amino acids but in a side-chain component bound either covalently or otherwise. We showed that gliadin contained some carbohydrate components and preliminary experiments suggested that these were involved in the toxic properties of gliadin. If this hypothesis were true then removal of carbohydrate should make these proteins non-toxic to coeliac patients. An enzyme system which would effect this cleavage was prepared from *Aspergillus niger*[11]. We have previously presented evidence which suggests that cleavage of glycosidic linkages in gliadin does markedly reduce its toxicity[12]. In this communication we present further morphological and biochemical evidence of reduced toxicity.

We have previously stated that because of the similarity between gliadin molecules, the possibility exists that the toxicity may reside in more than one gliadin molecule. If this argument is valid, then, since glutenin is obviously part of the same family of molecules (character-ized by high proline and glutamine content) it should also be toxic. We present evidence which shows that glutenin is toxic to coeliac patients.

If, as we suggest, more than one gliadin molecule is toxic, then chromatography of gliadin will result in the distribution of toxicity across the chromatographic profile, thus reducing the amounts of material available for feeding experiments. In this laboratory we are

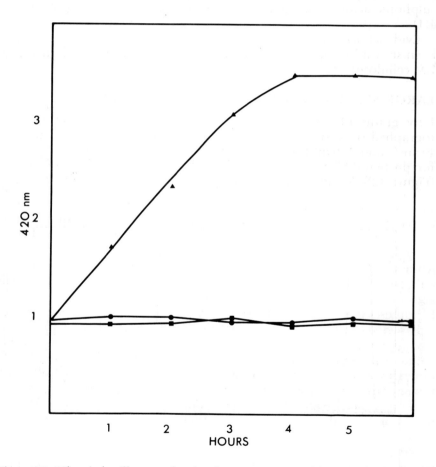

Figure 4.1 The circles illustrate the absorbance at 420 nm obtained where gliadin is reacted with TNBS[14] at hourly intervals. The squares illustrate the absorbance obtained while gliadin is being incubated with detoxifying enzyme, while the triangles illustrate the figures obtained when gliadin was incubated with pepsin

attempting to locate the toxic fractions by studying chromatographic changes catalysed by the detoxifying enzymes. Since we now possess three distinct detoxifying enzymes then only those changes catalysed by the three enzymes individually, will be considered relevant to the toxicity. In this communication we will outline the experimental approach adopted and will describe selected chromatographic changes which occurred on incubation of fractions with the detoxifying enzymes.

Gliadin was prepared and incubated with detoxifying enzymes as previously described[13]. When the digest was periodically examined for the appearance of amino groups with 2,4,6-trinitrobenzene sulphonic acid[14] proteolytic activity was found to be negligible (Figure 4.1).

Evidence for the conservation of the primary structure has already been shown by peptide mapping and by chromatography of gliadin on CM cellulose[12,13].

LARGE SCALE CHROMATOGRAPHY OF GLIADIN

Fifty grams of gliadin, *Triticum aestivum, (var quern)* were chromatographed on CM cellulose (55 cm × 7.5 cm) according to Patey and Evans[15] and 100 ml fractions were collected and the effluent examined for protein (280 nm) and for carbohydrate with phenol sulphuric acid (Figure 4.2). Some fractions containing up to 1 g of protein were treated

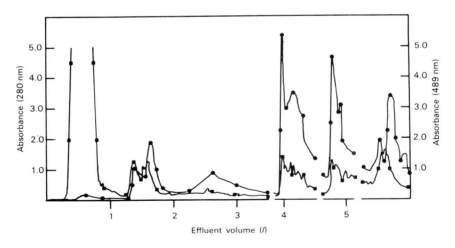

Figure 4.2 Large scale chromatography of 50 g of gliadin on a column of CM cellulose (55 × 7.5 cm) according to Patey and Evans[15]. The circles illustrate the absorbance at 280 nm and the squares the carbohydrate after phenol-sulphuric acid. Where the graph is not continuous, points with low readings have been omitted

individually while other fractions were mixed and pooled according to their carbohydrate content and were then dialysed and freeze-dried. Selected fractions from the four major peaks were digested simultaneously with elastase and chymotrypsin and trypsin (1% each) at pH 8.5 in ammonium bicarbonate. The peptides were chromatographed on a column of Biogel P6 (140 cm × 2 cm). The effluent was monitored for protein at 280 nm and 230 nm and for carbohydrate with anthrone and phenol-sulphuric acid. (Figure 4.3). The anthrone and phenol-sulphuric acid peaks always coincided, but the phenol sulphuric acid was more sensitive.

Each fraction was examined by high-voltage electrophoresis and tubes with similar peptide mixtures were pooled and concentrated by rotary evaporation. A portion of each fraction was then digested with a mixture of detoxifying enzyme at pH 4.5 and then the digested and undigested portions were compared by high voltage electrophoresis or by paper chromatography. The peptides were detected by ninhydrin and by chlorination according to Reindel and Hoppe[16].

Chromatographic changes were examined by monitoring for specific peptides as follows; p-dimethylamino benzaldehyde (tryptophan), the Pauley reagent for histidine and tyrosine, phenanthrene quinone for

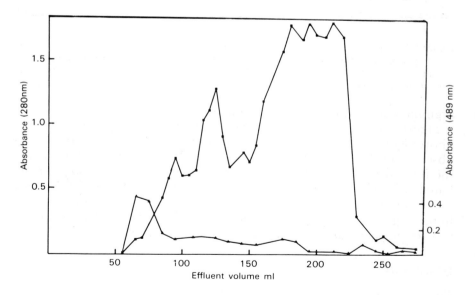

Figure 4.3 Chromatography of gliadin peptides on Biogel P6: approximately 500 mg of peptides were chromatographed on a column of Biogel P6 (140 cm × 2 cm) using 0.1 M ammonium acetate buffer pH 6.0 Protein was monitored at 280 nm and carbohydrate, using phenol-sulphuric acid at 489 nm

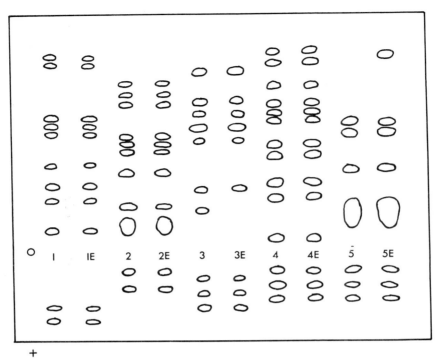

Figure 4.4 High voltage paper electrophoresis of peptides from Biogel columns (Figure 4.3) at pH 3.5. Columns 1,2 and 3 etc., represent the patterns obtained with fractions 1,2, and 3 from Biogel columns, while 1E, 2E, 3E, etc., represent the spots obtained after incubation with the detoxifying enzymes

arginine and isatin for amino-terminal proline.

Figure 4.4 is a diagramatic representation of the comparative electro-phoretograms of enzyme-treated and untreated peptides. The changes observed in Row 3E and Row 5E were catalysed by a mixture of each of the three detoxifying enzymes. When the peptides in row 5 were incubated with each detoxifying enzyme individually, it was apparent that only one of the enzymes catalysed the change seen in row 5E, indicating that this peptide is not involved in toxicity. In contrast to this result, the change in electrophoretic mobility of the spot in Row 3

DISCUSSION

Thus far, our initial approach to the characterization of the toxic fraction in gliadin has been to isolate three enzyme preparations which detoxify gliadin.

In the process, we have demonstrated that the toxicity is not an

was catalysed by each of the three detoxifying enzymes, as shown in Figure 4.5. In a single experiment, this reaction was also catalysed by a biopsy homogenate of normal patient. The structure of this peptide is being investigated.

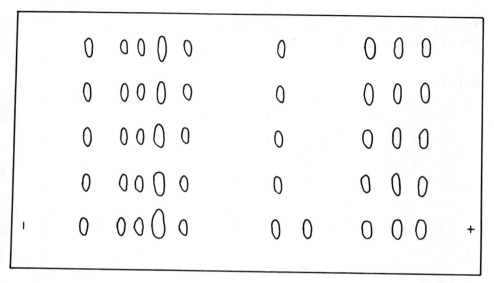

Figure 4.5 Column 1 shows the peptides from Figure 4.4, Row 3, electrophoresed for a longer period. Rows 2, 3 and 4 illustrate the removal of one spot under the influence of three detoxifying enzymes and Row 5 shows the same result with the homogenate of an intestinal biopsy from a normal patient

integral part of the amino acid sequence of gliadin but is a side-chain substituent, bound (covalently or otherwise) to gliadin. We have argued that, because of the lack of a reliable *in vitro* assay for toxicity, the task of finding the toxic fraction by successive feeding experiments, is unrealistic. We propose then to locate the toxic fraction by observing chromatographic changes catalysed by the detoxifying enzymes. The possibility of being misled by spurious reactions is reduced if a similar change is catalysed by all three detoxifying enzymes, as was shown in Figure 4.4, Row 5E, where no chromatographic change was seen with two detoxifying enzymes. In contrast to this result, the change in Figure 4.4, Row 3, was observed with all three detoxifying enzymes and the implication is that this peptide is involved in toxicity. The possibility also exists, that an enzyme common to all three enzyme preparations, such as a phosphatase, is catalysing the removal of a phosphate group, which is not involved in toxicity. The search for the toxic fragment, then, using detoxifying enzymes, can at best give only an indication of where toxicity resides and the conclusions drawn must be confirmed by feeding experiments.

ACKNOWLEDGEMENTS

This work is supported by grants from the Wellcome Trust and the Medical Research Council of Ireland. The authors are indebted to Sheila Baynes for technical assistance.

References

1. Dicke, W. K., Weijers, H. A. and Van de Kamer, J. H. (1953). An investigation into the injurious constituents of wheat in connection with their action on patients with coeliac disease. *Acta paediatr.*, **42**, 233

2. Dicke, W. K. (1950). Coeliakie, een onderzoek naar de nadelige invloed van sommige graansoorten op de lijder ann coeliakie. Thesis, Utrecht

3. Van de Kamer, J. H. and Weijers, H. A. (1955). Coeliac disease: some experiments on the cause of the harmful effect of the gliadin. *Acta Paediatr.* **44**, 465

4. Alvey, C., Anderson, C. M. and Freeman, M. (1957). Wheat gluten and coeliac disease. *Arch. Dis. Childh.*, **32**, 434

5. Frazer, A. C., Fletcher, R. F., Ross, C., Shaw, B., Sammons, H. G and Schneider, R. (1958). Gluten-induced enteropathy. The effect of partially digested gluten. *Lancet*, **ii**, 252

6. Van Roon, J. F., Haex, A. F. Ch., Seeder, W. A. and de Jong, J. (1960). Clinical and biochemical analysis of gluten toxicity. II. *Gastroenterologia*, **94**, 227

7. Bronstein, H. D., Haeffner, L. F. and Kowlesser, O. D. (1966). Enzymatic digestion of gliadin: the effect of the resultant peptides in adult coeliac disease. *Clin. Chem. Acta*, **14**, 141

8. Dissanayake, A. S., Jerrome, D. W., Offord, R.E., Truelove, S. C. and Whitehead, R. (1974b). Identifying toxic fractions of wheat gluten and their effect on the jejunal mucosa in coeliac disease. *Gut*, **15**, 931

9. Krainich, H. C. and Mohn, G. (1959). Weitere Untersuchunger uber den schadlichen Weizenmehleffect bei der Coeliakie 2. Die Wirkung der enzymatischen Abbauprocukte des Gliadin. *Helv. Paediat. Acta*, **14**, 124

10. Messer, M., Anderson, C. M. and Hubbard, L. (1964). Studies on the mechanism of destruction of the toxic action of wheat gluten in coeliac disease by crude papain. *Gut*, **5**, 295

11. Phelan, J. J. (1974). The nature of gliadin toxicity in coeliac disease. *Biochem. Soc. Trans.*, **2**, 1368

12. Phelan, J. J., Stevens, F. M., McNicholl, B., McCarthy, C. F. and Fottrell, P. F. (1974). The nature of gliadin toxicity in coeliac disease: a new concept. In: Coeliac Disease Hekkens, W. Th. M. and Peña, A. S. (eds.) pp.58–68 (Leiden: Stenfert Kroese)

14. Fields, R. (1972). Methods in Enzymology. In: Hirs, C. H. W. and Timasheff, S. N. (eds.) Vol. *XXVB*, pp. 464–468. (New York and London: Academic Press)

15. Patey, A. L. and Evans, D. J. (1973). Large scale preparation of gliadin proteins. *J. Sci. Food and Agric.*, **24**, 1229

16. Reindel, and Hoppe. (1969). In: *Data for Biochemical Research*, Dawson, R., Elliott, D., Elliot W. and Jones, K. (eds.), p. 528. (London: Oxford University Press)

5

Clinical demonstration of the reduction of gliadin toxicity by enzymic cleavage of a side-chain substituent

FIONA M. STEVENS, J. J. PHELAN, B. McNICHOLL,
F. R. COMERFORD, P. F. FOTTRELL and C. F. McCARTHY

The chemical nature of the toxic moiety in gluten is not known. No purified proteolytic enzyme has been shown to abolish toxicity. In Leiden, preliminary evidence was presented showing that the enzymic removal of surface carbohydrates from gliadin appeared to abolish toxicity without altering the protein backbone[1].

The study has since been enlarged. Six adult coeliac patients in remission have been fed either enzyme-treated gliadin, untreated whole flour, untreated gliadin or glutenin. Fifty grams of gliadin or the

Table 5.1   Patient data

Patient	Age	Sex	Duration of GFD (months)
1	21	F	14
2	19	M	34
3	22	M	20
4 a	52	F	8
4 b	53	F	8
5	51	F	4
6	33	M	7

equivalent amount of whole flour or glutenin was made into bread with gluten-free flour.

PATIENTS AND METHODS

The patients' age, sex and duration of gluten-free diet prior to study are shown in Table 5.1. An initial small intestinal biopsy (B_1) was performed no more than 36 hours before commencing fraction feeding. A subsequent biopsy (B_2) was performed after feeding. The time interval after commencing feeding and the amount of each particular fraction consumed prior to B_2 is shown in Table 5.2.

Table 5.2 Study details

Patient	Gliadin preparation	Duration of feeding (days)	Gliadin eaten (g)	Key to symbols
1	treated gliadin	2	15	----
2	treated gliadin	5	47	------
3	treated gliadin	5	47	----
4 a	treated gliadin	4	40	•·········•
4 b	Whole flour	3	15	•·········•
5	Untreated gliadin	2	15	•———•
6	Glutenin	4	30	•———•

Patient 4 has been fed two different materials. During the first study she was fed enzyme-treated gliadin and eight months later she was fed untreated flour.

Intestinal biopsies were obtained before and after feeding from the region of the ligament of Treitz with the Watson capsule (except in patient 1 in whom biopsies from the duodenal bulb were obtained with a duodenoscope). Part of the biopsy was wrapped in parafilm, stored at −20 °C until assayed for enzyme activity, as detailed elsewhere[2]. A further portion was examined under the dissecting microscope and processed for histology. Coded 5μm sections were examined and intra-epithelial lymphocyte (IEL) counts performed[1], and enterocyte heights measured[3].

RESULTS

The mucosal biopsy enzyme activities of lactase, sucrase and alkaline

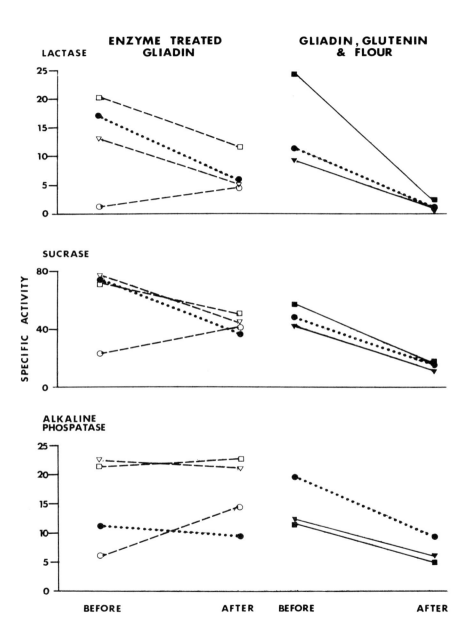

Figure 5.1 Changes in mucosal brush border enzyme activities of lactase, sucrase, and alkaline phosphatase after feeding 'gliadin' preparations

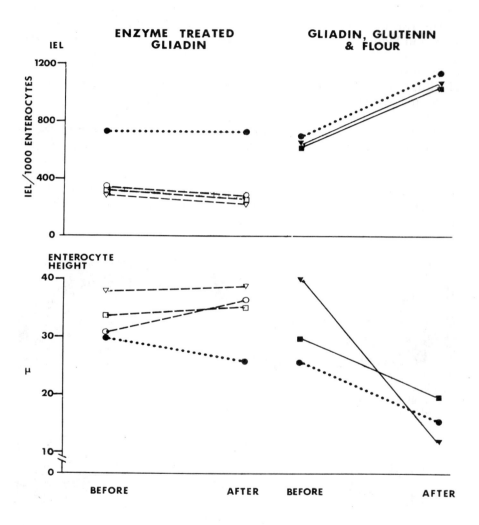

Figure 5.2 Changes in intraepithelial lymphocyte (IEL) counts and enterocyte heights after feeding 'gliadin' preparations

phosphatase before and after fraction feeding are shown in Figure 5.1. There was a fall in activity of all enzymes in the patients fed flour, untreated gliadin and glutenin. There was a fall in lactase and sucrase activity in three of the four patients fed enzyme-treated gliadin. However, there was no accompanying drop in alkaline phosphatase activity.

The IEL counts and enterocyte heights before and after feeding are shown in Figure 5.2. There is no rise in IEL counts after feeding treated gliadin in contrast to the marked rise after feeding the untreated fractions. A slight fall in enterocyte height was noted in patient 4 fed treated gliadin, but the fall was not as marked as that seen in the same patient when fed whole flour, or in the patients fed untreated gliadin or glutenin.

The histological sections from patient 4 before and after feeding enzyme-treated gliadin and untreated gliadin are shown in Figures 5.3 (a and b) and Figure 5.4 (a and b) respectively. There is no marked change in inflammatory cell infiltrate in the epithelium or lamina propria, nor is there a marked reduction in enterocyte height after feeding enzyme treated gliadin. However, after feeding whole flour there is damage to the epithelium and an increased inflammatory cell infiltrate

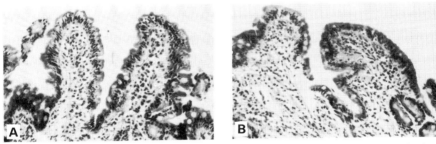

Figure 5.3 Small intestinal biopsies from patient 4 before (A) and after (B) feeding treated gliadin. There is shortening of villi and loss of enterocyte height after feeding treated gliadin. × 105

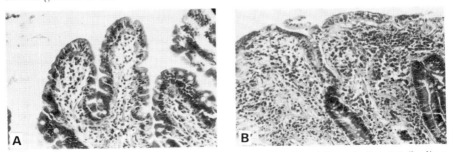

Figure 5.4 Small intestinal biopsies from patient 4 before (A) and after (B) feeding whole flour. Severe damage is shown after feeding flour with complete atrophy of villi and disruption of the epithelial cell layer. × 105

in the lamina propria.

Histological sections from patients 1, 2, 3 and 5 have been published elsewhere[3].

DISCUSSION

The feeding of toxic material to adult coeliac patients in remission produces a rapid fall in all mucosal brush border enzyme activities to exceedingly low levels,[4,5] and histological damage i.e. loss of entero-cyte height and increased inflammatory cell infiltrate in the epithelium and the lamina propria[5]. In the present study, untreated gliadin, flour and glutenin produced alterations in enzyme activity, IEL counts and enterocyte heights indicative of toxicity. When enzyme-treated gliadin was fed it produced a drop in lactase and sucrase with no corresponding drop in alkaline phosphatase activity; a slight fall in enterocyte height was noted in one patient, but in none of the four patients was there a rise in IEL count.

From these feeding studies, it appears that the gliadin toxicity has been markedly reduced by the enzymic removal of a side-chain sub-stituent of the protein backbone of gliadin.

ACKNOWLEDGEMENTS

We wish to acknowledge the support of the Wellcome Trust, The Medical Research Council of Ireland and The Western Health Board.

References

1. Phelan, J. J., McCarthy, C. F., Stevens, F. M., McNicholl, B. and Fottrell, P. F. (1974). The nature of gliadin toxicity in coeliac disease: a new concept. In: W. Th. J. M. Hekkens and A. S. Peña (eds.) *Coeliac Disease. Proceedings of the Second International Coeliac Symposium*, pp. 60–70, (Leiden: Stenfert Kroese)
2. Stevens, F. M., Lloyd, R., Egan-Mitchell, B., Mylotte, M. J., Fottrell, P. F., Wright, R., McNicholl, B. and McCarthy, C. F. (1975). Reticulin antibodies in patients with coeliac disease and their relatives. *Gut*, **16**, 598
3. Phelan, J. J., Stevens, F. M., McNicholl, B., Fottrell, P.F. and McCarthy C. F. (1977). Coeliac disease: the abolition of gliadin toxicity by enzymes from *Aspergillus niger*. *Clin. Sci. Mol. Med.* **53**, 35
4. Hekkens, W. Th. J. M., Van dem Aarsen, C. J., Gilliams, J. P., Lem-Van Kan, P. H. and Bouma-Frolich, G. (1974). α-Gliadin structure and degradation. In: W. Th. J. M. Hekkens and A. S.Peña (eds.) *Coeliac Disease. Proceedings of the Second International Coeliac Symposium*, pp. 39–45 (Leiden: Stenfert Kroese)
5. Dissanayake, A. S., Jerrome, D. W., Offord, R. E., Truelove, S. C. and Whitehead R. (1974). Identifying toxic fractions of wheat gluten and their effect on the jejunal mucosa in coeliac disease. *Gut*, **15**, 931

PAPER READ IN DISCUSSION BY F. R. COMERFORD

The ultrastructure of small bowel biopsies before and after challenge with treated gliadin and flour is shown in Figures 1–7.

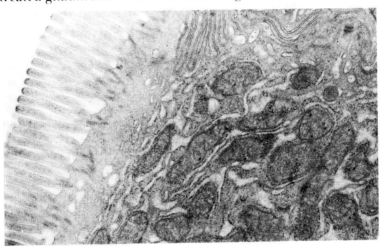

Figure 1   (Before treated gliadin). Enterocyte cytoplasm, × 17 000

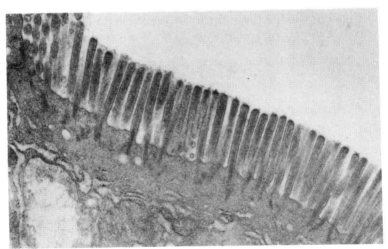

Figure 2   (Before treated gliadin). Microvilli with glycocalyx × 17 000

Four small bowel biopsies from the 52-year-old patient with coeliac disease described by Dr Stevens, were examined by electron microscopy. The first pair of biopsies were examined before and after exposure to treated gliadin, the second pair before and after exposure to flour. Each pair of specimens were processed together.

In the first control biopsy, the morphology was unremarkable. Enterocyte cytoplasmic structure appeared normal (Figure 1) as did the microvilli, (Figure 2). The biopsy obtained after the patient had ingested

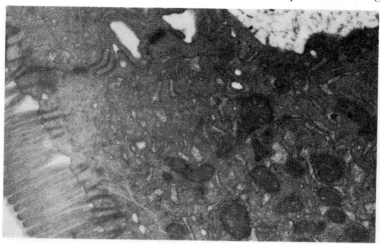

Figure 3 (After treated gliadin). Enterocyte cytoplasm. Note intercellular separation (upper centre and left) × 17 000

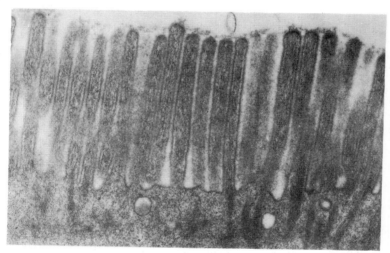

Figure 4 (After treated gliadin). Microvilli with glycocalyx × 33 000

treated gliadin did not differ significantly in ultrastructure from the control specimen. Some intercellular separation was noted (Figure 3) but the cytoplasm was otherwise normal. Microvilli were of normal dimensions with an intact glycocalyx (Figure 4).

The second set of biopsies were technically less satisfactory. In the control specimen, microvilli were normal in size and no significant cytoplasmic abnormalities were noted (Figure 5). In the specimen obtained

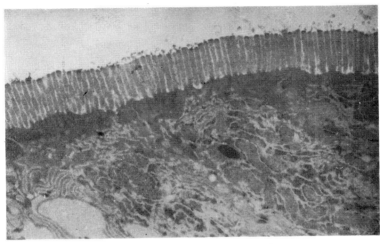

Figure 5 (Before flour). Microvilli and underlying cytoplasm × 7 250

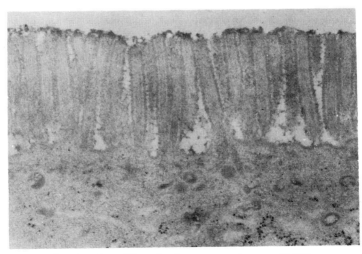

Figure 6 (After flour). Microvilli and adjacent cytoplasm × 19 000

after flour ingestion, areas with intact microvilli were observed (Figure 6). In other areas, there appeared to be focal damage to enterocytes with cytoplasmic abnormalities and distortion of microvilli (Figure 7). Changes thought to be indicative of vascular damage were also noted.

In conclusion, in this patient with coeliac disease, the ingestion of treated gliadin resulted in, at most, minor changes in small bowel ultra-structural morphology. In contrast, after flour ingestion, significant focal damage to enterocytes and perhaps also to blood vessels was observed.

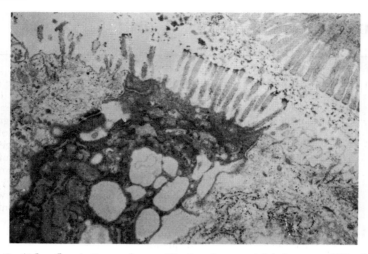

Figure 7 (After flour). Parts of two villi. One (upper right) does not differ from the control specimen. The second has a central enterocyte with vacuolated cytoplasm. The two adjacent cells are abnormal with loss of cytoplasmic organization and distorted microvilli, × 7 250

Discussion of chapters 4 and 5

Ferguson: Dr Hekkens started off this morning with a plea that we reach agreement about standardization of a test for gluten toxicity. I have the impression that the speed of damage produced by any fraction in the patient or in the *in vitro* cultures, is related to the degree of abnormality of the original biopsy. If the biopsy is absolutely normal, there seems to be greater resistance to tissue damage than if the biopsy is not absolutely normal. In Dr Stevens's subjects lymphocyte counts and disaccharidase activities were normal in three of the four patients given treated gluten, whereas they were abnormal in all patients challenged with untreated gluten. I would like to propose that *in vivo* challenges are carried out only on patients in whom the histology, disaccharidases and plasma counts are normal, and subsequent analysis should include disacchari-dase measurements and quantitative counts.

Stevens: If one were to challenge only coeliac patients in whom the biopsy has become completely normal, the challenge might have to be prolonged for months or years; especially if the toxicity had been reduced. Patient 4 has been fed with both treated gliadin and flour. The intraepithelial lymphocyte counts prior to feeding were almost identical in the two studies. Her mucosa was in a similar state at the commencement of feeding the two different fractions. The treated gliadin produced depression of lactase and sucrase and minor histological change, whereas flour produced severe enzyme and histological change and symptoms.

Douglas: I am very worried about the sensitivity of the test systems used. We are increasingly aware of the variability in responsiveness of patients when they are exposed to different amounts of gluten. This may underline the reason why even the so-called detoxified materials that have been studied by the Galway workers do not show any abnormalities in the short term. We are much more interested in what happens in the long term. We are getting very excited about what may be abnormal in the gluten and forgetting the abnormality in the patient. That is the primary abnormality that we should be involved with.

The same criticism applies to the beautiful work on this unique strain of wheat that Dr Kasarda has shown us. I'm rather disappointed, however, that in 1977 anybody can demonstrate toxicity by just referring to symptoms and changes in xylose without any reference to what happens to the intestinal biopsy. Even if he had shown us no change in the biopsies, I would still have said, you have got to go on feeding for a longer period of time.

Stevens	We have tried to overcome the problem of variable patient responsiveness to toxicity. On separate occasions two fractions have been fed to the same patient. Treated gliadin produced minimal changes whilst flour produced dramatic changes in toxicity.
Rey	I would like to stress the duration of the gluten-free diet in the patients studied by Dr Stevens. The length of the gluten-free diet is only six or seven months in the patients who were given untreated gluten, but it was two years in the patients given treated gliadin. It is well-known that relapse is more rapid when the length of the gluten-free diet is very short. You have a better correlation with the length of the gluten-free diet than with the type of gliadin.
Stevens	In our earlier studies, patients fed treated gliadin had been on gluten-free diets for much longer periods than the patient fed untreated gliadin. More recently, we have performed two studies on patient 4. The first challenge (treated gliadin) was conducted eight months after diagnosis and the commencement of a gluten-free diet. Following this study, the gluten-free diet was reintroduced. The subsequent challenge (flour) was performed after a further eight months.
McCarthy	I am also worried about the sensitivity of our assay system. However, I think it is hard to find a better assay system than giving the same patient two different fractions, each on a separate occasion.
Clarke	It is difficult to see some of the changes in histology, particularly where you are seeing only a single villus. I would have thought that you could have shown a significant change in brush border enzymes sucrase and lactase. They altered in both groups. Although the depression was not as much in the patients fed the so-called non-toxic fraction, the enzyme activity decreased in most of the patients studied. Perhaps you could explain how that happened?
Stevens	Depression of lactase and sucrase activity occurred in all but one patient. This might be the first sign of toxic change, and if we had prolonged the challenge with treated gliadin for a much longer period histological damage would have ensued. Originally, we suggested that the toxicity of gliadin had been abolished by enzyme treatment. Now we consider that the toxicity has been markedly reduced but not completely removed.
Holmes	Have you been able to isolate the carbohydrate radical and feed it alone, or mixed in with your detoxified gluten?
Phelan	We have not fed the diffusate after dialysis of the enzyme-treated gliadin, but we do have material prepared for feeding. We do not know the size of the side-chains, nor whether they will dialyse out.
Fielding	The results could equally be interpreted as showing that the treated gliadin was capable of priming the patient for the toxic response seen with the second substance.
Stevens	In the series where patients were primed prior to testing, I think this was done only weeks before the challenge. In this patient, the priming would have been eight months prior to the challenge. I do not know if the effect would be the same.
Kasarda	Because of Phelan's earlier work we examined our A-gliadin preparation for carbohydrate rather carefully. (Bernardin, *et al.*, *Cereal Chem.*, **53**, 612, 1976). We found carbohydrate at the level equivalent to 1 molecule of glucose for every 10 molecules of

protein (M.W. 36 000). This is a very low level. This could easily be explained by contamination. On the other hand, we know that our A-gliadin is not completely pure, there is certainly a few per cent of other proteins in it. If 1% of the preparation was a glyco-protein, we could end up with the carbohydrate levels that we find. The question is, could 1% impurity in the A-gliadin prepar-ation account for the toxicity? There is no answer to that question right now.

Phelan   I would like to substantiate Dr Kasarda's finding. After precipi-tating and resuspending the protein several times we find the carbohydrate level in gliadin is extremely low.

Rossipal   In coeliac disease, on electron microscopy, the cells down in the crypts may have a normal structure. Where did the cells you examined come from? Are they from the crypt, the neck of the crypt or the villi?

Comerford   We thought these cells were superficial.

Hekkens   Jim, you stated that no proteolytic enzyme could abolish toxicity. Could you make the same statement about your carbohydrase? Do you have a pure carbohydrase, and does it abolish toxicity? Is it only a crude preparation?

Phelan   No-one has found a purified proteolytic enzyme which abolishes toxicity.

We started deliberately with enzymes from *Aspergillus niger*. The enzymes had broad substrate specificity to cleave as many bonds as possible, but they were free of proteolytic activity. The enzymes abolish toxicity almost completely. Using these enzymes, we are trying to locate the toxic fraction. Once the toxic fraction is found, then we will be able to purify the enzyme. During prepar-ation of enzyme-treated gliadin, we were very careful not to unfold the gliadin molecule. The side-chain substituent on gliadin is probably added to the outside of the molecule after it is folded. There may be other aggregates in gliadin which prevent the enzyme from removing the last trace of toxicity.

Trier   Even if one only looks at the superficial zone, either a villus or surface epithelium, on electron microscopy one has a problem. The changes described are found frequently in normal tissue. As cells exfoliate from the intestine they undergo degenerative changes. Quantitation is extremely important. Dr Comerford, were the changes quantified, and were the electron microscopic studies performed on coded grids without foreknowledge if it was before or after treatment?

Comerford   We do not have quantitation as yet and the studies were not done on coded grids. The abnormal findings we described were not seen with an equal search on the pretreatment biopsy. The villus adjacent to the abnormal area showed a relatively normal struc-ture.

Douglas   Dr Holmes raised the point as to whether Dr Phelan had tried feeding the carbohydrate material. In the work that Dr Hekkens referred to earlier on the binding of fractions from gliadin to the mucosa, I showed that certain simple sugars were able to interfere with the interaction. This would be a very useful experiment if it were possible to carry it out.

6

A test of toxicity of bread made from wheat lacking α-gliadins coded for by the 6A chromosome

D. D. KASARDA, C. O. QUALSET, D. K. MECHAM,
D. M. GOODENBERGER and W. STROBER

TOXICITY OF α-GLIADINS

In 1950, Dicke[1] discovered that wheat grain was responsible for producing the symptoms of coeliac disease in susceptible individuals. Some other cereal grains were found subsequently to produce symptoms as well. Rye, barley and possibly oats (see discussion of Baker and Read[2]) were also toxic (in the sense of producing symptoms of the disease) whereas rice and maize were not. These species all belong to the grass family (Gramineae); their taxonomic relationships are shown in Figure 6.1 where it can be seen that rye is most closely related to wheat, followed by barley, whereas oats and rice are more distantly related to

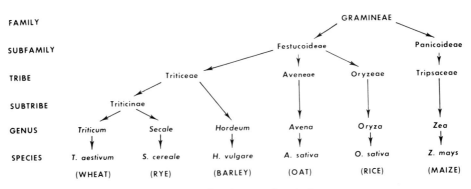

Figure 6.1   Taxonomic relationships of major cereal grains[3]

wheat according to this classification scheme[3].

In 1953, Van de Kamer *et al.*[4] showed that the gliadin proteins were the most toxic fraction of wheat grain. In 1970, Hekkens *et al.*[5] fractionated the complex mixture of gliadins to show that the α-gliadin fraction was toxic, and in 1972, Kendall *et al.*[6] provided some evidence that only the α-gliadin fraction may be toxic.

In earlier work at the Western Regional Research Laboratory[7,8], we had characterized a particular α-gliadin fraction which we now call A-gliadin[9]. Our method for preparation of A-gliadin was one of the methods used by Hekkens *et al.*[5] in their demonstration of α-gliadin toxicity. Falchuk *et al.*[10] found that A-gliadin inhibited the development of specific enzyme activities in organ cultures of tissue obtained by jejunal biopsy from patients with active disease.

RELATIONSHIP OF α-GLIADINS TO CHROMOSOMES

Bread wheats (*Triticum aestivum*) belong to a hexaploid species that incorporates three different genomes (designated A, B, and D) each of which contributes seven chromosomes (haploid number) to the polyploid genome. The species that contributed the A and B genomes are not known with certainty, whereas *Aegilops squarrosa* is accepted as the donor of the D genome. Several hypotheses have been advanced for the evolution of wheats; one of the most recent schemes, proposed by Konarev *et al.*[11] is shown in Figure 6.2.

In our studies of A-gliadin, we found that the genes coding for this fraction were located on chromosome 6A[12]. Shepherd[13] and Wrigley and Shepherd[14] had shown previously that the α-gliadins of the wheat

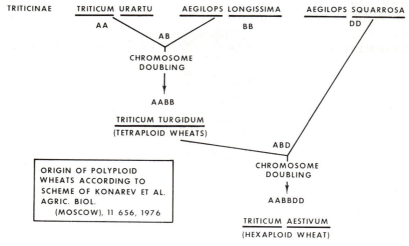

Figure 6.2 Origin of polyploid wheats from diploid grass species[11]

variety 'Chinese Spring' were coded for mainly by genes of chromosome 6A. Because A-gliadin was controlled by the 6A chromosome, and was toxic in coeliac disease, we thought it possible that the α-gliadins of 'Chinese Spring' might be equivalent toxic proteins although this has not been tested.

NULLISOMIC 6A-TETRASOMIC 6B 'CHINESE SPRING'

We were aware that Sears[15] had produced nullisomic–tetrasomic variants of Chinese Spring wheat in which particular chromosomes were completely missing (nullisomic) and compensated for by two extra doses of a homologous chromosome (tetrasomic). Kasarda *et al.*[12] proposed that the variants of 'Chinese Spring' that were missing chromosome 6A might be free of the toxic factor if gliadins coded by other chromosomes were not also toxic.

Sears[15] had developed both the nullisomic 6A–tetrasomic 6B variant (N6A–T6B) and the nullisomic 6A–tetrasomic 6D variant (N6A–T6D) of 'Chinese Spring'. Because some of the α-gliadin components of 'Chinese Spring' are controlled by genes located on chromosome 6D (Figure 6.3), and because we did not know if these gliadins were toxic (we hoped not), we decided to test the hypothesis that nullisomic-6A wheats were free of the toxic factor[12]. N6A–T6B produced less of the 6D α-gliadins than did N6A–T6D because N6A–T6B has the normal dose of two 6D chromosomes (although having four 6B chromosomes),

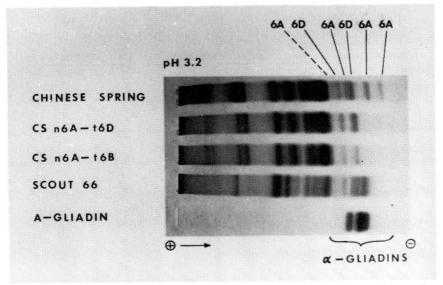

Figure 6.3 Electrophoretic patterns of gliadins and of A-gliadin obtained according to the procedure of Kasarda *et al.*[12]

whereas N6A–T6D has two extra 6D chromosomes beyond the normal two and synthesis of gliadin protein components is roughly proportional to the number of chromosomes coding for these components[16].

The electrophoretic patterns of gliadin proteins extracted from N6A–T6B and N6A–T6D are compared in Figure 6.3 with the gliadins of normal 'Chinese Spring', 'Scout 66' and of A-gliadin prepared from 'Scout 66'. As can be seen in Figure 6.3, the 6A α-gliadins are missing from the patterns of N6–T6B and N6A–T6D and the bands corresponding to the 6D α-gliadins are more intense in N6A–T6D than in N6A–T6B.

NULLI–6A BREAD

From their developer, E. R. Sears, we obtained a few seeds of each of the nullisomic–tetrasomic variants of 'Chinese Spring' that were missing chromosome 6A and increased the seed for three plant generations at the University of California, Davis, and at Tulelake, California. Special precautions were taken to prevent contamination by normal wheats. Although the agronomic characteristics of these variants (and of 'Chinese Spring' itself) were not as good as those of commercial wheat varieties, no important problems were encountered in producing enough wheat grain for testing[17]. Large quantities for use in a speciality bread could be produced with minimal difficulty under California field conditions.

The grain was milled into flour at the Western Regional Research Laboratory and bread was baked there from the N6A–T6B flour (nulli-6A bread). Again, elaborate precautions were taken to insure that no contamination took place from normal wheat flour residues in the mills, mixers, and other equipment used. The bread had good texture and excellent taste. It was stored in a cold room at –34 °C until needed.

TESTS WITH PATIENTS

So far, two patients have each been fed about 65 g of nulli–6A bread per day for a period of two weeks. This is equivalent to 1.8 to 2.0 g of gliadin per day. The clinical results are summarized in Figures 6.4 for one patient, who was challenged also with bread made from normal 'Scout 66' wheat for a brief period. Neither patient had any adverse reaction to the bread. On the basis of previous testing of these patients and of the past experience of the patients themselves, the amount of bread eaten should have produced a reaction.

DISCUSSION

We consider the results of our initial tests encouraging and worth con-

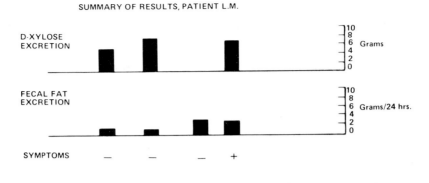

Figure 6.4 D-xylose excretion, faecal fat excretion, and symptomatic response data for patient L.M. Nulli–6A bread was fed from day 6 through day 19. 'Scout 66' bread was fed from day 26 through day 33

tinuing. At the least, the nulli-6A bread seems to be less toxic than normal bread; it may not be toxic at all. We are continuing the testing to answer that question.

We have noted[8,9] that some wheats, such as 'Scout 66' (from which we presently prepare A-gliadin), have more protein with the mobility of α-gliadins than others, such as 'Justin' and 'Chinese Spring'. We have not carried out any tests with the parent 'Chinese Spring'. Perhaps it is less toxic than other wheats; however, we are not aware of any solid information on the relative toxicity of different wheat varieties.

It would seem that the most direct course toward obtaining a non-toxic wheat would be to define the toxic factor exactly at the molecular level and then to analyse qualitatively and quantitatively for its presence in wheat and related species. The definition of the toxic factor has seemed to be almost within reach numerous times over the past twenty years, but it still has yet to be achieved. Characterization of the toxic factor at its most elemental molecular level will require much painstaking and imaginative chemistry carried out, ultimately, at the milligram level—unless considerably greater support than now seems to be available provides the means for scaling up those milligrams into grams. Testing milligram amounts presents some problems, although they can be overcome.

While working toward exact definition of the toxic factor, we think that considerable benefit might also be obtained from an examination of the toxicity of prolamines from diploid species related to wheat, particularly those that may have contributed genomes to polyploid wheats. In a preceding section, we pointed out that bread wheats combine three different genomes, each derived originally from a diploid grass species. The D genome was contributed, for example, by *Aegilops squarrosa* and, as we have seen, some of the α-gliadins of 'Chinese Spring' were contributed by the D genome. Are these α-gliadins toxic in addition to the α-gliadins contributed by the A genome? Is *Aegilops squarrosa* toxic? Answers to these questions could ease our way toward development of a non-toxic wheat.

If *Aegilops squarrosa* proved to be non-toxic, this would provide considerable support for the possibility that a non-toxic wheat could be achieved by genetic means of the sort we describe in this paper.

ACKNOWLEDGEMENTS

We thank E. R. Sears for providing us with seeds of the aneuploids, A. P. Mossman for milling the wheat, and M. M. Hanamoto for assistance in baking the bread.

References

1. Dickie, W. K. (1950). *Coeliakie*. M. D. Thesis (University of Utrecht, The Netherlands)
2. Baker, P. G. and Read, A. E. (1976). Oats and barley toxicity in coeliac disease. *Postgrad. Med. J.*, **52**, 264
3. Hitchcock, A. S. (1950). *Manual of grasses of the United States*. 2nd Ed. Revised by Agnes Chase, 1051 p. (US Dept. Agriculture, Miscellaneous Publication No. 200)
4. Van de Kamer, J. H., Weijers, H. A. and Dicke, W. K. (1953). Coeliac disease, IV. An investigation into the injurious constituents of wheat in connection with their action on patients with coeliac disease. *Acta Paediat.*, **42**, 223
5. Hekkens, W. Th. J. M., Haex, A. J. Ch. and Willighagen, R. G. J. (1970). Some aspects of gliadin fractionation and testing by a histochemical method. In: C. C. Booth and R. H. Dowling (eds.) *Coeliac Disease. Proc. Int. Symposium*, pp. 11–19. (London: Churchill Livingstone)
6. Kendall, M. J., Cox, P. S., Schneider, R. and Hawkins, C. F. (1972). Gluten subfractions in coeliac disease. *Lancet*, **ii**, 1065
7. Bernardin, J. E., Kasarda, D. D. and Mecham, D. K. (1967). Preparation and characterization of α-gliadin. *J. Biol. Chem.*, **242**, 445
8. Kasarda, D. D., Bernardin, J. E. and Nimmo, C. C. (1976). Wheat proteins. In: Y. Pomeranz (ed.) *Adv. Cereal Sci. Tech.*, **Vol. 1.**, pp. 158–236 (St. Paul, Minn.: American Assoc. Cereal Chemists)
9. Platt, S. G., Kasarda, D. D. and Qualset, C. O. (1974). Varietal relationships of the α-gliadin proteins in wheat. *J. Sci. Food Agric.*, **25**, 1555
10. Falchuk, Z. M., Gebhard, R. L., Sessoms, C. S. and Strober, W. (1974). An *in vitro* model of gluten sensitive enteropathy: the effect of gliadin on intestinal epithelial cells in organ culture. *J. Clin. Invest.*, **53**, 487
11. Konarev, V. G., Gavrilyuk, I. P., Peneva, T. I., Konarev, A. V., Khakimova, A. G. and Migushova, E. F. (1976). Nature and origin of wheat genomes based on data from the biochemistry and immunochemistry of wheat proteins. *Sel'skokhozyaystvennaya Biologiya*, **11**, 656
12. Kasarda, D. D., Bernardin, J. E. and Qualset, C. O. (1976). Relationship of gliadin protein components to chromosomes in hexaploid wheats (*Triticum aestivum L.*). *Proc. Natl. Acad. Sci. USA*, **73**, 3646

13. Shepherd, K. W. (1968). Chromosomal control of proteins in wheat and rye. In: K. W. Finlay and K. W. Shepherd (eds.) *Proc. 3rd Int. Wheat Genetics Symposium*, pp. 86–96 (Canberra: Australian Acad. Sci.)
14. Wrigley, C. W. and Shepherd, K. W. (1973). Electrofocussing of grain proteins from wheat genotypes. *Ann. N. Y. Acad. Sci.*, **209,** 154
15. Sears, E. R. (1954). The aneuploids of common wheat. *Res. Bull. 572.* 59p. (Columbia, Mo.: Missouri Agric. Exp. Sta.)
16. Mecham, D. K., Kasarda, D. D. and Qualset, C. O. (1977). Genetic aspects of wheat gliadin proteins. (In preparation)
17. Tucić, B., McGuire, P. E., Qualset, C. O. and Kasarda, D. D. (1977). Nullisomic–tetrasomic wheat for agronomic and nutritional studies. (In preparation)

Discussion of chapter 6

Cooke
Xylose absorption and faecal fast studies are, in my opinion, inaccurate tests of gluten toxicity and I wonder if you have done other more specific tests; with such highly and brilliant scientific work I found that as a clinician who really is just a cookery book sort of chap extremely disappointing. No doubt they have done cell counts and cell counting in our view is a very accurate way, though referees to gut do not seem to think so, and complement changes and other more specific and scientific methods than the crude xylose and the very, very crude fat absorption.

Dr Kasarda
This is very preliminary work. It took us three plant generations to get sufficient wheat to do a feeding experiment. We hope to do more elaborate tests, only xylose absorption and faecal fat absorption have been studied in these two patients I mentioned.

Section II
Gluten toxicity and organ culture

7

Organ culture model of gluten-sensitive enteropathy

Z. M. FALCHUK and A. J. KATZ

We have previously developed an *in vitro* model of gluten-sensitive enteropathy (GSE) using organ culture techniques[1,2]. This model relies on the observation that jejunal tissue obtained from patients with active enteropathy undergoes morphological and biochemical improvement when cultured in a gluten-free environment. Surface epithelial cells regain a more normal histological appearance and acquire more mature brush borders; this improvement is associated with dramatic increases of microvillar enzyme activity, most notably alkaline phosphatase. In contrast, no improvement occurs in these measurements if the tissue is cultured in the presence of gluten protein. Jejunal mucosa of patients with gluten-sensitive enteropathy in remission and normal controls cultured in similar fashion is not affected by the presence of gluten protein in the culture medium. The behaviour in organ culture of tissue from patients with active enteropathy is an *in vitro* model of the disorder because, in parallel with the manifestations of the disease *in vivo*, the biochemical and morphological changes are exquisitely gluten-dependent (Figure 7.1).

The lack of effect of gluten on tissues from patients in remission reflects the belief that gluten is not directly toxic to intestinal tissue of patients with the disease, but rather that gluten must first initiate a set of events *in vivo*, possibly related to the immune system, which in turn mediates the cytotoxic events.

We utilized this model to investigate two questions. In the first of these

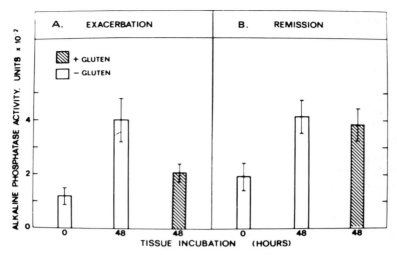

Figure 7.1 The *in vitro* model of gluten sensitive enteropathy (GSE). The effect of gluten peptides on alkaline phosphatase activity of intestinal mucosa after 48 hours in organ culture. A, Patients with GSE in exacerbation. Initial low alkaline phosphatase activity increases significantly in tissue cultured in the absence of gluten. The increase is inhibited by the addition of gluten peptides to the medium. The bars represent the mean ± 1 standard error of studies in 9 to 12 patients. B, Patients with GSE in remission. Alkaline phosphatase activity is not influenced by the presence or absence of gluten during the culture. This behaviour is indistinguishable from that of tissue from normal individuals. (From Katz, A. J. and Falchuk, Z. M. (1975). *Pediatric Clinics of North America,* **22,** 767)

we asked: what is the value of the intestinal organ culture model in differentiating GSE from other causes of the flat villous lesion? That is, is it possible to obviate the need for three biopsies to firmly establish the diagnosis of GSE[3]—a biopsy at the time of presentation to document mucosal damage, a biopsy at the time of clinical remission on a gluten-free diet to show mucosal morphological recovery, and a biopsy after a gluten challenge to show return of mucosal damage.

To address this question, we studied prospectively, patients coming to our clinics for evaluation of diarrhoea[4]. These patients were evaluated by conventional means as well as by intestinal biopsy. The biopsies were assessed morphologically and portions of the biopsies were placed into organ culture in the presence and absence of a peptic tryptic digest of gluten[5]. Under these conditions, gluten is detrimental to mucosa of patients with GSE as previously shown by us[1]. The morphological assessment of the biopsies revealed that 50% were completely normal.The remaining ones showed a flat villous lesion ranging from partial villous shortening to total absence of villi. Of the patients with a flat villous lesion, the organ culture model allowed us to differentiate the ones which were gluten-sensitive from those who were not in greater than 85% of the cases. These data will be published elsewhere.

In every case where gluten sensitivity was demonstrated *in vitro* the diagnosis of GSE was subsequently confirmed. No gluten sensitivity was demonstrated *in vitro* when the flat villous lesion was not due to GSE. The technique, if positive, can obviate the need for multiple biopsies and challenges to establish the diagnosis of GSE in patients with a flat villous lesion.

The second question we approached using the model was: does cortisol, an agent which prevents the effects of gluten *in vivo* in patients with GSE[6-8], prevent the deleterious effect of gluten *in vitro* on intestinal mucosa of patients with GSE? If so, can we gain insight into the mechanism of action of this agent in GSE? We studied a group of patients with documented GSE who were on a gluten challenge[9]. Biopsies were placed into culture in media with and without gluten and/or cortisol.

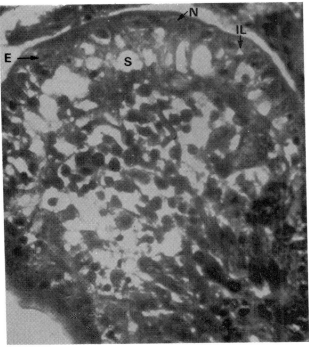

Figure 7.2 Intestinal biopsy specimen obtained from a patient with active gluten-sensitive enteropathy cultured for 24 h in the presence of gluten protein. The appearance is indistinguishable from the baseline (0 h) specimen. The epithelial cells (E) are cuboidal; the nuclei (N) are not basally oriented. Intraepithelial lymphocytes are noted (IL). Numerous intercellular spaces are seen (S). This is an *in vitro* perpetuation of the exacerbation state. (× 125). (From Katz, A. J., Falchuk, Z. M., Strober, W. and Shwachman, H. (1976). *N.Engl. J. Med.*, **295**, 131)

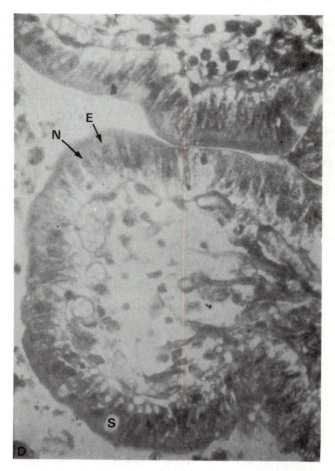

Figure 7.3 Intestinal biopsy specimen obtained from a patient with active gluten-sensitive enteropathy cultured for 24 h in the absence of gluten protein. Extruded cellular debris is seen on the surface (D). This specimen was cultured in the absence of gluten protein. As compared with the baseline appearance (see Figure 7.2), the epithelial cells (E) are columnar, nuclei (N) are basally oriented, and only occasional intercellular spaces (S) are present. This is an *in vitro* remission. (× 180). (From Katz, A. J., Falchuk, Z. M., Strober, W. and Shwachman, H. (1976). *N. Engl. J. Med.*, **295**, 131)

Cortisol was present in a concentration of 5 micromolar. This is the equivalent steroid concentration of the value achieved when 60 mg of prednisone are given to a 70 kg person. The tissues were harvested at the end of culture and assessed for morphology and alkaline phosphatase activity. The morphology after 24 hours of culture in a gluten containing medium is the same as that of the tissue prior to culture and shows cuboidal epithelial cells, infiltration with lymphocytes and plasma cells in the lamina propria, and increase in numbers of interepithelial lymphocytes (Figure 7.2) This is *in vitro* perpetuation of the exacerbation state. After 24 hours of culture in a gluten-free medium, the epithelial cells became columnar, the nuclear polarity became normal, and epithelial cell vacuoles nearly disappeared (Figure 7.3). This is *in vitro* remission. In contrast to the results of culture in a gluten–containing medium alone, with perpetuation of the exacerbation state, culture in the presence of gluten and cortisol dramatically inhibited the damage brought on by the gluten—the biopsy under these conditions reverted toward normal just as if gluten was omitted from the culture (Figure 7.4). The enzyme activities of these tissues paralleled

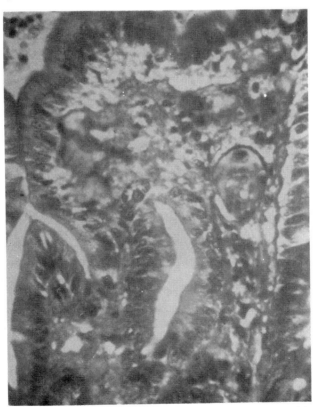

Figure 7.4 Intestinal biopsy specimen obtained from a patient with active gluten sensitive enteropathy cultured for 24 h in the presence of both gluten protein and $5 \mu M$ cortisol. The effect of gluten is completely abolished, with the histological appearance reverting toward normal. The tissue has the same appearance as that cultured in the absence of gluten. ($\times$ 130). (From Katz, A. J., Falchuk, Z. M., Strober, W. and Shwachman, H. (1976). *N. Engl. J. Med.*, **295**, 131)

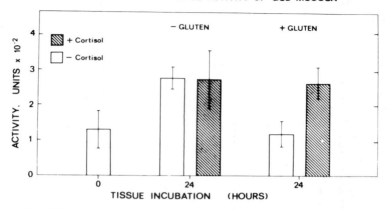

EFFECT OF CORTISOL AND GLUTEN ON
ALKALINE PHOSPHATASE ACTIVITY OF GSE MUCOSA

Figure 7.5 Alkaline phosphatase activity of jejunal mucosa from patients with active gluten-sensitive enteropathy. Cultures were carried out for 24 h in the presence or absence of gluten or cortisol. The hatched bars represent the values obtained in the presence of cortisol. In the absence of cortisol, gluten prevents the increase in activity of alkaline phosphatase. Addition of cortisol ablates this effect. Each bar represents the mean ± SE of eight studies done in duplicate. (From Katz, A. J., Falchuk, Z. M., Strober, W. and Shwachman, H. (1976). *N. Engl. J. Med.*, **295**, 131)

the morphological findings. Culture in the absence of gluten led to final alkaline phophatase activities of two-fold over baseline while culture in the presence of gluten abolished this rise: *in vitro* remission and exacerbation. Culture in the presence of gluten, but also in the presence of cortisol, on the other hand, led to final alkaline phosphatase values which were two-fold over baseline, thus eliminating the deleterious effect of gluten. Cortisol alone, in the absence of gluten, had no effect (Figure 7.5). Cortisol eliminates the deleterious effect of gluten *in vitro*.

Since cortisol interferes with certain immune phenomena,[10–13] we asked whether the salutory action of cortisol *in vitro* might be related to some effect upon the local immune system which we previously showed to have a possible role in the pathogenesis of the lesion of GSE[14]. Thus, patients with GSE have values for mucosal IgA synthesis 5–8 fold greater than values in normal subjects (Figure 7.6). Much of the mucosal immunoglobulin has antigluten antibody activity[14]. We examined the effect of cortisone in organ culture on mucosal IgA secretion by assessing the amount of ^{14}C-labelled IgA[15] secreted into the medium during a 24 h period of continous labelling by [^{14}C]leucine. The data show that cortisol has a striking effect on [^{14}C]IgA secretion by the tissue during the period of culture (Falchuk and Katz, unpublished observations). There is a 50% drop in the total secreted immunoglobulin in the presence of cortisol as compared to the absence of cortisol. We

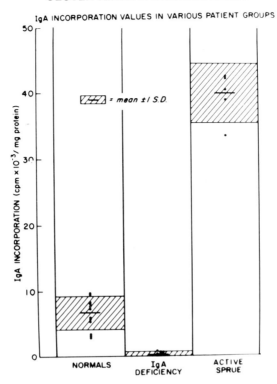

Figure 7.6 [14C] L-leucine incorporation into IgA. Values in normal individuals (12), patients with isolated serum IgA deficiency or panhypogammaglobulinaemia (8), and patients with sprue (5). The bar and shaded areas represent the mean ± 1 standard deviation. Each point was measured in duplicate. (From Falchuk, Z. M. and Strober, W. (1972). *J. Lab. Clin. Med.,* **79,** 1004)

believe that decreased secretion of IgA into the medium is related to a decreased synthesis of local immunoglobulin. We speculate that the beneficial effect of cortisone in this situation is in some way related to the decreased immunoglobulin production.

We hope to use the techniques we developed to shed further light on the pathogenic events in gluten sensitive enteropathy.

ACKNOWLEDGEMENTS

Supported in past by NIH grants AM17684, AM07121. Dr Falchuk is a recipient of Public Health Service Research Career Development award AM00210. Dr Katz is a recipient of the Basil O'Connor Award from the National Foundation—March of Dimes.

References

1. Falchuk, Z. M., Gebhard, R. L., Sessoms, C. and Strober, W. (1974). An *in vitro* model of gluten-sensitive enteropathy. *J. Clin. Invest.,* **53,** 487
2. Browning, T. H. and Trier, J. S. (1969). Organ culture of mucosal biopsies of human small intestine. *J. Clin. Invest.,* **48,** 1423
3. Visakorpi, J. S. (1974). Definition of coeliac disease in children. In: W. Th. J. M. Hekkens and A. S. Peña (eds.) *Proceedings of the Second Coeliac Symposium,* p. 10
4. Katz, A. J. and Falchuk, Z. M. (1977). Intestinal organ culture: the definitive diagnosis of gluten-sensitive enteropathy. *Paediatr. Res.,* **11,** 445
5. Frazer, A. C., Fletcher, R. F., Ross, C. A. C. *et al.* (1959). Gluten induced enteropathy. The effect of partially digested gluten. *Lancet,* **ii,** 252
6. Adlersberg, D., Colcher, H. and Drachman, S. R. (1951). Studies on the effects of cortisone and pituitary adrenocorticotropic hormone (ACTH) in the sprue syndrome. *Gastroenterology,* **19,** 674
7. Taylor, A. B., Wollaeger, E. E., Comfort, M. W. *et al.* (1952). The effect of cortisone on non-tropical sprue (idiopathic steatorrhea). *Gastroenterology,* **20,** 203
8. Wall, A. J., Douglas, A. P., Booth, C. C. *et al.* (1970). Response of the jejunal mucosa in adult coeliac disease to oral prednisolone. *Gut,* **11,** 7
9. Katz, A. J., Falchuk, Z. M., Strober, W. and Shwachman, H. (1976). Gluten-sensitive enteropathy. Inhibition by cortisol of the effect of gluten protein *in vitro. N. Engl. J. Med.,* **295,** 131
10. Nowell, P. C. (1961). Inhibition of human leukocyte mitosis by prednisolone *in vitro. Cancer Res.,* **21,** 1518
11. Balow, J. E. and Rosenthal, A. S. (1973). Glucocorticoid suppression of macrophage migration inibitory factor. *J. Exp. Med.,* **137,** 1031
12. Heilman, D. H., Gambrill, M. R. and Leichner, J. P. (1973). The effect of hydrocotisone on the incorporation of tritiated thymidine by human blood lymphocytes cultured with phytohaemagglutinin and pokeweed mitogens. *Clin. Exp. Immunol.,* **15,** 203
13. Wahl, S. M., Altman, L. C. and Rosenstrech, D. L. (1975). Inhibition of *in vitro* lymphokine synthesis of glucocorticoids. *J. Immunol.,* **115,** 476
14. Falchuk, Z. M. and Strober, W. (1974). Gluten-sensitive enteropathy. Synthesis of antigliadin antibody *in vitro. Gut,* **14,** 947
15. Falchuk, Z. M. and Strober, W. (1972). Increased jejunal immunoglobulin synthesis in patients with non-tropical sprue as measured by a solid phase immunoabsorption technique. *J. Lab. Clin. Med.,* **79,** 1004

Discussion of chapter 7

Cluysenaer   I am amazed at the high number of non-coeliacs in your group with mucosal abnormalities: one-third of all patients with a flat mucosa did not have gluten-sensitive enteropathy. This is extremely peculiar. Most authors, and also our own experience, indicate that a flat mucosa is nearly pathognomic for coeliac sprue. Could it be due to your method of biopsying, being a sampling error, or an omittance of orienting the biopsies?

Falchuk   No, I think it is not due to any of the factors you mention, I think it is due to the peculiar patient population referred to us. We have a referral centre to which are sent most of the patients with diarrhoea that have been worked up elsewhere and for which no solution has been found. Of the patients who have had lesions, 14 of them had diseases that were clearly identified as being able to produce flat villous lesions, not due to gluten sensitivity, so I think it is just a question of the type of patient referred to us.

Challacombe   There is some evidence that coeliac disease in childhood is in fact dose-related to the amount of gluten. In your experiments did you find that the activity of alkaline phosphatase was at any time related to the dose of gluten in your medium?

Falchuk   Early in our work we discovered that the gluten preparation we used was non-specifically toxic if we used enough of it, so we did careful dose titration curves to arrive at a dose that doesn't produce toxicity in normal mucosa, or as demonstrated by these studies a mucosa which is not gluten-sensitive. I think that is a critical question, and anybody using this kind of technique for assessment of toxicity must do that kind of a study.

Asquith   With respect to your reduction of immunoglobulin synthesis by cortisol. In previous studies you have shown that about 70 or 80% of the immunoglobulin produced was specific antigluten antibody. Do you think it is possible that most of the suppression that you are showing by cortisol is of non-specific antibody production. Have you shown specificity of IgA antibody for gluten?

Falchuk   I think that is a very critical question, Peter. I'd like to point out to you that what we demonstrated previously is that up to 75 or 80% of the increment in immunoglobulin synthesis by patients who are challenged, has antigluten specificity. It is not 75 or 80% of a total immune globulin. With cortisol there is a decrement of approximately 50% of total immunoglobulin. The critical question is the one that you raise and that is, at the same time that we are diminishing total immunoglobulin synthesis, are we also eliminating specific antigluten antibody activity? We haven't examined this as of yet. I would predict that we are.

73

8

Isolation and characterization of the toxic fraction of wheat gliadin in coeliac disease

J. JOS, L. CHARBONNIER, J. F. MOUGENOT, J. MOSSE and J. REY

INTRODUCTION

The pathogenesis of coeliac disease has not yet been entirely cleared up but organ culture methods have greatly helped to clarify it, so that the enzymatic hypothesis is now practically excluded[1]. Biopsy specimens from untreated coeliac patients improve after only 24 hours of culture in a gluten-free environment[2], whereas the morphologic and enzymatic restoration is prevented by the addition of a peptic–tryptic digest (PT digest) of gliadin to the medium[3,4]. On the other hand, in cultured specimens from treated patients, i.e. after normalization of the intestinal histology, the cytotoxic effect is no longer observed[3,5]. It seems, therefore, that gluten peptides *per se* are not directly toxic to coeliac mucosa but require the participation of an 'endogenous effector mechanism', as is suggested by the fact that a cytotoxic effect is observed in biopsy specimens from treated patients when they are cultured in the presence of specimens from untreated patients (mixed culture) in a gluten-containing medium[6]. Furthermore it was demonstrated that cortisol partially prevents the harmful effect of gluten in the *in vitro* system, as well as *in vivo*[7], and that a migration inhibition factor (MIF) is secreted into the culture medium when biopsy specimens from untreated patients are cultured in the presence of α-gliadin[8].

Since our previous publications[4,5], considerable progress has been made in the isolation and characterization of the toxic components of wheat gluten by further *in vitro* experiments using the organ culture method and lymphocyte stimulation assays. In the present report, we describe the results of these additional studies.

MATERIAL AND METHODS

Patients

Biopsies were taken at the duodeno-jejunal flexure with the Crosby paediatric capsule from 58 children with active coeliac disease. Of these, 39 had never been treated before, 6 had been on a gluten-free diet for less than 7 days and 15 were in relapse after the reintroduction of gluten in the diet for at least one year; all had subtotal or total villous atrophy. Thirteen children with colitis or transient diarrhoea but without malabsorption or abnormal jejunal mucosa were taken as controls. Informed consent of the parents was obtained in every case.

For lymphocyte stimulation assays, 14 patients with coeliac disease were selected, all having been on a gluten-free diet for at least three months at the time of testing; 6 children with cow's milk intolerance and 8 without any gastrointestinal disorder or immunodeficiency were chosen as controls.

Preparation and fractionation of gliadin

Gliadin was prepared from defatted flour of Capitole wheat by extraction with a 55% ethanol solution followed by precipitation with a 1.5% NaCl solution[9].

Large-scale preparation of gliadin fractions was carried out by ion exchange chromatography using a modification of the method previously described[9,10]. A column of sulfopropyl-Sephadex G-50 (90 × 7 cm) was equilibrated with eluting buffer (2 M urea, 0.04 M ethylenediamine, 0.08 M HCl, pH 3.1 with acetic acid). It was loaded with a 5% gliadin solution in buffer (200 ml) and was first eluted with 2000 ml of

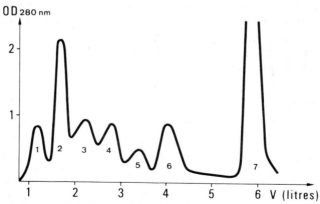

Figure 8.1   Isolation of gliadin fractions from Capitole wheat by chromatography on sulfopropyl-Sephadex G-50 (see text)

buffer and then with the same buffer containing 0.5 M sodium acetate instead of acetic acid. The flow rate was 60 ml/h and 20 ml fractions were collected (Figure 8.1). Pooled fractions were dialysed against 0.05 M acetic acid at +4 °C and freeze-dried.

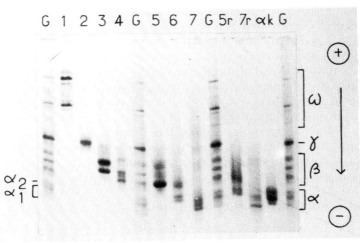

Figure 8.2 Starch gel electrophoresis pattern of gliadin fractions separated on sulfo-propyl-Sephadex G-50 (G=total gliadin, 1 = ω-gliadins, 2 = γ-gliadins, 3 and 4 = β-gliadins, 7r = α_1-gliadin isolated from fraction 7 by chromatography on Sephadex G-100 and αK = Kasarda's α-gliadin)

The composition of each fraction was assessed by starch gel electrophoresis (Figure 8.2). Fraction 1 (ω-gliadins), fraction 2 (γ-gliadins) and fractions 3 and 4 (β-gliadins) were used for the *in vitro* experiments. Electrophoretic diagrams showed that these fractions were not contaminated by α-gliadin components. Fraction 7, which contained α-gliadin, albumins and a low molecular weight glutenin fraction, was further fractionated by chromatography on Sephadex G-100. The recovered α-gliadin which was used in the *in vitro* tests was pure as shown by electrophoresis.

Preparation of PT digests

A PT digest of gliadin was prepared as Frazer' fraction III[11] with some modifications[4]: 10 g of gliadin and 200 mg of 3 × recrystallized pepsin (NBCo, Cleveland, Ohio) were added to 100 ml of 0.1 N HCl (pH 1.8) and hydrolysis was carried out with continuous stirring at 37 °C for 4 h. The digest was then adjusted to pH 7.8 with 1 N NaOH, 100 mg of twice-recrystallized trypsin (NBCo) were added and hydrolysis was continued for 4 h at 37 °C. After filtration and adjustment of pH to 7, the proteolytic activities were destroyed by immersing the flask in boiling water for 30 minutes.

PT digests of casein, glutenin, α_1-, β-, γ- and ω-gliadins were prepared under similar conditions.

Fractionation of PT digests

After dilution with an equal volume of saline, PT gliadin digests were first fractionated by ultrafiltration at +4 °C in an Amicon 50 milli-litre cell equipped with a PM 10 membrane (Amicon Ltd., High Wycombe, UK) in an oxygen-free atmosphere. The residue (fraction G1) was dialysed against normal saline for 48 h using an 8/32 cellu-lose membrane (Visking Co., Chicago, Ill.). The ultrafiltrate, after concentration on an UM 2 Amicon membrane, was further fraction-ated by dialysis for 96 h at +4 °C against normal saline using an 18/32 Visking membrane. This dialysis yielded two fractions: the dialysed ultrafiltrate (G2) and the liquid of dialysis (G3) which was subsequently concentrated on a UM 2 membrane.

Since the exclusion limit of both PM 10 Amicon membrane and 8/32 Visking tube is a molecular weight of about 10–12 000, fraction G1 may be considered as containing large peptides (M.W > 12 000). On the other hand, membrane calibration, according to Craig and King[12], showed that 18/32 Visking membrane was permeable to glucagon (M.W. = 4000) and B-chain from insulin (M.W. = 3600) but not to insulin (M.W. = 5700). It was therefore expected that fraction G2 contained medium-sized peptides with a molecular weight between 5000 and 10 000 daltons and fraction G3 small peptides (M.W. < 5000). In fact, preliminary results of chromatography on Sephadex G-50 showed that G2 mainly contains peptides with a M.W. of about 7000 daltons and G3 peptides with a M.W. of between 2000 and 3000 daltons.

Starting from 100 ml of PT gliadin digest (5 g of soluble peptide material), this fractionation procedure yields about 2.5 g of fraction G1 (50%), 0.5 g of fraction G2 (10%) and 1 g of fraction G3 (20%). One gram of starting material (20%), which consists of amino acids and small peptides not exceeding 1000 daltons, was lost in the process of concen-tration on the UM 2 membrane.

PT digests of casein and α-gliadin were also fractionated respectively into C1, C2 and C3 and αG1, αG2 and αG3 subfractions using the same procedure.

The protein digests and their subfractions were sterilized by millipore filtration (0.45 μm filter) and kept frozen at −20 °C in small aliquots until use.

Analysis and characterization of gliadin components and their fractions

Starch gel electrophoresis was carried out in aluminium lactate buffer (pH 3.2) as described elsewhere[9]. Amino acid analyses were performed on a Phoenix K 8000 amino acid analyser after hydrolysis by 6 N HCl at 110 °C for 24 h in evacuated pyrex tubes[10]. Protein and peptide concentrations were determined by the method of Lowry et al.[13] and nitrogen contents by the micro-Kjeldahl technique.

Organ culture

Organ culture was carried out as previously reported[5] with slight modifications. Briefly, well-oriented biopsy specimens were cut into three or four pieces; one of them was fixed immediately and processed for light and, in some instances, for electron microscopy. The others, villous side up were placed, within 5 minutes of being obtained, onto special stainless grids in Falcon culture dishes. The central well of the dish was filled with sufficient culture medium just to reach the cut surface of tissue sample. The plates were then covered and incubated at 37 °C for 48 h in an atmosphere of 95% O_2 and 5% CO_2. The culture medium, which was changed after 24 h, contained 65% Trowel T–8 medium, 20% NCTC 135 medium, 15% fetal calf serum (previously heated at 56 °C for 1 hour) and a mixture of antibiotics. Human albumin peptides which were added in previous experiments[4] were omitted in the present study.

Morphological studies

For light microscopy, mucosal samples, just after excision and after 48 hours of culture, were fixed in Carnoy's solution, dehydrated, embedded in paraffin and serially sectioned.

For electron microscopy, they were fixed for one hour in ice cold s-collidine buffered osmium tetroxide, dehydrated in increasing concentrations of ethanol and embedded in epon. Tissue blocks were cut on a Reichert ultramicrotome. Sections one μm thick were stained with toluidine blue. Ultra-thin sections were cut with a diamond knife, stained with uranyl acetate and lead citrate and examined in a Siemens Elmiskop 101 electron microscope.

Lymphocyte stimulation

Twenty ml of venous heparinized blood were diluted with Hanks solution and centrifuged at 400 g through a Ficoll Hypaque solution[14]. Mononuclear cells, banding at the interface, were harvested, washed twice and adjusted to a concentration of 10^6 cells/ml with culture medium containing RPMI 1640, antibiotics and 20% heat inactivated

(56 °C for 30 min) human blood-group AB serum.

Doubling dilutions of test substance were made in normal saline. Aliquots of 0.1 ml of each dilution were added in triplicate to 1 ml of lymphocyte suspension and incubated at 37 °C in a humidified atmosphere (5% CO_2, 95% air) 0.1 ml of medium containing 1 μ Ci [^{3}H] methyl thymidine (specific activity 100 mCi/mmol, C.E.A., Saclay, France) was added after 5 days of culture. Twenty-four hours later, the tubes were harvested on glass-fibre filter papers. Samples were dried and counted on a liquid scintillation counter.

Results were expressed as a stimulation index, namely the ratio of counts in test cultures to the counts in antigen-free 'control' cultures.

Concentrations of proteins and peptides in culture media

The PT digests of gliadin, glutenin, casein, α-, β-, γ- and ω-gliadins were added to the organ culture medium at a concentration of 0.5 mg/ml. For lymphocyte-stimulation assays, the same digests were tested at four distinct concentrations: 0.4, 0.8, 1.6 and 3.2 mg/ml.

The subfractions of PT gliadin digests (G1, G2 and G3), PT casein digests (C1, C2 and C3) and PT α-gliadin digests (αG1, αG2 and αG3) were added to the organ culture medium, usually at a concentration of 0.25 mg/ml and, in some instances as otherwise stated, at a concentration of 0.12 or 0.50 mg/ml. In addition, the response to G2 and G3 was studied in lymphocyte stimulation assays at three distinct concentrations: 0.3, 0.6 and 1.2 mg/ml.

RESULTS

Organ cultures

PT digests of gliadin, glutenin and casein

The PT digests of gliadin exerted a clear *in vitro* cytotoxic effect at a concentration of 0.5 mg/ml (but not at lower concentrations) on mucosa from children with active coeliac disease. They did not only inhibit epithelial restoration but also produced evident mucosal change in 11 cultured samples, including 7 with extensive necrosis; in most cases surface epithelium was severely injured and overlaid with a thick layer of necrotic desquamated cells.

In contrast, casein and glutenin digests did not inhibit epithelial restoration in 6 out of 9 flat biopsies cultured in the presence of glutenin peptides and in 13 out of 18 cultured in the presence of casein peptides respectively. Evidence of cellular damage was only observed in one explant in the presence of glutenin digests, whereas casein digests did not produce any severe change in cultured samples.

In addition, most specimens from controls were not affected by culture for 48 h in the presence of the PT digests of gliadin or casein. Only one sample cultured in the presence of casein digest underwent obvious alterations of villi and epithelial cells (Table 8.1).

Table 8.1   *In vitro* toxicity of PT digests from gliadin, casein, glutenin and gliadin components

				P.T. digests of				
	0	Glutenin	Casein	Gliadin	α_1	β	γ	ω
Coeliac patients (33 flat biopsies)								
Reparation	9	13	6				2	2
No reparation	1	4	3	1	3	1	1	3
Impairment		1		4	5	3	2	
Extensive necrosis				7	7	3	1	
Controls (5 normal biopsies)								
No change			3	3	3			
Slight change				1				

PT digests of gliadin components

The PT digests of α_1-and β-gliadins at a concentration of 0.5 mg/ml also induced a noxious effect in flat mucosa from untreated coeliac patients. Severe changes were observed in 12 out of 15 cases (including 7 with extensive necrosis) in the presence of α_1-gliadin digests and in 6 out of 7 cases (including 3 with necrosis) in the presence of α-gliadin digests. γ-Gliadins appeared to be somewhat less noxious (three experiments with toxic effects—including one with necrosis—and three others without clear deleterious effect). ω-Gliadins proved to be the less toxic components since, in two *in vitro* experiments, their digest did not inhibit epithelial restoration and, in three explants, surface epithelium was only slightly damaged after culture (Table 8.1).

Subfractions

The subfractions prepared from the PT digests of gliadin, α-gliadin and casein were tested in additional *in vitro* experiments. Fractions G1 and especially G2 and αG2 exhibited a clear *in vitro* cytotoxicity on the mucosa from children with active coeliac disease, while fractions G3 and αG3, as well as the three casein subfractions (C1, C2 and C3) were harmless. Fraction G2 appeared to have the most damaging effects *in vitro*. At a concentration of 0.25 mg/ml in culture medium, it consistently inhibited the improvement of flat mucosa from coeliac patients

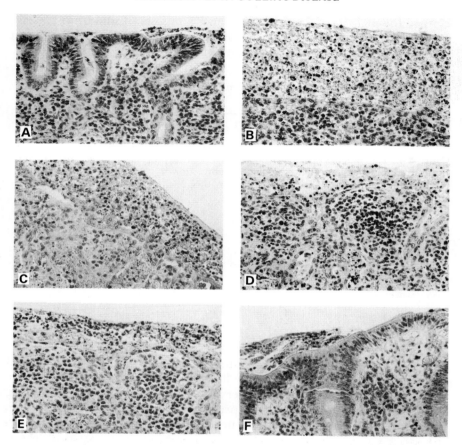

Figure 8.3 Mucosa samples obtained from children with active coeliac disease and cultured for 48 hours in the presence of various PT digests.
A. With glutenin digests, the surface epithelium is almost normal. B. With gliadin digests, the surface epithelium is severely injured and overlaid with a thick layer of necrotic material. C. With α_1-gliadin digests; these show the same damaging properties as gliadin digests. D. With β-gliadin digests, the deterioration of surface epithelium is evident. E. With γ-gliadin digests; the toxic effects are also noticed. F. With ω-gliadin digests; no deleterious effect is observed on this light micrograph ($\times$ 112).

and determined either severe change (10 cases) or extensive necrosis (6 cases) of surface epithelium. In two other cultures, there was also clear evidence of epithelial impairment though G2 was added at a concentration of 0.12 mg/ml to the culture medium. Two ultrastructural studies of coeliac mucosa cultured in the presence of G2 (0.25 mg/ml) revealed a considerable change in the surface epithelial cells which appeared flat, undifferentiated, with sparse short damaged microvilli,

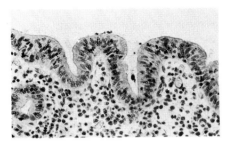
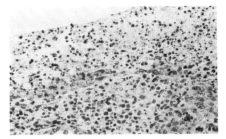

Figure 8.4 Flat mucosa specimens from a child with untreated coeliac disease after 48-hour culture in the presence of gliadin subfractions (0.25 mg/ml). A. With G3 the surface epithelium appears near normal. B. With G2; this micrograph shows a severe impairment of surface epithelium (× 112).

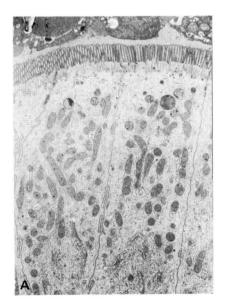
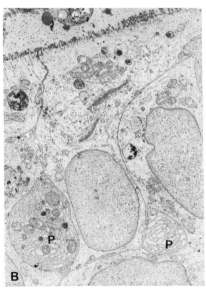

Figure 8.5 Electron micrographs of biopsy specimens obtained from a child with active coeliac disease and cultured for 48 hours in the presence of gliadin subfractions (0.25 mg/ml). A. With G3, the absorptive cells closely resembled those seen in normal biopsies. B. With G2, the epithelial cells are grossly injured with especially sparse short microvilli, large lysosomes, a disorganized terminal web and, in some intercellular spaces, cells with cisternae of endoplasmic reticulum typical of plasma cells (P) (× 1650)

large lysosomes and a disorganized terminal bar; in addition, many large lymphocytes and plasma cells with extensively developed cisternae were present in the lamina propria and occasionally in surface epithelium (Figure 8.5B). On the contrary, G3 produced no light or electron microscopic observable toxic effects at the concentration of 0.25 or

0.5 mg/ml (Figure 8.5A).

On the other hand, in most samples from controls no damaging effect was observed after culture in the presence of G1, G2 or G3 as well as C2 and αG2 (Table 8.2).

Table 8.2 In vitro toxicity of subfractions obtained from casein (C), gliadin (G) and α-gliadin (αG)

				PEPTIDES				
	MW>10 000		5000	<MW	<10 000		MW<5000	
	C1	G1	C2	G2	αG2	C3	G3	αG3
Coeliac patients								
(25 flat biopsies)								
Reparation	2	2	2			3	4	2
No reparation	4	2	3			1	1	
Impairment		2		12	2			
Extensive necrosis		1		6	2			
Controls								
(8 normal biopsies)								
No change		1	4	7	1			
Slight change			1	1				

Lymphocyte stimulation assays

Peripheral blood lymphocytes from children with coeliac disease were not reproducibly stimulated by the PT digests of gliadin, glutenin, α_1-, β-, γ- and ω-gliadins. In addition, they did not give any proliferative response to G3 and other dietary proteins including α-lactalbumin and β-lactoglobulin.

In contrast, they were consistently stimulated by G2 subfraction provided that lymphocytes were obtained from coeliac patients treated by a gluten-free diet for at least three months. Maximum response was observed with a concentration of 0.6 mg/ml of G2.

Finally, no proliferative response was given by lymphocytes from normal controls cultured in the presence of wheat antigens and particularly G2 subfraction. The same results were obtained in children with cow's milk intolerance except in one lymphocyte stimulation assay which showed a proliferative response to G2 and G3 (Figure 8.6).

Amino acid compositions of gliadin components

Partial results of amino acid analyses are given in Table 8.3. They are expressed as the number of residues/1000 total residues. They confirm that ω-gliadins differ considerably in overall amino acid composition from the other gliadin components (α-, β- and γ-gliadins). Omega-

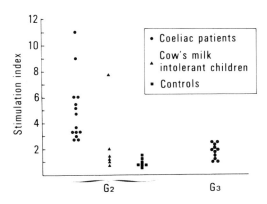

Figure 8.6 Stimulation index of lymphocytes cultured with G3 and G2 (0.6 mg/ml)

gliadins particularly contain much more glutamine, proline and phenylalanine. On the contrary, α_1-, β- and γ-gliadins afford similar amino
acid analyses but glutamine and proline contents decrease slightly from
γ- to α-gliadins.

Table 8.3 Partial amino acid compositions of gliadin fractions used
for *in vitro* tests
(numbers of residues/1000 recovered residues)

	ω	γ	β	α
Total of basic amino acids	20	32	36.4	50
Serine	34	48	55	52
Glutamine	501	391	378	370
Proline	229	181	165	151
Alanine	5.7	30.2	30	28
Cystine	3.6	25	26	26
Valine	5.3	42	48	47
Methionine	1	12.5	11	8.2
Leucine	34	66	68	77
Phenylalanine	91	49	39	39

DISCUSSION

Gluten is a complex mixture of gliadins, glutenins, albumins and globulins[15] and only gliadins are regarded as toxic to coeliac patients[16].
'Gliadin', the alcohol-soluble fraction of gluten, consists of about 40
different components which can be divided into four groups (α-, β-,
γ- and ω-gliadins) according to mobility on starch gel electrophoresis,
the α-gliadins having the fastest mobility and the ω-gliadins the
slowest[9]. Since several studies have disclosed genetic heterogeneity
with distinct differences in protein composition among most wheat

varieties, we used gliadin obtained from a single pure flour, as starting material.

The question of which component of gliadin is responsible for the toxic effects in coeliac disease remains controversial. It was supposed that the toxic part of gliadin was its protein fraction, but some recent studies have suggested that its carbohydrate moiety might share the toxic properties[17]. On the other hand, it has been claimed that only α-gliadins are damaging to coeliac patients and that not all gliadin components are toxic[18]. It has even been said that removal of α-gliadin components by genetic manipulations may yield an innocuous wheat[19].

However, if the properties of α-gliadins have been the subject of many investigations, those of the other gliadin components were studied little or not at all; furthermore the toxicity of gliadin components was generally assessed under unsuitable conditions; in most cases, a very small number of experiments were carried out (frequently only one or two) and feeding tests which require large quantities of test material were done for too short a period; investigations using the oral xylose technique to check the toxicity of α-gliadin[18] can hardly be regarded as reliable; *in vitro* tests performed in two organ culture experiments[3] are not conclusive, since undigested α-gliadins were added to the culture medium at a concentration considerably exceeding its solubility; finally, studies which established the damaging properties of α-gliadins using instillation tests in combination with repeated intestinal biopsies[20] have not demonstrated that other fractions—especially β- and γ-gliadins—were harmless.

Contrariwise, since α-, β- and γ-gliadins have closely similar amino acid compositions and share some common peptide sequences, and since they probably derived from a common ancestral gene by successive duplications[21], it could be expected that β- and γ-gliadins would also be toxic[1].

In fact, the present *in vitro* investigation demonstrated that the α-gliadin fraction was not the unique toxic component and that β- and, to a less degree, γ-gliadins exhibited also damaging effects. Only ω-gliadins appeared to be completely harmless. These differences of toxicity between ω-gliadins and the other three gliadin components are not surprising and could have been predicted from their very different amino acid composition, especially from the much higher proline, glutamine and phenylalanine contents of ω-gliadins.

It is well-known that pepsin and trypsin do not split peptide bonds when one of the two linked amino acids is proline. Therefore, in the PT digests of gliadins, the size of peptides probably depends on their proline content, the peptides with the higher proline content having the higher molecular weight. On the other hand, the less toxic gliadin components appear to have the highest proline contents, so that there may be a connection between the size of gliadin peptides, their proline content and their toxicity.

Further fractionations of the PT digests of gluten on the basis of molecular size were recently achieved. A fraction B which mainly contains peptides with a molecular weight of 8000[22] and its subfraction B2[23] proved to share the toxic properties of whole gluten digest. In addition, the B2 subfraction has been found to stimulate the lymphocytes of patients with coeliac disease, but not those of healthy control subjects[24], and to give positive Arthus-type skin reactions in coeliac patients following intradermal injections[25].

Our *in vitro* observations are consistent with these results. Our fraction G2, containing mainly peptides of about 7000 daltons, exhibited a clear mucosal toxicity *in vitro* at a very low concentration. Moreover peripheral blood lymphocytes from children with treated coeliac disease were consistently stimulated by G2. These data suggest that B2 and G2 subfractions are closely related regarding their peptide and amino acid compositions. It is however of importance to stress that our subfractions were prepared from gliadins extracted from a single pure flour and not from commercial gluten resulting from a blend of wheats[26]. Furthermore, preliminary tests using the subfractions of α-gliadin digests suggest that αG2 has the same damaging properties as G2. Therefore it would be advisable in further attempts to isolate the toxic component of gluten to use α- or β-gliadins instead of gliadin or gluten, as starting material.

However different G2 and B2 may be, these results confirm that the toxicity of gliadin peptides is dependent on their molecular size. In addition, they give evidence of a good correlation between lymphocyte reactivity to a gluten subfraction and its potential toxicity to coeliac mucosa and provide further data suggesting that lymphocyte sensitization and cell-mediated immune reactions may be involved in the pathogenetic mechanism of coeliac enteropathy.

ACKNOWLEDGEMENTS

This work was supported by a grant from the INSERM (Contract No. 75 50 237).

We are indebted to Dr D. D. Kasarda for giving a sample of A-gliadin and checking the purity of our gliadin fractions.

We thank Miss A. Dellon, Miss C. Demarteau and Miss M.-F. de Tand for their excellent technical assistance, J. C. Huet for the amino acid analysis and M. Sallantin for carrying out the starch gel electrophoresis.

References

1. Jos, J. and Rey, J. (1975). L'apport de la culture organotypique à l'étude pathogénique de la maladie coeliaque. *Arch. Fr. Mal. App. Dig.,* **64**, 461
2. Trier, J. S. and Browning, T. H. (1970). Epithelial cell renewal in cultured duodenal biopsies in coeliac sprue. *N. Engl. J. Med.,* **283**, 1245
3. Falchuk, Z. M., Gebhard, R. L., Sessoms, C. and Strober, W. (1974). An *in vitro* model of gluten-sensitive enteropathy. Effect of gliadin on intestinal epithelial cells of patients with gluten-sensitive enteropathy in organ culture. *J. Clin. Invest.,* **53**, 487
4. Jos, J., Lenoir, G., de Ritis, G. and Rey, J. (1975). In vitro pathogenetic studies of coeliac disease. Effects of protein digests on coeliac intestinal biopsy specimens maintained in culture for 48 hours. *Scand. J. Gastroenterol.,* **10**, 121
5. Jos, J., Lenoir, G., de Ritis, G. and Rey, J. (1974). In vitro culturing of biopsies from children. In: W. Th. J. M. Hekkens and A. S. Peña (eds.) *Coeliac Disease. Proceedings of the Second International Symposium,* pp. 91–105. (Leiden: Stenfert Kroese)
6. Strober, W., Falchuk, Z. M., Rogentine, G. N., Nelson, D. L. and Klaeveman, H. L. (1975). The pathogenesis of gluten-sensitive enteropathy. *Ann. Int. Med.,* **83**, 242
7. Katz, A. J., Falchuk, Z. M., Strober, W. and Shwachman, H. (1976). Gluten-sensitive enteropathy. Inhibition by cortisol of the effect of gluten protein in vitro. *N. Engl. J. Med.,* **295**, 131
8. Ferguson, A., McDonald, T. T., McClure, J. P. and Holden, R. J. (1975). Cell-mediated immunity to gliadin within the small-intestinal mucosa in coeliac disease. *Lancet,* **i**, 895
9. Charbonnier, L. (1973). Etude des protéines alcoolosolubles de la farine de blé. *Biochimie,* **55**, 1217
10. Charbonnier, L. (1974). Isolation and characterization of ω-gliadin fractions. *Biochim. Biophys. Acta,* **359**, 142
11. Frazer, A. C., Fletcher, R. F., Ross, C. A. C., Shaw, B., Sammons, H. G. and Schneider, R. (1959). Gluten-induced enteropathy; the effect of partially digested gluten. *Lancet.* **ii**, 252
12. Craig, L. C. and King, T. P. (1962). Dialysis. In: D. Glick (ed.). *Methods of Biochemical Analysis.* Vol. X, pp. 175–199 (New York: Interscience Publishers)
13. Lowry, O. H., Rosebrough, N. J., Farr, A. L. and Randall, R. J. (1951). Protein measurement with the Folin phenol reagent. *J. Biol. Chem.,* **193**, 265
14. Bøyum, A. (1968). Separation of leucocytes from blood and bone marrow. *Scand. J. Clin. Lab. Invest.,* **21**, (Suppl. 97), 1
15. Patey, A. L. (1974). Gliadin: the protein mixture toxic to coeliac patients. *Lancet,* **i**, 722
16. Van de Kamer, J. H., Weijers, H. A. and Dicke, W. K. (1953). Coeliac disease. IV. An investigation into the injurious constituents of wheat in connection with their action on patients with coeliac disease. *Acta Paediatr.,* **42**, 223
17. Phelan, J. J., Stevens, F. M., McNicholl, B., Fottrell, P. F. and McCarthy, C. F. (1977). Coeliac disease: the abolition of gliadin toxicity by enzymes from Aspergillus niger. *Clin. Sci. Mol. Med.,* **53**, 35
18. Kendall, M. J., Cox, P. S., Schneider, R. and Hawkins, C. F. (1972). Gluten subfractions in coeliac disease. *Lancet,* **ii**, 1065
19. Kasarda, D. D., Bernardin, J. E. and Qualset, C. O. (1976). Relationship of gliadin protein components to chromosomes in hexaploid wheats (*Triticum aestivum* L.) *Proc. Nat. Acad. Sci. USA,* **73**, 3646
20. Hekkens, W. Th. J. M., Haex, A. J. Ch. and Willighagen, R. G. J. (1970). Some aspects of gliadin fractionation and testing by a histochemical method. In: C. C.

Booth and R. M. Dowling (eds.) *Coeliac disease. Proc. Int. Coeliac Symposium,* pp. 11–19 (Edinburgh: Churchill Livingstone)

21. Kasarda, D. D., Bernardin, J. E. and Nimmo, C. C. (1976). Wheat proteins. In: Y. Pomeranz (ed.). *Advances in Cereal Science and Technology,* pp. 158–236 (St. Paul, Minn.: American Association of Cereal Chemists)

22. Dissanayake, A. S., Jerrome, D. W., Offord, R. E., Truelove, S. C. and Whitehead, R. (1974). Identifying toxic fractions of wheat gluten and their effect on the jejunal mucosa in coeliac disease. *Gut,* **15,** 931

23. Anand, B. S., Offord, R. E., Piris, J. and Truelove, S. C. (1977). Isolating the component of gluten which causes the mucosal damage in coeliac disease. (Abstract). *Gut,* **18,** 408

24. Sikora, K., Anand, B. S., Truelove, S. C., Ciclitira, P. J. and Offord, R. E. (1976). Stimulation of lymphocytes from patients with coeliac disease by a subfraction of gluten. *Lancet,* **ii,** 389

25. Anand, B. S., Truelove, S. C. and Offord, R. E. (1977). Skin test for coeliac disease using a subfraction of gluten. *Lancet,* **i,** 118

26. Jos, J., Rey, J., Charbonnier, L., Mossé, J. and Mougenot, J. F. (1976). Stimulation of lymphocytes from patients with coeliac disease by subfraction of gluten. (Letter to the editor). *Lancet,* **ii,** 630

Discussion of chapter 8

Jos

I think that the toxic effect is clearly demonstrated in 48 hours, whereas after 24 hours sometimes the toxic effect is not obvious. I believe that crypt cells are also affected by the toxic fractions.

Hauri

I have a question concerning the comparison of the morphology *in vivo* and *in vitro*. With gliadin digests you have shown that you obtained a complete necrosis *in vitro* which does not correspond to the *in vivo* picture. Do you think that what you have tested is really the toxicity of gliadin which is comparable to the *in vivo* situation?

Jos

When we obtain a toxic effect with gliadin digests such as Frazer's fraction III, we see damaged epithelial cells, with a thick layer of desquamated cells and the lamina propria is infiltrated with many cells. When a non-specific toxic effect occurs i.e. with casein digests at a high concentration, we only observed the disappearance of cells in the lamina propria, therefore the thick layer of desquamated cells is probably characteristic of a specific toxic effect.

Strober

Am I right in assuming that all of your fractions were first subjected to peptic/tryptic digestion?

Jos

Yes.

Strober

Have you studied purified fractions that are not subjected to digestion?

Jos

No, because gliadin fractions, as well as gliadin, have a very low solubility. If we use such fractions they form a suspension in the culture medium and produce non-specific toxic effects.

Strober

We have been successful in using alpha gliadin in these test systems and finding it toxic. We dissolve the protein in acid at low pH and at a high concentration. It is then diluted in buffer and brought to a physiological pH, thus allowing use of native protein instead of digested protein. I think your data are very impressive, and I believe you are getting toxicity in culture certainly with beta gliadins and frequently with gamma, but I would suggest that you also use the undigested proteins.

9

In vitro assessment of gluten toxicity by organ culture of human duodenal mucosa

G. FLUGE and L. AKSNES

Gluten toxicity has been assessed *in vitro* by comparison of biopsies cultured in a gluten-free medium to specimens cultured in the presence of gluten. Jos[1] has supplied histological examination and electron microscopy, while Falchuk and Strober[2] measured the brush border enzyme alkaline phosphatase in their studies. We have performed organ culture of human duodenal mucosa by the method described by Browning and Trier[3] with the modification of Jos[1]. The aim of our study has been to compare biopsies cultured in a gluten-free medium to specimens exposed to either α-gliadin, Frazer's fraction III or to a gel- and ultrafiltrate of Frazer's fraction III with molecular weight between 500 and 10 000.

MATERIAL AND METHODS

Twenty-six biopsies from coeliac patients in different phases of the disease and 9 specimens from non-coeliac controls (prolonged diarrhoea) in the paediatric age group were cultured. The biopsies were obtained with a Watson paediatric capsule. Each biopsy was cut into three or more pieces of equal size before culture. [³H]thymidine (specific activity 5 Ci per mmol, 2 μCi per ml medium) was usually added to the culture medium during the first 12 hours of the culture period. In 13 culture experiments L-[¹⁴C]leucine (specific activity 330 mCi per mmol, 1 μCi per ml medium) was added during the whole culture period to give an estimate of protein synthesis. At the end of

91

the culture period mucus covering the biopsy surface was carefully removed under a dissecting microscope before fixation. The biopsies were fixed in ice-cold 2% glutaraldehyde in 1 M cacodylate buffer, post-fixation in 1% osmium tetroxide in 1 M cacodylate buffer, dehydration and embedding in Epon. In a few experiments Carnoy's solution 2 was used as fixative and the tissue was embedded in paraffin. Serial sections of 1 μm thickness were taken throughout the entire biopsy 30 to 40 μm apart to avoid recounting of the same cells. Sections were either stained with toluidine blue for light microscopy, or processed for auto-radiography by the dipping method using Ilford K5 emulsion with 4 weeks' exposure time. Label indices were expressed as number of label-led cells per 1000 crypt cells. In total 2000 to 5000 crypt cells were counted per biopsy.

The quantity of immunoglobulin secreted into the culture medium and into the mucus was estimated by rocket immunoelectrophoresis using commercial rabbit anti-immunoglobulin preparations, Dakopatts A/S, Denmark. The mucus was either examined separately or added to the culture medium after homogenization.

To show that immunoglobulin synthesis had taken place during the culture period, autoradiograms of the immunoprecipitates after [14C]leucine incorporation was obtained with 3 M medical X-ray film, type HL, and 21 days' exposure time. As shown in Figure 9.1, the auto-radiogram of IgA rockets gave a precise image of the original rockets. The standard dilutions, which are not radioactive, gave no autoradio-grams. Precipitates of IgG and IgM gave similar autoradiograms. Secretory components gave very weak precipitations, but the autoradio-grams indicated that synthesis must have taken place.

Scintillation counting of the culture medium after [14C]leucine in-corporation showed good correlation of counts per min per biopsy to the quantity of IgA secreted, but not to the other immunoglobulins measured.

RESULTS

In cases of untreated coeliac disease marked improvement of the histo-logical picture was observed after 24 hours' culture with gluten-free medium (Figure 9.2, A and B). The enterocytes were higher, more regu-lar and with basically oriented nuclei. In the presence of α-gliadin an obvious toxic effect was noted (Figure 9.2C). The whole thickness of the biopsy was reduced compared to the specimens contained in gluten-free medium. The epithelium was lower and had become more irregu-lar. The crypts were partly dilated. In some areas there was necrosis. The biopsy surface was covered by a thick layer of mucus and desquamated material. Frazer's fraction III was somewhat less toxic than α-gliadin.

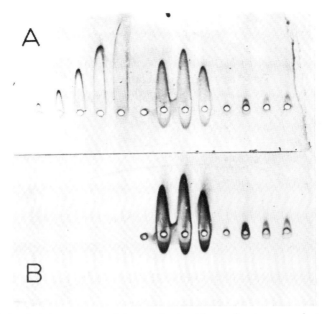

Figure 9.1 A IgA immunoprecipitates obtained by rocket immunoelectrophoresis of medium and mucus after 24 hours' organ culture. Rockets of standard dilutions are seen to the left. B. Corresponding autoradiograms of the immunoprecipitates showing incorporation of L-[14C]leucine into immunoglobulins. The standard dilutions gave negative autoradiograms, as expected

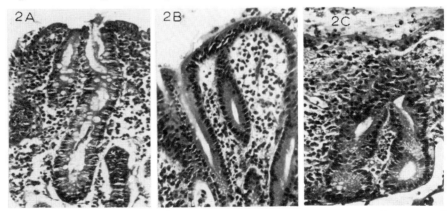

Figure 9.2 Histological section of duodenal mucosa from a patient with untreated coeliac disease. A. Before organ culture with typical findings of flat mucosa. B. After 24 hours' organ culture in a gluten-free medium the epithelium has reverted towards normal and low villi are now present. C. In the presence of α-gliadin the epithelium has become more irregular and lower. Small areas of necrosis are noted underneath the surface epithelium. The biopsy surface is covered by mucus and desquamated material (H+E, × 160).

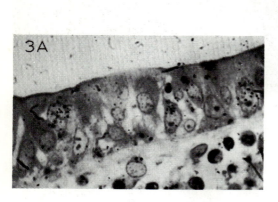
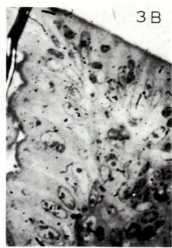

Figure 9.3 Histological section (autoradiogram after [³H]thymidine incorporation) of duodenal mucosa from a coeliac patient in silent relapse (flat mucosa). A. After 24 hours in a gluten-free medium the epithelium is well preserved. Some enterocytes are labelled. The mucus covering the surface has been removed. B. In the presence of α-gliadin no obvious toxic effect is noted (Toluidine blue, × 600)

However, in other phases of coeliac disease these fractions, except for a few cases, had a minimal or no toxic effect as assessed histologically. This was so even in patients with a silent relapse and a flat mucosa due to a normal diet for several years (Figure 9.3, A and B).

Autoradiograms of biopsies from active coeliac disease showed high labelling indices. DNA synthesis in crypt cells seemed to be stimulated by α-gliadin, as measured by higher label indices after exposure to this fraction (Figure 9.4, A and B).

The labelling indices in different categories of coeliac disease are shown in Figure 9.5. The highest labelling indices were found in untreated coeliac disease and in patients with silent relapse. In these biopsies a marked rise in labelling index was usually observed with α-gliadin exposure, while Frazer's fraction III showed no stimulation in a patient in silent relapse. During gluten challenge after gluten-free diet for 2 years, a high labelling index was noted and this was augmented by α-gliadin. In remission patients there were low labelling indices, of the same order as in normal mucosa, and there seemed to be no stimulating effect of α-gliadin. In a non-coeliac mucosa with partial villous atrophy due to prolonged diarrhoea a high labelling index was noted, but there was no stimulating effect by α-gliadin.

The quantity of IgA secreted by coeliac biopsies into the medium during successive culture periods of 12 hours was estimated to give an

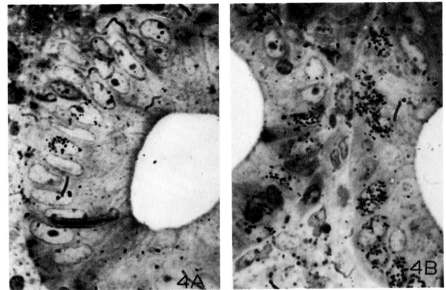

Figure 9.4 Autoradiogram after [³H]thymidine incorporation during the first 12 hours of a 24 h organ culture period. Same patient as shown in Figure 9.3. In a gluten-free medium (A) some crypt cells are labelled, while numerous cells are labelled in the presence of α-gliadin (B) (Toluidine blue, × 750)

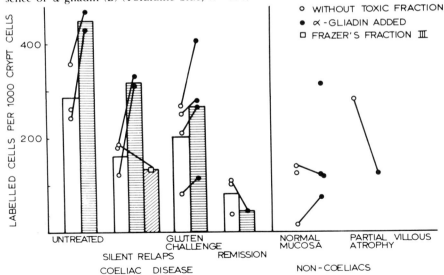

Figure 9.5 Label index of human duodenal crypt cells after organ culture (24 h) following [³H]thymidine incorporation during the first 12 h of the culture period. Individual label indices after culture over a gluten-free medium and after exposure to gluten fractions are connected with lines. The bars represent the mean values in each group (see text)

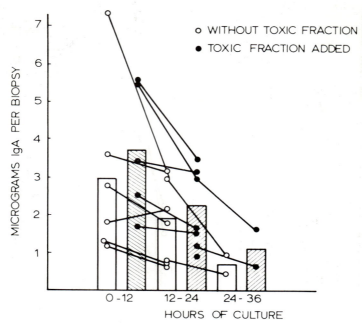

Figure 9.6 Quantity of IgA secreted into the culture medium by duodenal biopsies from coeliac patients during successive 12 h culture periods. The open bars represent the mean values in the absence of gluten fractions. Hatched bars represent mean values after exposure to gluten fractions. Values obtained in individual experiments are connected with lines

impression of the rate of immunoglobulin synthesis. As shown in Figure 9.6, the greatest quantity was secreted during the first 12 hours, averaging between 3 and 4 μg per biopsy. There was a decline during the rest of the culture period, and this was most marked in those with high initial values, while those with a low IgA synthesis rate showed a more steady state synthesis during 36 hours. The quantity of IgA from biopsies exposed to toxic fractions was somewhat higher than from those kept in a gluten-free medium.

IgA secreted into the medium and mucus during 24 hours' culture was estimated in different categories of coeliac biopsies and in controls with and without addition of toxic fractions (Figure 9.7). The highest concentration was found in untreated coeliac disease with stimulation by Frazer's fraction III. Two patients in this group had IgA deficiency and there was no detectable IgA secreted. In silent relapse the quantity was somewhat lower, but most often there was a rise in IgA quantity in the presence of α-gliadin while Frazer's fraction III had no such stimulating effect on the biopsies. The same pattern was noted both in

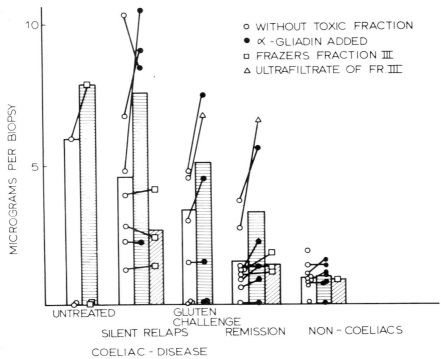

Figure 9.7 Quantity of IgA secreted into mucus and medium during 24 h organ culture. The individual observations in the absence and with addition of gluten fractions are connected with lines. Open bars represent the mean values in the absence of toxic fractions. Hatched bars show the mean values after exposure to α-gliadin and gel filtrate of Frazer's fraction III and to Frazer's fraction III

gluten challenge patients and in remission patients. The gel filtrate of Frazer's fraction III seemed to be a potent stimulus to IgA synthesis.

In normal mucosa the IgA quantity was about 1 μg per biopsy per 24 hours, and there was no stimulating effect of toxic fractions. As no stimulation by toxic fractions seemed possible in patients with IgA deficiency, the zero values have not been calculated into the mean values.

IgG has been quantified in a smaller number of patients. The highest quantity was found in untreated coeliac disease and in silent relapse, but there was no regular stimulation by α-gliadin.

The highest IgM rockets were obtained in untreated coeliac disease as shown in Figure 9.8. In silent relapse, although the patients had been on a normal diet for several years with a flat mucosa, there was no detectable IgM. The same pattern was noted in remission mucosas, whereas gluten challenge biopsies gave rockets, and again possible stimulating effect by α-gliadin. It is noteworthy that a non-coeliac patient with partial villous atrophy also showed a high level of IgM secretion.

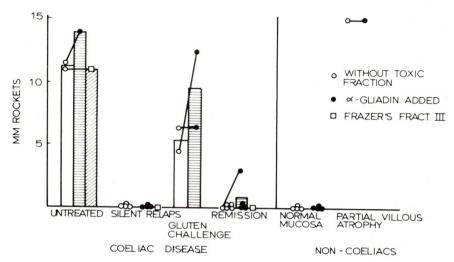

Figure 9.8 Height of IgM immunoprecipitates (rockets) after 24 h organ culture of duodenal biopsies from coeliac patients and controls. Values obtained in individual experiments are connected with lines. Open bars represent the mean values in the absence of toxic fractions. Hatched bars show the mean values after exposure to α-gliadin and to Frazer's fraction III

DISCUSSION

Histological examination showed toxic effect by α-gliadin and Frazer's fraction II only in untreated coeliac disease. Mucosa from patients in silent relapse, during gluten challenge and in remission was most often resistant to the toxic fractions. These observations could possibly reflect the *in vivo* observation that patients in silent relapse had minimal or no symptoms of the disease and the absorptive function of the small intestine seemed to be affected to a much lesser degree than in untreated cases. Patients on a gluten-free diet usually become more tolerant to gluten exposure the longer the period of gluten-free diet treatment.

Labelling indices after incorporation of radioactive thymidine and quantitation of IgA secreted into the mucus and the medium seemed to be more sensitive parameters than histology.

Frazer's fraction III seemed to be less potent than α-gliadin both in causing histological damage and in stimulating IgA synthesis.

Our filtrate of Frazer's fraction III probably corresponds to the B2 fraction which Sikora and co-workers[4] found potent in stimulating lymphocytes *in vitro* and giving positive skin tests in coeliac patients.

This fraction probably has a higher concentration of toxic peptides. We have few observations with this fraction so far, but in our experiments it seems that the filtrate of Frazer's fraction III has a more potent stimulating effect on IgA synthesis than the less homogeneous fraction III. It also seems to have a more potent deleterious effect on the histological picture of coeliac mucosas other than those from patients with untreated coeliac disease.

References

1. Jos, J., Lenoir, G., de Ritis, G. and Rey, J. (1974). In vitro culturing of biopsies from children. In: W. Th. J. M. Hekkens and A. S. Peña (eds.) *Coeliac disease. Proceedings of the Second International Coeliac Symposium,* pp. 91–105. (Leiden: Stenfert Kroese)
2. Falchuk, Z. M., Gebhard, R. L., Sessoms, C. and Strober, W. (1974). An in vitro model of gluten-sensitive enteropathy. *J. Clin. Invest.,* **53,** 487
3. Browning, T. H. and Trier, J. S. (1969). Organ culture of mucosal biopsies of human small intestine. *J. Clin. Invest.,* **48,** 1423
4. Sikora, K., Anand, B. S., Truelove, S. C., Ciclitira, P. J. and Offord, R. E. (1976). Stimulation of lymphocytes from patients with coeliac diseases by a subfraction of gluten. *Lancet,* **ii,** 389

Discussion of chapter 9

Asquith	Do you think the differnt effects shown may be due to different mechanisms, that you may in fact be having a cell-mediated reaction, where there is not a toxic effect as shown by lack of IgA production? In other words it is a humoral reaction in the exacerbation situation. In your silent relapses it is a cell-mediated one maintaining the flat mucosa.
Fluge	Such factors could possibly be involved, but we haven't results so far to give a definite answer to that question. Perhaps if one goes further into these problems and tries to find specific antibodies, one could find humoral factors implicated.
Hauri	I would like to ask whether or not IgA release is specifically related to gluten. What happens if you use casein?
Fluge	We haven't used casein as a control. The concentration of toxic fractions was 0.5 mg of culture media. This is the same concentration as Jos has used and casein in this concentration gave no unspecific effect in his experiments. In our further experiments we will try other factors which should probably be non-toxic and compare these by IgA release and other parameters.
Watson	I suppose a problem with a tissue culture method is that when you take that piece of tissue you separate it from a reservoir of renewable material and that reservoir may well contain toxic factors, or at least complementary factors which then fall out of the challenge system. I wonder if you could comment on that?
Fluge	Of course that is a problem when you are testing these fractions; I think the problem to be solved mainly is to find out which other factors, humoral or whatever, that effect the enterocytes in addition to the toxic fractions. I think this could be tried in *in vivo* systems too.
Rosekrans	What is your definition of the patients in silent relapse?
Fluge	These patients have none or minimal symptoms on a gluten-containing diet. All our patients are coeliac patients who have been treated with gluten-free diet for two or three years. Their doctor has then put them on a normal diet, and they have continued on a normal diet from the age of three or four years until the age of twelve to fourteen years. They have been exposed to gluten, but at least α-gliadin and Frazer's fraction III seem to have non-significant toxic effects as judged by histological examination.
Rosekrans	It is certain that these patients are real coeliacs?
Fluge	Yes, they have a flat mucosa on normal diet and those which we have re-biopsied after one or two years on a gluten-free diet show remission, so I think they are definitely coeliacs.

10

Organ culture of small intestinal mucosa from coeliac children: absence of cytotoxicity of various gluten preparations

H. P. HAURI, M. KEDINGER, K. HAFFEN, H. GAZE, B. HADORN and W. Th. J. M. HEKKENS

INTRODUCTION

Organ culture of flat intestinal mucosa from patients suffering from active coeliac disease has been proposed as a tool for the assessment of toxicity of gluten fractions. In this system toxic fractions were reported to inhibit regeneration of the surface epithelium[1-3] observed in control cultures without gluten. The aim of the present study was to further elucidate the mechanism of gluten toxicity in organ culture using four different gluten fractions, three of which had been shown to be toxic *in vivo*.

PATIENTS, MATERIAL AND METHODS

Flat intestinal biopsies from 23 children (1 to 10 years old) with acute coeliac disease were included in this study. All patients had received gluten-containing food on the days previous to the test. Biopsies (10–30 mg wet weight) were taken with a paediatric-sized Watson capsule at the ligament of Treitz and transfered into the culture medium immediately after excision. One quarter of the biopsy was photographed and processed for routine histology. The remainder of the biopsy was cut into 3 to 6 pieces for organ culture. Organ culture was performed essentially according to Browning and Trier[4] in RPMI 1640 medium containing 10% heat-inactivated fetal calf serum and antibiotics[5]. The following gluten fractions were tested:
1. A peptic–tryptic digest prepared from gliadin (Fluka, Switzerland)

according to Cornell *et al.*[6]: PT-gliadin. The final digest was neutralized with HCl and centrifuged for 20 min at 2000 g. The resulting supernatant was immersed into a boiling water bath for 15 min to destroy trypsin activity and was lyophilized.

2. A peptic–tryptic digest of gluten from the wheat variety Scout 66 following the exact Frazer *et al.* procedure[7]: Frazer fraction III. The fraction was heat-inactivated prior to lyophilization.
3. Alpha-gliadin from Scout 66[8].
4. Alpha-GT-18'000, a tryptic fraction of *α*-gliadin[8]. Residual trypsin activity was inhibited by soya bean trypsin inhibitor (Sigma).

Electron microscopy was performed as previously described[5]. In order to obtain an overall impression 1 μm thick sections were cut and stained with toluidine blue prior to the analysis of ultra thin sections.

RESULTS

Different fragments of each individual biopsy obtained from children with active coeliac disease were cultured in the presence or absence of gluten fractions for 24 or 48 h (Table 10.1) and were analysed in a comparative manner by light and electron microscopy. Non-cultured specimens fixed immediately after excision always lacked villi, had increased intra-epithelial lymphocyte counts and showed elongated crypts. However the severity of enterocyte damage at the surface of the biopsy varied considerably from one individual to another (Figure 10.1a, b). The epithelium of less injured biopsies at excision remained essentially unchanged when maintained *in vitro* with the exception of a

Table 10.1 Behaviour in organ culture of flat intestinal biopsies from 20 children with acute coeliac disease or with coeliac disease in remission after a subsequent gluten challenge of 30 days. 'Regeneration', 'unchanged' or 'damage' respectively characterize the appearance of the epithelial ultrastructure after culture with or without (control) gluten when compared to the non-cultured fragment of the same biopsy. In no case was a difference observed between specimens cultured in the presence and absence of the four gluten fractions.

	Gluten fractions			
	PT-gliadin (Fluka) (1 and 2 mg/ml)	Frazer fraction III (1 mg/ml)	α-Gliadin (1 and 2 mg/ml)	α-GT-18'000 (1 mg/ml)
Hours in culture				
24 : regeneration	5	3*	2	2
unchanged	1	0	1	0
damage	0	0	0	0
48 : regeneration	3	n.d.	n.d.	n.d.
unchanged	1			
damage	2**			

* Cultures without fetal calf serum. ** Unspecific necrosis in both the culture with PT-gliadin and the control. n.d. = not done.

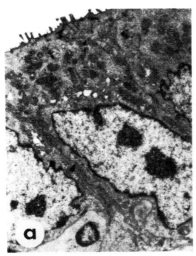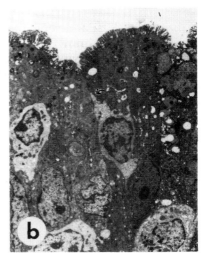

Figure 10.1 Non-cultured flat intestinal biopsies. Electron micrographs illustrating the variability of surface enterocyte damage. (a) Almost complete absence of microvilli. (b) moderately injured enterocytes. × 5200 and × 2900

decreased number of intra-epithelial lymphocytes in the cultured fragment. Severely injured biopsies underwent a remarkable regeneration which was characterized by the appearance of almost normal enterocytes at the surface with a well-developed brush border (Figure 10.2a). The occasional presence of small areas with heavily damaged enterocytes suggests that not all injured cells had been sloughed off during culture.

Surprisingly none of our four tested gluten fractions proved to be toxic *in vitro* (Table 10.1). The same histological and ultrastructural improvement of the surface epithelium was observed regardless of the presence or absence of gluten in the culture medium (Figure 10.2b, c). The crypts always remained healthy (Figure 10.3). In the rare cases with extended tissue necrosis after culture both the fragments with and without gluten were affected.

The absence of cytotoxicity was confirmed for Frazer fraction III by measuring brush border enzyme activities before and after culture. The specific activity of alkaline phosphatase, sucrase, maltase, lactase and glucoamylase determined in tissue homogenates after 24 hours' culture was essentially the same with or without this fraction (Figure 10.4).

DISCUSSION

The absence of *in vitro* toxicity from all tested gluten fractions was

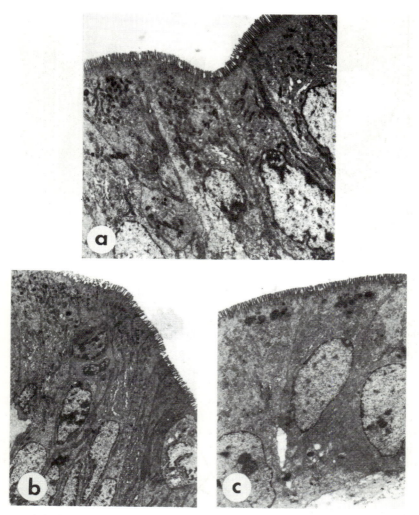

Figure 10.2 Representative areas of ultrastructural improvement observed after 24 hours of culture in control medium (a), in serum-free medium containing 1 mg/ml Frazer fraction III (b), and after 48 hours of culture in medium containing 2 mg/ml PT-gliadin (c). × 4200, × 2500 and ×3350.

surprising since it does not corroborate the observations reported so far[1-3]. The absence of toxicity of PT-gliadin cannot be attributed to a thorough digestion, a possibility mentioned by Jos *et al.*[3]. Furthermore these authors suggested that a culture time of 24 h may not be sufficient for the detection of gluten toxicity, since they obtained cell damage only after 48 h culture. In our experimental conditions however, prolong-

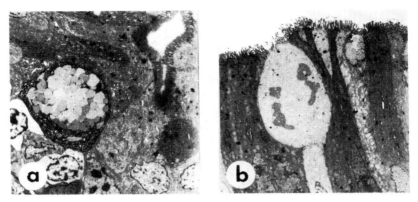

Figure 10.3 Ultrastructural aspect of crypt cells after 24 hours culture in medium containing 1 mg/ml α-GT-18'000.
(a) Cross section near the crypt mouth. Note the presence of well developed microvilli. × 1930
(b) Lower part of crypt with cell in mitosis. × 2250.

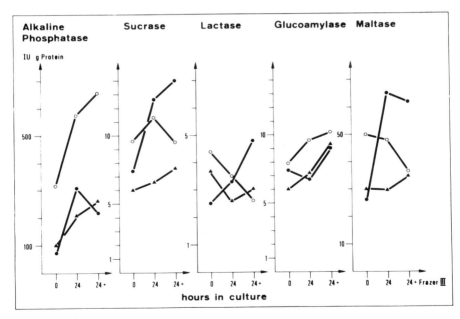

Figure 10.4 Brush border enzyme activities in mucosal homogenates of three flat intestinal biopsies before and after a 24 h culture in RPMI 1640 with 10% fetal calf serum. Each biopsy was cut into three fragments, two of which were cultured, one in the presence and one in the absence of 1 mg/ml of peptic–tryptic digested gluten (Frazer fraction III).

ation of the culture period up to 48 h did not alter the results obtained after 24 h, but showed that areas of non-specific cell necrosis were more frequent than after 24 h regardless of the presence or absence of PT-gliadin. Since, for ethical reasons, we could only test the *in vivo* toxicity of the undigested gliadin and not of PT-gliadin itself a direct *in vivo–in vitro* comparison was not possible for this particular fraction. We therefore extended our studies to gluten preparations with established *in vivo* toxicity. This is the case for Frazer fraction III[7] (and W. Th. J. M. Hekkens, unpublished), α-gliadin[9] and α-GT-18'000[8]. The absence of toxicity in organ culture of α-gliadin may be explained by its partial solubility in the culture medium. More difficult to explain is the lack of *in vitro* toxicity of Frazer fraction III and of α-GT-18'000, a soluble tryptic fragment of α-gliadin. Fetal calf serum which may have a certain capacity to bind toxic proteins[10] was not responsible for the lack of cytotoxicity, since biopsy cultures in serum-free medium for 24 h were not affected by Frazer fraction III.

Falchuk *et al.*[2] have shown that the regeneration of flat mucosa *in vitro* is accompanied by an increase in brush border enzyme activities, mainly of alkaline phosphatase, which could be inhibited by the presence of gliadin. Our experiments confirm the increase of alkaline phosphatase activity but we were unable to demonstrate any significant difference in brush border enzyme activities between cultures with and without Frazer fraction III. This discrepancy is as yet inexplicable since the culture technique, the medium, and the preparation of gluten were essentially the same.

Organ culture has proved in our hands to represent a valuable method for the study of protein synthesis[5], biosynthesis and turnover of brush border enzyme glycoproteins[11,12]. However its use as an *in vitro* test system for the assessment of gluten toxicity towards flat intestinal biopsies is questioned by the present results.

ACKNOWLEDGEMENTS

This work was supported by grants numbers 3.915.72 and 3.676-0.75 from the Swiss National Science Foundation and by grants from the D.G.R.S.T. No. 737.1630, I.N.S.E.R.M. and C.N.R.S. (France).

We are grateful to Mrs C. Ryser for secretarial assistance.

References

1. Townley, R. R. W., Bhathal, P. S., Cornell, H. J. and Mitchell, J. D. (1973). Toxicity of wheat gliadin fractions in coeliac disease. *Lancet*, **i**, 1362
2. Falchuk, Z. M., Gebhard, R. L., Sessoms, L. and Strober, W. (1974). An in vitro model of gluten-sensitive enteropathy. Effect of gliadin on intestinal epithelial cells of patients with gluten-sensitive enteropathy in organ culture. *J. Clin. Invest.*, **53**, 487

3. Jos, J., Lenoir, G., Ritis, G. de and Rey, J. (1975). In vitro pathogenetic studies of coeliac disease. Effects of protein digests on coeliac intestinal biopsy specimens maintained in culture for 48 hours. *Scand. J. Gastroenterol.*, **10**, 121

4. Browning, T. H. and Trier, J. S. (1968). Organ culture of mucosal biopsies of human small intestine. *J. Clin. Invest.*, **48**, 1423

5. Hauri, H. P., Kedinger, M., Haffen, K., Grenier, J. F. and Hadorn, B. (1975). Organ culture of human duodenum and jejunum. *Biol. Gastroenterol., (Paris)*, **8**, 307

6. Cornell, H. J. and Townley, R. R. W. (1973). Investigation of possible intestinal peptidase deficiency in coeliac disease. *Clin. Chim. Acta*, **43**, 113

7. Frazer, A. C., Fletcher, R. F., Ross, C. A. C., Shaw, B., Sammons, H. G. and Schneider, R. (1959). Gluten-induced enteropathy. The effect of partially digested gluten. *Lancet*, **ii**, 252

8. Hekkens, W. Th. J. M., Van den Aarsen, C. J., Gilliams, J. P., Lems-van-Kan, Ph. and Bouma-Frölich, G. (1974). -gliadin structure and degradation. In: W. Th. J. M. Hekkens and A. S. Peña (eds). *Coeliac Disease. Proceedings of the Second International Coeliac Symposium*, pp. 39–45 (Leiden, Stenfert Kroese)

9. Hekkens, W. Th. J. M., Haex, A. J. Ch. and Willighagen, R. G.J. (1970). Some aspects of gliadin fractionation and testing by histochemical method. In: C. C. Booth and R. H. Dowling (eds.) *Coeliac Disease. Proceedings of the First International Coeliac Symposium*, pp. 11–19. (Edinburgh: Churchill Livingstone)

10. Hudson, D. A., Cornell, H. J., Purdham, D. R. and Rolles, C. J. (1976). Non specific cytotoxicity of wheat gliadin components towards cultured human cells. *Lancet*, **i**, 339

11. Hauri, H. P., Kedinger, M., Haffen, K., Freiburghaus, A., Grenier, J. F. and Hadorn, B. (1977). Biosynthesis of brush border glycoproteins by human small intestinal mucosa in organ culture. *Biochim. Biophys. Acta*, **467**, 327

12. Hauri, H. P., Kedinger, M., Haffen, K. and Hadorn, B. (1977). Biosynthesis of brush border glycoproteins by human small intestinal mucosa in organ culture. *Experientia*, **33**, 820

Discussion of chapter 10

Falchuk I find the results interesting although I have some questions and maybe possible explanations for the differences observed. Early on we also noted that some individuals didn't respond to peptic/tryptic digests of gluten as far as toxicity went in the organ culture and we came up with a number of different possibilities to account for this. Historically the first one had to do with the observation that the patients who were in remission didn't demonstrate any toxicity to the gluten in culture. Toxicity was present only in patients who were in exacerbation. On looking at your pictures the initial histology prior to challenge in culture looked pretty good to begin with. The question would be how sure are you that the patients are under challenge and are active, because if they aren't in a significant state of activity it will be difficult to demonstrate *in vitro* toxicity. The other point has to do with the observation that we also made some time ago, and this is that there is a difference in the sensitivity *in vitro* to gluten depending on the patient's histocompatibility status. We have now expanded our studies in that sphere and find a very definite correlation with *in vitro* gluten sensitivity and HLA B8. The patients who have B8 have a much higher correlation with *in vitro* sensitivity than the patients who do not.

Trier I think to paraphrase what Dr Falchuk really wants to know is how long were your patients on a gluten-containing diet? Have they been challenged?

Hauri Our patients are children; most of them are only a few years old. They came into our hospital, and had a gluten-containing diet between some months and some years. They had an initial flat biopsy and 80% at least proved to be coeliac patients afterwards. That is to say when they were two years on gluten-free diet and then re-challenged they demonstrated adverse effects. The second point I can't answer because we didn't do HLA typing.

Strober I want to reiterate the second point that Dr Falchuk made, that the HLA status of the patients is very important in predicting the response in organ culture. The HLA B8 negative patients in our hands are not as responsive in culture as the HLA B8 positive patients, I am aware of the fact that in the area of the world your studies originate the incidence of HLA B8 in the patients is far lower than elsewhere. Of the three patients—as judged by change in alkaline phosphatase, one responded and two did not. Now, it would be very interesting to know whether or not the two who

	didn't were in fact HLA B8 negative, and the one that did respond was HLA B8 positive.
Hauri	We have to test this. At least we can say that the system is not useful in our hands, since we have only false negatives.
Jos	I think that the preparation of the peptic–tryptic digest is very important. It is important to take care about the duration of digestion and especially we find heating to inactivate proteolytic activity is a critical step. If you autoclave it for more than 10 or 15 minutes it is possible to inactivate the digest, and also filtration of the fraction, I think, can also inactivate some digests. If the gliadin is dialysed and left in contact with acid solution for long term, inactivation may occur. I think that is because of deamidation. How did you destroy proteolytic activity?
Hauri	This is indeed very important. We destroyed trypsin activity of our first fraction by boiling for 15 minutes. The fact still remains that Frazer's Fraction III which was also inactivated by heat was toxic *in vivo* but not *in vitro*.
Watson	Dr Dick Hamilton in Toronto has shown that in children particularly, the earlier you start treatment with a gluten-free diet and the longer you have them on it, the more nearly to normal does the tissue become. I think we have to accept that the children you have studied may well have been almost normal, and therefore take longer to respond to the re-introduction of gluten. Such patients do not respond as acutely as the untreated or the more chronic patients.
Hauri	Theoretically I agree; in practice I do not agree since the biopsies we studied clearly were completely flat.

11

Sequential biochemical studies in coeliac disease using jejunal organ culture techniques

P. E. JONES, C. L'HIRONDEL AND T. J. PETERS

INTRODUCTION

The ultrastructural abnormalities of the enterocyte in coeliac disease have been well described [1-4] and, elsewhere in this symposium[5], the enterocyte organelle pathology has been described quantitatively using analytical subcellular fractionation combined with enzymic microanalysis. There have however been few *in vitro* studies of enterocyte function in coeliac disease. Such studies would be expected to indicate how the malabsorption is induced and might also yield important clues on the mechanism of gluten damage.

An organ culture technique[6] has been used to measure the protein, DNA and alkaline phosphatase synthesis rates in jejunal biopsies from seven patients with untreated coeliac disease and to follow sequentially these parameters during treatment by gluten withdrawal.

A technical problem with organ culture techniques is that there is a progressive loss of tissue from the biopsy during culture and thus the expression of results related to tissue protein[7,8] at the end of the culture period may be misleading. It has been shown that total DNA in the culture tube, i.e. tissue + medium, remains constant during the culture and is therefore a more reliable reference parameter for the expression of results.

PATIENTS AND METHODS

Seven adult patients with untreated coeliac disease were studied before and after treatment with a gluten-free diet. In all seven patients there was an improvement in absorption tests and microscopic evidence of villous regeneration. Jejunal biopsies were obtained with the Watson–

Crosby capsule and processed for histology or organ culture as previously described[6].

Protein was determined by a micromodification of the method of Lowry *et al*[9]. with bovine serum albumin (Armour Pharmaceuticals) as standard. DNA was determined by the method of Le Pecq and Paoletti[10] with calf thymus DNA (Koch-Light Laboratories Ltd., Colnbrook, Bucks., UK) as standard.

Protein synthesis was measured by culturing mucosa for 24 h with 2μCi L-[^{14}C] leucine (50μCi/mg, The Radiochemical Centre, Amersham). Protein was precipitated from the tissue homogenate and medium with trichloracetic acid and the radioactivity determined. Results are expressed as total (tissue + medium) cpm/μg total DNA.

Alkaline phosphatase synthesis was determined during 24h culture; alkaline phosphatase activity in the tissue homogenate and medium were measured fluorimetrically with 4-methyl umbelliferyl phosphate as substrate[10]. Synthesized alkaline phosphatase was calculated by subtracting basal levels from total activity after 24 h culture. DNA synthesis was determined as described previously[12].

RESULTS

Protein content of cultured biopsy

The decrease in protein content of cultured pieces of jejunum from four control subjects and four untreated coeliac patients after varying periods of culture is shown in Table 11.1. There is a progressive and approximately linear loss of protein throughout the period of culture so that by 24 h approximately one-third of the protein has been lost.

Table 11.1 Protein content of control and coeliac mucosa after varying periods of culture

Time(h)	Protein (μg)
0	290 ± 60
3	274 ± 70
6	255 ± 50
24	200 ± 50

Mean $\pm$ SE. Thirteen pieces of mucosa were assayed at each time point

DNA content of cultured biopsy

Since there is no detectable DNA in the culture medium the DNA content of the biopsies and of the culture medium was assayed in 52 specimens from nine patients (five control subjects and four patients with coeliac disease). Figure 11.1 shows that the fall in tissue DNA after various periods in culture is followed by an increase in medium DNA so that

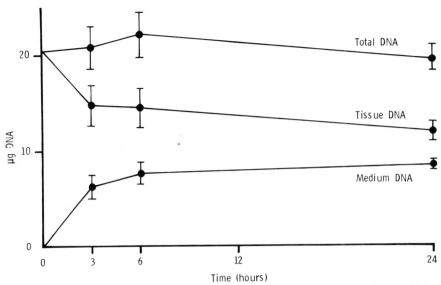

Figure 11.1 DNA content of tissue and of medium in cultured pieces of jejunal biopsy from both control and coeliac mucosa. Results show mean values ± SE of 13 determinations at each time point. Reproduced from Ref. 6

total (tissue + medium) DNA remains constant during 24 h culture. In order to compare DNA loss from normal and untreated coeliac mucosa the piece/medium DNA ratios were calculated after 24 h culture for normal and untreated coeliac mucosa. Figure 11.2 shows the piece/medium DNA ratio for mucosa from untreated coeliac patients is significantly less than for normal mucosa.

DNA, protein and alkaline phospatase synthesis by cultured biopsies

Studies on groups of patients (Figure 11.3) have shown that untreated coeliac mucosa exhibits an increased rate of protein synthesis, median 4480 cpm/μg DNA (95% confidence limits 3270–6270) compared to normal mucosa 1500 cpm/μg DNA (1000–2700, $p < 0.01$), decreased alkaline phosphatase synthesis, 0.31 mU/μg DNA (0,25–0.42) compared to normal, 1.46 mU/μg DNA (1.12–2.06, $p < 0.01$) and an increased DNA synthesis 78 cpm/μg DNA (40–230) compared to normal 15 cpm/μg DNA (5–25, $p < 0.01$).

These three parameters of enterocyte function have been measured in seven patients with untreated coeliac disease before and after varying periods of time on a gluten-free diet. Protein synthesis decreased significantly in all seven patients, from a mean of 4960 c.p.m./μg DNA to one of 2130 cpm/μg DNA (Figure 11.4). Alkaline phosphatase synthesis

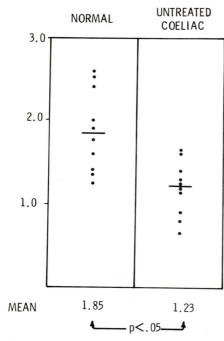

Figure 11.2 Piece/medium DNA ratio after 24 h culture for mucosa from normal subjects and patients with untreated coeliac disease. Statistical analysis by Wilcoxon rank and sum test

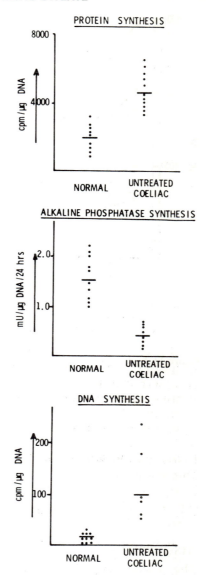

Figure 11.3 Protein, alkaline phosphatase and DNA synthetic rates by cultured jejunal biopsies from normal subjects and patients with untreated coeliac disease

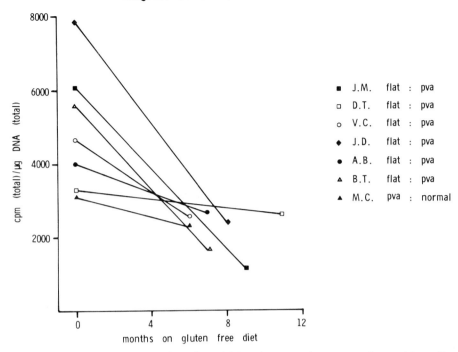

Figure 11.4   Protein synthesis by cultured jejunal mucosa in seven patients with coeliac disease before and after varying periods of gluten withdrawal. The morphology of the jejunal mucosa is shown: flat — subtotal villus atrophy; pva — partial villus atrophy; normal — finger-like villi

increased in all seven patients from a mean of 0.49 mU/μg DNA to 0.95 mU/μg DNA (Figure 11.5). DNA synthesis was measured in five patients. In four patients DNA synthesis before treatment was increased and fell after gluten withdrawal; one patient who had a low rate of DNA synthesis before treatment did not show significant alteration after treatment. The mean fall in DNA synthesis for the five patients was from 72 c.p.m./μg DNA to 19 c.p.m./μg DNA.

DISCUSSION

The marked reduction in tissue protein during 24 h culture and the greater loss of tissue from untreated coeliac mucosa questions the validity of tissue protein for use as a reference parameter in organ culture experiments. The total, i.e. tissue + medium, DNA remains constant during 24 h culture giving an accurate measurement of the amount of tissue at the start of culture and avoids inaccuracies due to differing rates of tissue loss into the medium.

Autoradiographic studies[6] indicate that the increased protein

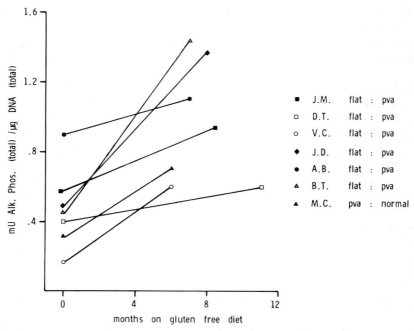

Figure 11.5 Alkaline phosphatase synthesis by cultured jejunal mucosa in seven patients with coeliac disease before and after varying periods of gluten withdrawal. Legend as Figure 11.4

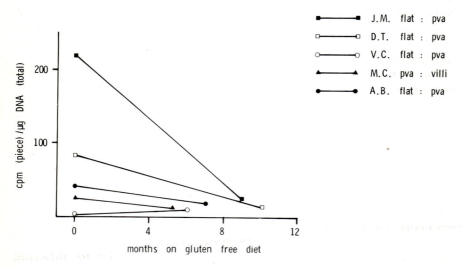

Figure 11.6 DNA synthesis by cultured jejunal mucosa in five patients with coeliac disease before and after varying periods of gluten withdrawal. Legend as Figure 11.4

synthesis shown by untreated coeliac mucosa is mainly due to an increase in protein synthesis by the enterocytes and enteroblasts. This increase in protein synthesis and the decrease in alkaline phosphatase synthesis could reflect either the immaturity of the enterocytes or a direct or indirect toxic action of gluten or its products on these cells. When complete villous regeneration has occurred after the removal of gluten from the diet the mean protein and alkaline phosphatase synthetic rates return towards the normal range. There is, however, a wide variation in alkaline phosphatase synthesis in the seven patients after treatment and this does not appear to be related to the length of time on a gluten-free diet. Furthermore, the one patient who achieved normal villous morphology (MC) showed after treatment a rate of alkaline phosphatase synthesis which was below the normal range. The reason for this variable response of alkaline phosphatase synthesis to gluten withdrawal remains to be determined.

DNA synthesis is an index of enterocyte production since autoradiographic studies have shown that [³H]thymidine is taken up predominantly by the enteroblasts[6]. In the five patients in whom DNA synthesis was measured before treatment a wide range in synthetic rate is seen. Four of the patients showed a DNA synthetic rate above the normal range and in these patients DNA synthesis fell to within the normal range after treatment. This is consistent with an increased enterocyte production rate in the untreated coeliac mucosa which returns to normal when villous regeneraton has occurred[13]. One patient (VC) showed a low DNA synthetic rate before treatment and this did not alter significantly with treatment, despite the observation that the jejunal mucosa did show villous regeneraton. It is likely therefore that this patient did not have a greatly enhanced enterocyte shedding rate and was therefore able to regenerate villi despite a relatively low enterocyte production rate.

These studies indicate how organ culture techniques can be used to investigate certain aspects of enterocyte function in coeliac disease. The use in models of coeliac disease is discussed elsewhere in this volume (Chapter 8, 9 and 10). Immunological mechanisms[7,8] and the effect of hormones[8] can be readily studied with this technique. Elsewhere[12] we have shown how responsive and non-responsive patients with coeliac disease can be distinguished using organ culture techniques.

ACKNOWLEDGEMENTS

We would like to thank Professor C. C. Booth for his continued encouragement and Ms. Jean de Luca for typing the manuscript. This work is supported by the Medical Research Council and The Wellcome Trust.

References

1. Trier, J. S. and Rubin, C. E. (1965). Electron microscopy of the small intestine: a review. *Gastroenterology, 47, 574*

2. Rubin, W., Ross, L. L., Sleisenger, M. H. and Weser, E. (1966). An electron microscopic study of adult coeliac disease. *Lab. Invest., 15, 1720*

3. Shiner, M. (1967). Ultrastructure of jejunal surface epithelium in untreated idiopathic steatorrhoea. *Br. Med. Bull., 23, 223*

4. Shiner, M. (1974). Electron microscopy of jejunal mucosa. *Clin. Gastroenterol.. 3, 33*

5. Peters, T. J., Jones, P. E., Jenkins, W. J. and NIcholson, J. A. (1978). Analytical subcellular fractionation of jejunal biopsy specimens from control subjects and patients with coeliac disease. *Ibid*

6. L'Hirondel, C., Doe, W. F. and Peters, T. J. (1976). Biochemical and morphological studies on human jejunal mucosa maintained in culture. *Clin. Sci. Mol. Med., 50, 425*

7. Falchuk, Z. M., Gebhard, R. L., Sessoms, C. and Strober, W. (1974). An *in vitro* model of gluten-sensitive enteropathy. Effect of gliadin on intestinal epithelial cells of patients with gluten-sensitive enteropathy in organ culture. *J. Clin. Invest., 53, 487*

8. Katz, A. J., Falchuk, Z. M., Strober, W. and Schachman, H. (1976). Gluten-sensitive enteropathy. Inhibition by cortisol of the effect of gluten protein *in vitro. New Engl. J. Med., 295, 131*

9. Lowry, O. H., Rosebrough, N. J., Farr, A. C. and Randall, R. J. (1951). Protein measurement with Folin-phenol reagent. *J. Biol. Chem., 193, 265*

10. Le Pecq, J-B. and Paoletti, C. (1966). A new fluorimetric method for RNA and DNA determination. *Anal. Biochem., 17, 100*

11. Peters, T. J. (1976). Analytical subcellular fractionation of jejunal biopsy specimens: methodology and characterisation of the organellas in normal tissue. *Clin. Sci. Mol. Med., 51, 557*

12. Jones, P. E. and Peters, T. J. (1977). DNA synthesis by jejunal mucosa in responsive and non-responsive coeliac disease. *Br. Med. J., 1, 1130*

13. Barry, R. E. and Read, A. E. (1973). Coeliac disease and malignancy. *Q. J. Med., 42, 665*

Discussion of chapter 11

Hauri	I would like to comment on alkaline phosphatase. First you speak about alkaline phosphatase synthesis, but what you measure is the activity before and after culture. This is not synthesis, this is an increase. Secondly it has been shown that alkaline phosphatase is more active when it is dilipated, so if alkaline phosphatase molecules diffuse into the glycocalyx, and are dilipated they may become more active, and so decrease in alkaline phosphatase as a sign of toxicity is still open to question. In addition we have shown that this corresponds to the results shown at the beginning of first session by Dr Stevens that alkaline phosphatase didn't decrease when there was a decrease in other enzyme activities, so although alkaline phosphatase is a membrane marker, it may not be the best marker for toxicity.
Jones	Well, your first point, is this increase true synthesis, in fact we haven't done these experiments but they have been done by other workers. The increase in alkaline phosphatase is blocked by protein synthesis inhibitor, so we believe that it is synthesis. We haven't considered your second point. All I can say is that alkaline phosphatase activity in the untreated coeliac tissue increases by 60% after the culture period. We also have no alkaline phosphatase activity at all in the medium at the beginning of culture and 70% of the total alkaline phosphatase activity at the end of culture is in the medium. I don't think that that kind of increase could be accounted for by an alteration in the physico-chemical environment of the enzyme. Your third point about whether alkaline phosphatase is a good marker for toxicity is not something that I have gone into on this data. It is part of ongoing experiments, and we would like to hold those results for a while.
Hauri	Maybe we should discuss it because most of the toxicity work is based on alkaline phosphatase.
Jones	Well, all I can say is that perhaps we may be able to give you an answer in about six months.
Fielding	You carefully told us that the return was towards normality. Have you had any further opportunity to study these patients subsequently, and whether that trend has continued and whether it has been arrested, and if continued whether it has continued towards normality still, or reached normality.
Jones	You are talking in terms of the alkaline phosphatase?
Fielding	Any of the three.
Jones	The protein and the DNA synthesis does in fact return to within the normal range. As yet, of the patients in whom we have measured it the alkaline phosphatase synthesis has still not returned

to the normal range, so there does appear to be a separation of the protein and DNA from the alkaline phosphatase at this stage in our studies.

Cluysenaer   One of your patients had a low DNA activity when he was un-treated and he did not react on gluten withdrawal. What happened to the patient clinically? Was he a case of refractory sprue?

Jones   Right, this lady actually had a low rate of DNA synthesis as you say. Now we had her on a gluten-free diet for six months and her jejunal morphology did show subjective improvement, and I stress subjective. Subjectively this improvement did not appear to be as marked as in the other patients. Before we could confirm this we have got to assess it formally in terms of villous volume measurements and so on. So whether this patient is not as good a responder as the others, at this stage we can't say. I would stress that when we measure DNA synthesis I think we have got good evidence now that this is a measurement of enterocyte production. Whether or not you get villous regeneration depends on the balance between enterocyte production and enterocyte loss. We are looking at one half of the system. We have not in these patients been able to measure the other side.

Section III
Genetic markers

12

B-cell alloantigens in coeliac disease

E. ALBERT, K. HARMS, R. BERTELE, A. ANDREAS, A.
McNICHOLAS, B. KUNTZ, S. SCHOLZ, B. SCHIEßL, H.
WETZMÜLLER, P. REISSINGER and CH. WEESER-KRELL

INTRODUCTION

Earlier investigations of our group[2] have demonstrated that in the
South German and Austrian population the frequency of HLA-B8 in
coeliacs is considerably lower (56%) than was found in England[10] and
Holland[8] (83%). After it had become clear that the HLA-D-locus antigen HLA-DW3 is also very significantly increased in coeliac disease
(CD)[3], the question arose, whether there would be a similar situation as
for HLA-B8.

HLA-D locus antigens can—by definition—be detected by typing
reactions with homozygous typing cells using the mixed leucocyte
culture test[5]. More recently, methods have become available to define
by serologic means B-cell specific antigens, which are very highly associated if not identical with HLA-D locus alleles. Accordingly, the HLA-
DW3 associated B-cell antigen (now officially named HLA-DRW3) has
also been found in a very high frequency among patients with CD[3]. It
was therefore the objective of this study to determine the frequency of
HLA-DRW3 in patients with CD from Southern Germany and to follow
their inheritance in families.

MATERIALS AND METHODS

A total of 42 unrelated patients and their families were tested for
HLA-A and B antigens as well as for HLA-DRW3 and DRW7. Diagnosis
of CD was based on the finding of a subtotal villous atrophy of the small
bowel mucosa and clear morphological and/or clinical improvement
with a gluten free diet.

Supported by DFG-A192/9/10, SFB37,TP-B1,2, and DFG Ha846/2

Typing for HLA-A and B was done using routine procedures; the testing of B-cell alloantigens was performed using a cytotoxicity test after B-cell enrichment according to van Rood et al. (1975). Antisera for B-cell typing were procured as described previously[1]. The specificity of the B-cell sera was assessed by crosstesting with 22 families tested in the VII International Histocompatibility Workshop (1977). For the definition of HLA-DRW3 eight sera and for DRW7 four sera were used. The presence of an antigen was assumed when 75% of the relevant sera reacted positively and where the relevant antigen segregated properly in the patient's family.

As a control for the frequency of the HLA-DRW3 and 7 antigens the 44 unrelated parents of 22 healthy families were used. For the HLA-A and B antigens 1142 unrelated healthy individuals of the Munich area formed the controls.

Table 12.1 Phenotype frequency of HLA-A and B antigens in 185 patients with coeliac disease and 1142 controls (143 from Harms et al. (1974) and 42 new patients)

Antigen	Patients Number positive	Patients Percent	Controls Percent
A1	104	56a	26
A2	80	43	49
A3	39	21	33
A9	32	17	19
A10	15	8	12
A11	11	6	9
A28	10	5	6
A29	11	6	5
AW30	10	5	3
AW31	2	1	3
AW32	20	11	3
B5	23	12	14
B7	14	8a	30
B8	103	56a	18
B12	41	22	23
B13	33	18a	7
B14	11	6	3
B15	19	10	11
BW16	9	5	4
B17	12	6	8
B18	13	7	8
BW21	6	3	4
BW22	2	1	3
B27	13	7	7
BW35	23	12	17
B40	12	6	13

a: $p \ll 0.0005$

RESULTS

HLA-A and B antigens

The pattern of frequencies of the HLA-A and B antigens in the 42 patients follows very closely that found in our earlier study[2]: HLA-A1 increased to 59%, B8 increased to 55% and B7 strongly decreased to 12%. Interestingly B13 is quite frequent (28%) in this new group of 42 patients and clearly confirms the trend observed in our earlier report. Thus HLA-B13 has now been significantly increased in two consecutive studies. In Table 12.1 are listed the combined HLA-A and B frequencies of 185 patients (143 from Harms et al.[2] and 42 new patients).

B-cell alloantigens HLA-DRW3 and DRW7

The antigen HLA-DRW3, which is highly associated with HLA-B8 has been found in 27 of 42 patients (64%) as compared to 20% in the normal population (chi-square=15.21; $p<0.0005$). The antigen HLA-DRW7 is in the normal population weakly associated with HLA-B13 and was found in 20 of 42 patients (48%) in contrast to a frequency of 25% in the controls (chi-square=3.84; $p<0.05$), an increase which has just reached the border of statistical significance. The analysis of DRW3 and 7 shows that 36 of 42 patients possess either DRW3 or 7 or both, where the DRW3/7 heterozygote state is quite frequent (11/42; chi-square=6.25; $p<0.05$). Taken together, the antigens DRW3 and 7 account for 60% of the gene frequency at the DRW locus of the 42 patients (DRW3: 36% and DRW7: 24%).

Table 12.2 lists the significantly increased HLA antigens with the level of significance and the relative risk as a measure of the degree of association. It can be seen that B8 and DRW3 convey a very significant relative risk 5.7 and 7.0 respectively) while B13 and DRW7 are more weakly associated with coeliac disease. An important finding seems to be that the presence of DRW3/7 heterozygotes appears to convey a higher

Table 12.2 Relative risks associated with different HLA-B or DRW antigens

| Antigen | CD patients | | Controls | | |
	Number positive	Percent	Percent	p value	Relative risk
B8 (N 185)	103	56	18	<0.0005	5.7
B13 (N 185)	33	18	7	<0.0005	2.9
DRW3 (N=42)	27	64	20	<0.0005	7.0
DRW7 (N=42)	20	48	25	0.05	2.7
DRW3/7 (N=42)	11	26	5	<0.05	7.45

relative risk than DRW3 alone, indicating a kind of a superdominance phenomenon, where alleles of the same locus cooperate in providing the genetic disposition to disease.

Family segregation

In order to validate the data from the unrelated patient population, a segregation analysis was performed in which informative backcross families (+/− × −/−) are investigated as to whether the patients and the healthy siblings show the expected partition of 50% positive and 50% negative. A significant deviation from this in the patients reflects an association. As can be seen in Table 12.3 all four previously discussed antigens HLA-B8, B13, DRW3 and DRW7 show significant deviations in the sense of an overrepresentation of these antigens among the patients.

The glyoxalase (GLO) polymorphism

A new genetic marker has recently been added to the HLA linkage group on chromosome 6 (Kömpf et al., 1976[4]: the polymorphism of GLO-1 is located between HLA-D and PGM_3 (Pretorius et al., 1976) at a distance from HLA-B of approximately 4–5% recombination frequency (Albert et al., unpublished data). Since this polymorphism is therefore located in the vicinity of HLA-D, two alleles of which are highly associated with CD, it was a logical step to investigate whether there would be any differences in allele frequencies in patients with CD. A total of 40

Table 12.3 Segregation analysis of HLA-B8, B13, DRW3 and DRW7 in 42 families of patients with coeliac disease

	Patients		Healthy siblings	
	Positive	Negative	Positive	Negative
HLA-B8	101	18	60	58
	Chi-square	57.9	Chi-square	0.00,n.s.
	$p<0.0005$			
HLA-B13	27	6	17	13
	Chi-square = 13.3		Chi-square = 0.53, n.s.	
	$p<0.0005$			
HLA-DRW3	30	1	22	14
	Chi-square = 27.12		Chi-square = 1.77, n.s.	
	$p<0.0005$			
HLA-DRW7	20	0	15	10
	Chi-square= 20.0		Chi-square = 1.0, n.s.	
	$p<0.0005$			

n.s. = not significant

patients and their families was tested for the presence of GLO-1 and GLO-2 using the methods published by Pretorius et al. (1976) The 116 parents of 58 normal families served as a control. Among the 40 CD patients a gene frequency of 0.39 for GLO-1 and 0.61 for GLO-2 was determined by gene counting, which is identical with the frequencies of 0.39 and 0.61 respectively found in the control group. Thus there is no indication for any involvement of GLO alleles in an association with CD.

DISCUSSION

One of the important aims of the continued study of the HLA association with CD is to attempt to identify the gene which is responsible for the disease susceptibility. It has become clear that the antigen HLA-B8 is in itself certainly not involved in the pathogenesis, which is borne out by the fact that one allele of a closely linked locus—HLA-D—has been found to be more strongly associated with CD. The association was in some studies[3] so strong that almost all patients were positive for the HLA-DW3 antigen, which might (again) suggest that this antigen could be directly involved in the pathogenesis of the disease. The results presented here however seem to rule out this possibility: in the South German population, the association between CD and the B-cell antigen HLA-DRW3 (which is equivalent to HLA-DW3) is by no means as striking as for example in the Dutch population tested by Keuning et al. (1976) and in the Norwegian population[9]. This finding is parallelled by our previous observation[2] of a much lower frequency of HLA-B8 in CD patients from Southern Germany and Austria. A varying degree of association in different populations is of course what one would expect to find if the association is the result of linkage disequilibrium between alleles of two closely linked loci. Thus, our data strongly support the concept of closely linked genes and at the same time indicate that HLA-DRW3 is probably not the gene directly involved in the pathogenesis of CD. In addition, by demonstrating the absence of any association with GLO alleles, we have shown that the linkage disequilibrium does not extend all the way out to the GLO marker gene.

Another surprising result of this study is the finding of a second HLA-DRW antigen in association with CD, although this might have been expected on the basis of our previous study[2], where an increase in HLA-B13 was found both in the population and the family analysis. Our present data confirm this increase of HLA-B13 very clearly. It is somewhat surprising that this has to our knowledge not been observed by any other group investigating CD. This might be explained by the fact that an association of this relatively moderate degree can only be demonstrated in a larger series of patients. Alternatively the differing ethnic background of the patients in the various CD studies could be used as an explanation, although it must be stated that the B13 frequency does not differ strongly between Holland and Southern Germany.

The relatively recently defined B-cell antigen DRW7 shows in the normal population a slight association with HLA-B13 and this association is even more pronounced in the 42 CD patients, where all B13 positive haplotypes also carry DRW7. In addition DRW7 is frequently found on B12 positive haplotypes. It is therefore possible that DRW7 is associated or identical with the LD12a specificity, which was found to be increased[11] in patients with dermatitis herpetiformis.

With these new antigens associated with CD the question arises whether all the CD-associated antigens could themselves be associated with the same disease susceptibility gene. If this was the case, one would have to assume a recessive action of the susceptibility gene since there is a considerable number of DRW3/ DRW7 heterozygotes, which would under this hypothesis then have to be homozygous for the disease susceptibility gene. A recessive mode of action however would lead to an increased number of DRW3 and DRW7 homozygotes. This however is clearly not the case so that one alternatively has to consider two or more HLA-associated genes which interact in the determination of disease susceptibility. This concept is also supported by our earlier observation[2] that HLA-B7 is disproportionately strongly decreased among CD patients, which is felt to indicate a B7 associated gene which exerts some protective effect, a phenomenon also observed in juvenile diabetes mellitus. The possible interaction between two different HLA-associated genes is strongly suggested by the finding of the very high number of DRW3/ DRW7 heterozygotes and the increased relative risk conveyed by this type. The question however remains open, whether the three HLA-associated genes, which influence the disease susceptibility for CD (one DRW3-, one DRW7- and one B7- (or DRW2?) associated gene) are alleles of the same or of different loci. Since it has become unlikely that the HLA-DRW- or HLA-DW antigens are directly involved in pathogenesis, it will be a challenge for the future to find genes that are even more strongly associated with CD than are DRW and DW antigens. The genes for complement polymorphisms C_2, C_4 and Bf are obvious candidates, which should be tested in CD patients of different ethnic background, as this study has once more underlined.

References

1. Albert, E. D., Andreas, A., McNicholas, A., Scholz, S. and Kuntz, B. (1977). B- and T- cell specific alloantigens in man. *Scand. J. Immunol.*, **6**, 427
2. Harms, K., Granditsch, G., Rossipal, E., Ludwig, H., Polymenidis, Z., Scholz, S., Wank, R. and Albert, E. D. (1974). In: *Coeliac Disease*, (W. Tu, J. M. Hekkens, and A. S. Peña, eds.) pp. 215–228. (Leiden: Stenfer Kroese)
3. Keuning, J. J., Peña, A. S., van Leeuwen, A., van Hooff, J. P. and van Rood, J. J. (1976). HLA-DW3 association with coeliac disease. *Lancet*, **i**, 506
4. Kompf, J., Bissbort, S. and Schunter, F. (1976). Confirmation of linkage between the loci for HL-A and glyoxalase I. *Human Genet.*, **32**, 197
5. Mempel, W., Grosse-Wilde, H., Albert, E., and Thierfelder, S. (1973). Atypical MLC reactions in HL-A typed related and unrelated pairs. *Transplant. Proc.*, **5**, 401
6. Pretorius, A. M. G., Scholz, S., Kuntz, B. and Albert, E. D. (1976). Investigations of the red cell glyoxalase (GLO) in recombinant families. *Eur. J. Immunol.*, **6**, No. 10, 759
7. Rood, J. J. van, Leeuwen, A. van, Keuning, J. J. and Bussé van Oud, Alblas, A. (1975). The serological recognition of the human MLC determinants using a modified cytotoxicity technique. *Tissue Antigens*, **5**, 73
8. van Rood, J. J., van Hooff, J. P. and Keuning, J. J. (1975). Disease predisposition, immune responsiveness and the fine structure of the HL-A supergene. *Transplant. Rev.*, **22**, 75
9. Solheim, B. G., Ek, J., Thune, P. O., Baklien, K., Bratlie, A., Rankin, B., Thoresen, A. B. and Thorsby, E. (1976). HLA antigens in dermatitis herpetiformis and coeliac disease. *Tissue Antigens*, **7**, 57
10. Stokes, P. L., Asquith, P., Holmes, G. K. T., Mackintosh, P. and Cooke, W. T. (1972). Histocompatibility antigens associated with adult coeliac disease. *Lancet*, **ii**, 162
11. Thomsen, M., Platz, P., Marks, J., Ryder, L. P., Shuster, S., Svejgaard, A. and Young, S. H. (1976). Association of LD-8a and LD-12a with dermatits herpetiformis. *Tissue Antigens*, **7**, 60

13

B-cell alloantigens and the inheritance of coeliac disease

A. S. PEÑA,* D. L. MANN, N. E. HAGUE, J. A. HECK, A. VAN LEEUWEN, J. J. VAN ROOD and W. STROBER

INTRODUCTION

Coeliac disease is associated with the histocompatibility antigen HLA-B8. Another closely linked antigen, HLA-DW3 known to be in linkage disequilibrium with HLA-B8, has recently been found to be primarily associated with coeliac disease[1]. When the patients and controls were divided into B8 positive and B8 negative subgroups, and these subpopulations tested for association of coeliac disease and DW3, a significant strong correlation was found. Because the genes that control the immune response in laboratory animals appear to be the same as those that are coded by the HLA-D locus antigens, the primary association of coeliac disease with an allele of the HLA-D locus, i.e. HLA-DW3, suggests the involvement of an immune response gene in the pathogenesis of the disease. The fact that not all coeliac patients carry the HLA-DW3 antigen, and the fact that there are DW3-positive relatives of coeliac patients who do not suffer from coeliac disease suggest that DW3 is not the gene itself but rather is in close association with an immune response gene.

Mann et al.[2] found that coeliac disease was strongly associated with a specific B-lymphocyte surface antigen recognized by maternal antisera. With serum B-1 not one of the 37 controls, including 8 who were HLA-B8 positive, were found to be positive. This makes it extremely unlikely that the B-1 and B-cell antigens DW3 were identical. A relationship between these cell surface specificities has not been previously studied, although such a relationship seems unlikely *a priori* because of differences in frequency in normal populations.

* Dr. Peña performed this work during his tenure as a fellow of the International Agency for Research on Cancer, Lyon, France, World Health Organization

The HLA gene and the specific B-cell antigen recognized by maternal antisera may act in a complementary fashion in the pathogenesis of coeliac disease.

We therefore investigated the B-lymphocyte antigen DW3 and the B-1 specificity in coeliac patients as well as in a control population. Furthermore some families of unrelated patients with coeliac disease were studied.

PATIENTS, CONTROLS AND METHOD

Eighteen unrelated patients with coeliac disease, 17 control Caucasians and 36 members of seven unrelated families with coeliac disease were studied.

Purified mononuclear white cells, macrophage depleted, were labelled with radioactive chromium and washed three times. B-cells were separated from other cells lacking surface immunoglobulins by differential adhesion to plastic surfaces coated with purified anti-Fab antibody. After removal of non-B cells, test serum and complement were added. The cell mixture was incubated at 37 °C for 45 min. The supernatant fluid containing ^{51}Cr released as a result of cytotoxicity was removed and the wells washed with 0.2 N NaOH. Both the supernatant fluid and NaOH wash fluid were counted in a gamma counter. The percentage of chromium release resulting from exposure of cells to test serum was compared to percentage of chromium release in controls.

Serum B-1 was obtained from the mother of two children with coeliac disease. To type for HLA-DW3, serum Mo was used. When properly absorbed, this antiserum has been shown to react only with cells that do not respond in the mixed leucocyte reaction to homozygous DW3 typing cells (van Rood et al[3]). Both serum B-1 and serum Mo were absorbed with platelets having the HLA specificities of the husbands of the alloantisera donors.

RESULTS

Table 13.1

Group	HLA-DW3 positive	HLA-DW3 negative	B-1 positive	B-1 negative
Coeliac disease	15	3	11	7
Controls	6	11	1	16
X^2 for significance	8.17		11.50	
p 0.004 19			0.001	

Table 13.1 shows that both HLA-DW3 and B-1 specificity is significantly more common in coeliac disease patients than in control individuals.

The family study showed that there were 8 positive individuals for HLA-DW3 and negative for B-1, and vice versa, there were 6 individuals positive for B-1 and negative for HLA-DW3. Furthermore five out of seven couples of parents of coeliac children were positive for B-1 specificity. In several instances B-1 segregated differently to DW3.

DISCUSSION

These studies provide evidence for the concept that two distinct, separately inherited genes are necessary for the occurrence of coeliac disease. The 'multigene' hypothesis for this disease was presaged by the work of Falchuk et al.[4], van Rood et al.[5], and by a segregation analysis made by Meera Khan and Volkers in this symposium[6].

It is unclear at present whether the gene products resulting from the separate genes involved function independently or cooperatively in the production of the disease. It is attractive to postulate that the two genes involved are coding for proteins which make up a single structure on the surface of B-lymphocytes. Such a structure could be a receptor site for gliadin.

SUMMARY

Coeliac disease is strongly associated with the HLA-DW3 antigen and more specifically with a different B-cell antigen recognized by maternal alloantisera. This study supports the hypothesis that coeliac disease has a multigenic basis. It is speculated that these B-cell alloantigens may code for a receptor for gliadin which is important to the initiation of the disease.

References

1. Keuning, J. J., Peña, A. S., van Leeuwen, A., van Hooff, J. P. and van Rood, J. J. (1976). HLA-DW3 association with coeliac disease. *Lancet*, **i**, 506
2. Mann, D. L., Katz, S. I., Nelson, D. L., Abelson, L. D. and Strober, W. (1976). Specific B-cell antigens associated with gluten-sensitive enteropathy and dermatitis herpetiformis. *Lancet*, **i**, 110
3. van Rood, J. J., van Leeuwen, A., Keuning, J. J. and Blussévan Oud Alblas, A. (1975). The serological recognition of the human MLC determinants using a modified cytotoxicity technique. *Tissue Antigens*, **5**, 73
4. Falchuk, Z. M., Rogentine, G. N. and Strober, W. (1972). Predominance of histocompatibility antigen HL-A8 in patients with gluten-sensitive enteropathy. *J. Clin. Invest.*, **51**, 1602
5. van Rood, J. J., van Hooff, J. P. and Keuning, J. J. (1975). Disease predisposition, immune responsiveness and the fine structure of the HLA supergene. *Transplant. Rev.*, **22**, 75
6. Peña, A. S., Rosekrans, P. C. H., Volkers, W. S., Meera Khan, P., Hekkens, W. Th. J. M. and Haex, A. J. Ch. (1977). Genetics of coeliac disease. This volume.

Discussion of chapters 12 and 13

Asquith

I accept that positive DW3s and B8s account for the vast majority of your coeliacs but there is still a small proportion of both of your series that are neither DW3- nor B8-positive. Should we be looking for another marker? The second point is what importance would you give to the reduction of the incidence of B7 that you have found in Leiden and have confirmed in your bigger series? The third point is could you explain how a disease specific gene would fit in with the heterogeneity of clinical manifestations of coeliac disease?

Albert

The first question related to the people who have coeliac disease but don't have DW3 or HLA-B8; I think we are looking for another marker gene that would be more closely associated with the disease. The way we are doing this is by testing populations of different ethnic backgrounds. If we find differing genetic markers—say in the Irish or German coeliacs—we know we are not really at the marker gene yet. If we don't find differences any more, then we are at the point where we are either directly next to it, or we have found it. We are looking for the gene that would be highly associated and may be 100% associated with the disease in all populations tested. The second question was about the low incidence of HLA-B7 and we have said before that we feel that the decrease for B7 is disproportionate. We have to expect some decrease because if some alleles are high then other alleles must be low, and the decrease must be spread out over all the alleles according to their frequencies. The decrease in incidence of B7 is greater than one would expect, so that indicated to us that there must be a protective role for B7 and perhaps BW2. The same claim has been made independently for the diabetics by Danish colleagues who found a decrease in B7 amongst their diabetic patients, and we have also found likewise. This is a concept that should be followed up. It is very difficult to assess this disproportionate decrease. Your third question. I don't think that we will come up with one single gene that determines the susceptibility. We are quite sure that there must be different genes. For one thing there must be something that is related to sex. Sex is determined genetically or course, and may act by modulating hormonal levels which then interact with environmental factors. So sex is certainly one genetic factor that we can include and other genetic factors are under discussion as Dr Peña has said, so I would very much hesitate to come up with one

	single gene which covers all susceptibilities. That is really very highly unlikely.
Douglas	A brief question for Dr Peña. In the family studies you show, I presume that filled-in circles were the coeliac and the white symbols were the non-coeliacs. How did you know that? Did you biopsy everybody?
Peña	No, unfortunately we have not biopsied everybody. We have two families only that have had complete biopsy studies.
Douglas	How do you know that the white circles don't have coeliac disease?
Peña	I agree with you. I think we have to do biopsies first. Nevertheless, if you study the segregation analysis of all the families that have been published up till now, and we have made a study of three hundred and ten families that have been published in the literature you cannot expect that all of the children are going to have the disease. I think that at this stage, it is reasonable to accept that the whites in this context are normal but I take your criticism.
Albert	You claim that the B-cell antigens Bi, BJi and the third one I have forgotten are really reflecting genes. Do you have any family studies that would show the distribution in the population, studies that would show the inheritance, studies that would show the absence of recessive patterns for this antigen, in other words families where you have positive children but negative parents, and do you have any evidence for the fact that the serum might be multispecific, and do you have any evidence that the serum might be detecting some antigen that is stuck on to the cell, which is not an inherited character?
Peña	There are several questions here. First of all, many mothers have been tested and so far we have found only four mothers that react with B-cells of coeliac patients. We know these mothers are all DW3-positive, so it is very unlikely that they are producing antibodies linked to the HLA system. The second point, in one family we showed that three children were positive, both parents positive, and one child was negative. If you call the capital A the dominant gene and the little b the recessive, and if both parents are heterozygotes, then according to Mendel a quarter do not have this antigen, so that family supports this. This should be done in the normal population, but because this test is time-consuming and very difficult we don't have the evidence yet.
Kasarda	Dr Peña, when you speak of a recessive gene for one of these antigens, it makes me wonder if we think of a gene as expressing a protein, so it is possible that we could look at a recessive characteristic as the absence of a protein antigen as opposed to the present where you require two doses. Just turn it around and look at the characteristics perhaps representing absence rather than the presence.
Strober	I agree with that, but I don't think that this is the only possibility because it may depend on the density of receptors on the cell surface. If these specificities are coding for receptor sites on the surface of either lymphoid cells or epithelial cells, then the density of receptor may determine whether or not disease develops, so I think it is a possibility but it is not the only possibility. I would like to take this opportunity to ask a question. The point was made strongly by Dr Albert that it is not likely that the HLA-B8 itself is

important to this disease and I would tend to agree with that, but there is one piece of data that Dr Falchuk and I have developed over the past several years, which tends to go against that point. We have no way of explaining this data except by saying that there is some direct contribution of HLA-B8 itself. I refer to the fact that there is a difference in the organ culture susceptibility to gliadin damage between HLA-B8 positive and HLA-B8 negative patients, and furthermore this difference crosses DW3 lines; hence it would seem that HLA-B8 is playing some role. So I would not at this point want to rule out completely that HLA-B8 doesn't play some direct role in the causation of the disease.

14

HLA antigens in coeliac disease and a control population in the West of Ireland

FIONA M. STEVENS, B. EGAN-MITCHELL, D. W. WATT, S. H.
BAKER, B. McNICHOLL and C. F. McCARTHY

In 1973, we reported a high prevalence of coeliac disease in the West of Ireland[1], and our recent results confirm this prevalence (Figure 14.1).

The frequency of HLA-B8 antigen in patients with coeliac disease shows marked geographic variability, being lower in Central Europe (56% Germany/Austria[2]) than in North America (75% USA[3]) or Northern Europe (80% England[4] and 90% Finland[5]).

It has been suggested that HLA-B8 negative coeliac patients have a higher frequency of HLA-B12 antigen than expected[6]. A decreased frequency of HLA-B7 antigen has been noted in coeliac patients[2], perhaps implying some protection imparted by the presence of this antigen.

A study of the HLA-A and B locus antigens has been undertaken in coeliac patients, their relatives and an indigenous control population in the West of Ireland, to determine if the coeliac patients are similar to those in Northern Europe and if a high frequency of HLA-B8 exists in the community contributing to the prevalence of coeliac disease.

PATIENTS AND METHODS

One hundred and seventeen unrelated coeliac patients were studied. In 64 patients (36 female and 28 male) symptoms indicative of coeliac disease occurred before the age of 12 years ('childhood coeliac disease', CCD) and in 53 patients (43 female and 10 male) characteristic symptoms developed after the age of 12 years ('adult coeliac disease', ACD).

Thirty-six first degree relatives of coeliac patients have been studied.

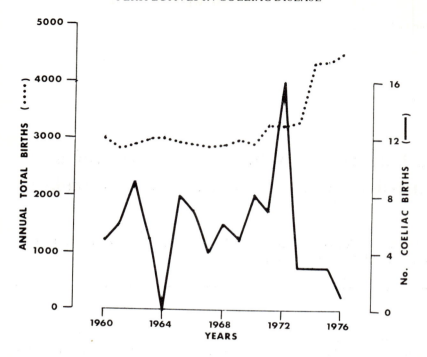

Figure 14.1 Incidence of childhood coeliac disease in County Galway (1960–1976)

All had a normal small intestinal biopsy. There were 30 parents and six children of coeliac patients.

One hundred and five unrelated healthy adults with no known coeliac relative were studied. All controls were at least third generation West of Ireland stock. All had a normal haemoglobin (>11 g/dl) and a normal serum iron (>10 μmol/l). There were 50 females and 55 males, with a mean age of 28.6 years and a range of 19–64 years.

HLA-A and B locus antigens were tested for by the two-stage micro-lymphocytotoxicity test[7]. Fifteen A locus specificities and 16 B locus specificities were sought.

In the results, A9 covers the specificities A9, AW23 and AW24, and A11 encompasses A11, AW25 and AW26. Results are statistically analysed by the chi-square (x^2) test. (Although x^2 : 3.841–10 yield $p<0.005$, the p value is no longer significant after the application of the Bonferroni correction for inequality[8]. Thus, only x^2 >10 are considered statistically significant).

Table 14.1 HLA antigens in 117 unrelated coeliac patients

Antigen	Coeliacs Onset < 12 years n = 64 No. positive	Coeliacs Onset >12 years n= 53 No. positive
A1	35	37
A2	31	16
A3	14	10
A9	5	13
A10	5	6
A11	9	6
A29	4	2
AW31	2	2
AW32	3	3
B5	6	1
B7	12	13
B8	47	42
B12	17	20
B14	5	6
B18	2	4
B27	4	2
BW15	1	1
BW16	2	1
BW17	2	1
BW21	1	1
BW35	6	0
BW37	1	0
BW40	8	2

RESULTS

The frequency of the HLA-A and B locus antigens in 64 CCD patients and 53 ACD patients is shown in Table 14.1. Differences in frequency of HLA antigens A1, A2, A9, BW35 and BW40 were noted, but none of the differences reach statistical significance. The frequency of haplotypes not having HLA-B8 or B12 or HLA-A1 or B8 or B12 is shown in Table 14.2 (x^2 <3.841, p = NS).

As there is no statistically significant difference between the two groups of coeliac patients, for the rest of the study all the coeliac patients are considered as a single group.

The frequency of HLA-A and B locus antigens in 117 unrelated coeliac patients and 36 first-degree relatives with normal biopsies is shown in Table 14.3. The pattern of HLA antigens is similar in the two groups, apart from an increased incidence of HLA-A11 and HLA-BW15

Table 14.2   HLA haplotype in 117 unrelated coeliac patients

Antigens	Coeliacs onset <12 years n = 64	Coeliacs onset >12 years n = 53
	Number	Number
Not having B8 or B12	12	6
Not having A1 or B8 or B12	10	2

Table 14.3   HLA antigens in coeliacs and their relatives

Antigen	Coeliacs n = 117	Relatives n = 36
	No. positive	No. positive
A1	72	18
A2	47	19
A3	24	6
A9	18	6
A10	11	4
A11	15	8
A28	0	1
A29	6	0
AW31	4	2
AW32	6	0
B5	7	3
B7	25	7
B8	89	25
B12	37	8
B13	0	1
B14	11	3
B18	6	0
B27	6	3
BW15	2	5
BW16	3	2
BW17	3	1
BW21	2	2
BW35	6	3
BW37	1	0
BW40	10	2

Table 14.4 HLA A antigens in coeliacs and controls

Antigen	Coeliacs n = 117 No. positive	Controls n = 105 No. positive
A1	72	51
A2	47	41
A3	24	17
A9	18	18
A10	11	19
A11	15	22
A28	0	5
A29	6	2
AW30	0	4
AW31	4	0
AW32	6	5
B5	7	5
B7	25	36
B8	89	45
B12	37	31
B13	0	1
B14	11	14
B18	6	7
B27	6	9
BW15	2	5
BW16	3	7
BW17	3	6
BW21	2	2
BW22	0	2
BW35	6	8
BW37	1	0
BW40	10	7

Table 14.5 HLA haplotypes in coeliacs, relatives and controls

Antigens	Coeliacs n = 117 No. positive	Relatives n = 36 No. positive	Controls n = 105 No. positive
A1 + B8	63	14	37
B8 + B12	27	4	10
A1 + B8 + B12	19	1	7

in relatives ($x^2 < 3.841$, p=NS). No increase in HLA-B7 was noted in coeliac relatives.

The frequency of HLA-A and B locus antigens in 117 coeliac patients and 105 unrelated healthy controls is shown in Table 14.4. No statistically significant differences were noted in A locus antigen frequencies, although HLA-A10, A11 and A28 were found more commonly and HLA-A29 less commonly in controls. HLA-B7 occurs more frequently in controls (34.3%) than in coeliac patients (21.4%), (x^2=4.009, p=NS). HLA-B8 was found in 76% of coeliac patients and 43% of controls. The difference is statistically highly significant, (x^2=24.14, p<0.00062).

The frequency of various combinations of HLA antigens in 117 coeliac patients, 36 relatives and 105 controls is shown in Table 14.5. No significant differences were found between coeliacs and relatives or relatives and controls. HLA-AI and B8 occur together in 53.8% of coeliacs and 35.2% of controls (x^2=7.007, p=NS). The difference in frequency of HLA-B8 and B12 (x^2=6.37) and HLA-A1, B8 and B12 (x^2=4.022) fails to reach statistical significance.

In HLA-B8 negative patients HLA-B12 was found in 10 (8.5%) whereas HLA-B12 without B8 was found in 21 (20%) of controls (x^2=4.446). Only 18 (15.4%) of coeliac patients had neither HLA-B8 nor B12 compared with 39 (37%) of controls (x^2=12.61, p=0.0213).

The frequency of HLA-A and B locus antigens in relatives with normal biopsies would be expected to fall between those of the coeliac patients and controls. This was found with most of the antigens except HLA-A2, AW31, BW15 and BW21.

DISCUSSION

The incidence of HLA-B8 in controls in this study is higher than that reported elsewhere [2-4,9]. The frequency of HLA-B8 in coeliac patients in the West of Ireland is similar to that in England[4] and the USA[3].

The comparison of coeliacs with their relatives with normal biopsies revealed a higher frequency of HLA-BW15 in relatives than in coeliacs. It is possible that the presence of HLA-BW15 imparts some protection against developing coeliac disease. A protective role had been ascribed to a gene associated with HLA-B7[2]. Our control data would support this theory, but in the family data, the frequency of HLA-B7 in coeliacs and their normal relatives is almost identical.

When the frequency of the HLA antigens is compared in childhood and adult coeliac disease, no statistically significant differences were found. No evidence has been found to support the hypothesis of two subpopulations in coeliac disease.

The high frequency of HLA-B8 in the indigenous population in the West of Ireland helps explain the high prevalence of coeliac disease in the community. When the results of HLA-DRW3 and B lymphocyte surface antigen are available, it may be that these antigens will also be particularly common in the West of Ireland.

Acknowledgements

We wish to acknowledge the support of the Wellcome Trust, the Medical Research Council of Ireland and the Western Health Board, and the supply of antisera by N.I.H.

References

1. Mylotte, M., Egan-Mitchell, B., McCarthy, C. F. and McNicholl, B. (1973). Incidence of coeliac disease in the West of Ireland. *Br. Med. J.*, **i,** 703
2. Harms, K., Granditsch, G., Rossipal, E., Ludwig, H., Polymenidis, Z., Scholz, S., Wank, R. and Albert, E. D. (1974). HL-A in patients with coeliac disease and their relatives. In W. Th. J. M. Hekkens and A. S. Peña (eds.) *Coeliac Disease. Proceedings of the Second International Coeliac Symposium* pp. 215–236, (Leiden: Stenfert Kroese)
3. Falchuk, Z. M., Rogentine, G. N. and Strober, W. (1972). Predominance of histocompatibility HL-A 8 in patients with gluten-sensitive enteropathy. *J. Clin. Invest.*, **51,** 1602
4. Stokes, P. L., Asquith, P., Holmes, G. K. T., Mackintosh, P. and Cooke, W. T. (1972). Histocompatibility antigens associated with adult coeliac disease. *Lancet*, **ii,** 162
5. Solheim, B. G., Baklien, K. and Er, J. (1974). Association of coeliac disease with HL-A antigens and MLC-antigens. In: W. Th. J. M. Hekkens and A. S. Peña (eds). *Coeliac Disease. Proceedings of the Second International Coeliac Symposium*. p. 232 (Leiden: Stenfert Kroese)
6. Scott, B. B., Losowsky, M. S. and Rajah, S. M. (1974). HL-A8 and HL-A12 in coeliac disease. *Lancet*, **ii,** 171
7. Terasaki, P. I. and McCellelland, J. D. (1964). Microdroplet assay of human serum cytotoxins. *Nature (London.)*, **204,** 298
8. Miller, R. G. (1966). *Simultaneous Statistical Inference*. p. 8 (New York: McGraw Hill)
9. Murtagh, T. J., Reen, D. J. and Greally, J. (1976). HL-A A1 and B8 in coeliac disease. Presented at the *First International Symposium on HLA and Disease*. June 23–25, Paris, France

Discussion of chapter 14

Histocompatibility antigen involvement in coeliac disease population from the East of Ireland

	Coeliac Disease—(50)		Controls—(175)		
HLA-A1	74%		49%		$p<0.001$
HLA-B8	70%		33.1%		$p<0.001$
HLA-B8					
England	88%	(49)	25.9%	(80)	
Scotland	—		30.7%	(140)	
Germany	66%	(53)	19%	(442)	
France	—		11%	(127)	
Japan	—		0%	(129)	
Italy			13.5	(104)	

Total numbers of patients in brackets ( )

Weir
: The table gives the results of a similar survey which we did with Dr Greally in the East of Ireland as opposed to the West. There is a high incidence of HLA-8 in the coeliac population. On the other hand our incidence of HLA-8 in the controls is 33.1% against the incidence in the West of Ireland which was 47%. This incidence of 33% is higher than most other reports but probably not significantly so. It suggests that the East of Ireland is a mixture of English and Irish and in the West there is a pure Celtic culture.

Rey
: I think that your data are very interesting because you have shown that there is practically no difference between your coeliacs and non-coeliac relatives and the frequency of HLA-B8, and I think this is a strong indication that there is only a correlation between HLA and coeliac disease, which is a reflection of a linkage disequilibrium, and is not a direct causal relationship.

Stevens
: The actual figures are that 76% of all our coeliacs are B8 positive and 64.5% of the 48 relatives. This is not statistically significant.

Albert
: I would like to ask a question about inbreeding in the families that you have studied. You might have many parents who are HLA-B8 homozygous and then all the children are positive for B8 and for that reason this difference might turn out to be smaller than one would expect.

Stevens
: There is no evidence in recent generations that there is inbreeding. In the population of the West of Ireland over many thousand years, yes, but not in recent times.

144

McNicholl   The evidence that we have does not tend to support the suggestion of inbreeding in the West of Ireland. Our incidence of cystic fibrosis is much the same as throughout the remainder of Europe, and in fact the incidence of pyloric stenosis in infancy was slightly lower. Both conditions are recessively inherited and might be expected to have a high incidence if there was a lot of inbreeding.

Cluysenaer   I'd like to ask what is the use of looking for a genetic marker if you have proven discordance in monozygotic twins. A second point is, is it not nicer to look for environmental factors especially in this region (i.e. Galway). What happened in 1964 and what happened in 1971 to account for the variation in incidence? And that brings me to a third point, perhaps if there are environmental factors it was not wise to organize a coeliac symposium here!

Stevens   I don't know what happened in 1964. At the last meeting Dr Wauters was said to have no coeliacs born in that year in Utrecht, but he tells me now that he does have some who were born in 1964. Really we should be seeing what happened in 1972 when such a large number were born.

15

Coeliac disease. A family study in The Netherlands

P. C. M. ROSEKRANS, A. S. PEÑA, W. Th. J. M. HEKKENS,
R. R. P. de VRIES and A. J. Ch. HAEX

INCIDENCE OF COELIAC DISEASE AMONGST RELATIVES

There is an increased incidence of coeliac disease amongst first-degree relatives of patients with that condition[1]. Studies based on jejunal biopsy data show an incidence which varies between 5.5 and 18.3%.

Table 15.1 Reports of coeliac disease in first-degree relatives diagnosed by jejunal biopsy

Year	Authors and ref.	No. biopsied	No. CD	Disease %
1965	MacDonald et al.[2]	62	7	11.2
1971	Robinson et al.[3]	29	3	10.3
1972	Mylotte et al.[4]	87	9	10.3
1972	Shipman et al.[5]	131	14	10.6
1974	Rolles et al.[6]	72	4	5.5
1974	Asquith et al.[7]	120	22	18.3
1974	McCarthy et al.[8]	133	16	12
	Total	634	75	11.8

We studied 19 unrelated families of propositi with biopsy-proven coeliac disease. Nine additional coeliacs were detected in the 42 first-degree relatives who had intestinal biopsies done. All biopsies showed the typical mucosal changes and the enzyme levels in the mucosa were low. On a gluten-free diet all the new coeliac patients showed a remarkable improvement. The incidence of coeliac disease in first-degree relatives who had a biopsy in our families was 21.4%. The total number of first-degree relatives in these 19 families was 70 (Table 15.2).

In some cases, a selection was made of family members in which an intestinal biopsy was done. More individuals with suboptimal health were biopsied. The HLA typing, the gliadin antibody titre and the serum folic acid values were also sometimes a reason for jejunal biopsy. Whether we could find more coeliacs if we biopsied all 70 family members is speculative.

Table 15.2 Patients with coeliac disease detected in 19 families

9 C.D. in 42 biopsied first-degree relatives	= 21.4%
9 C.D. in total 70 first-degree relatives	= 12.8%

The total incidence is probably between 12.8% and 21.4%. The pedigrees of the five families in which we found new coeliac patients are shown in Figure 15.1.

RELATION BETWEEN COELIAC DISEASE AND HLA ANTIGENS

Studies on histocompatibility antigens in coeliac disease in The Netherlands[9,10] reported the same high incidence of HLA-B8 as in other studies[11]. Falchuk et al.[12] found 88% HLA-B8 in coeliac patients and van Hooff et al.[15] found 83% HLA-B8.

Table 15.3 Incidence of HLA-B8 in coeliac disease

Year	Author	No. of patients	B8 positive patients	%
1972	Falchuk et al. [12]	24	21	88%
1972	Stokes et al. [11]	117	94	80%
1973	McNeish et al. [13]	30	23	77%
1974	Harms et al. [14]	143	80	56%
1974	van Hooff et al. [15]	40	33	83%
1974	Solheim et al.[16]	28	21	75%

The incidence of the B8 antigen in the general population is approximately 20%.

From the HLA phenotypes of the family members we deduced the haplotypes (genotypes) of the 28 coeliac patients in the 19 families. Three patients were non-B8 (10.7%), whereas 89.3% of the coeliac patients had a HLA-B8 antigen (Table 15.4).

More interesting is the HLA-B8 antigen frequency in the family group who had a biopsy-proven coeliac disease. Sixty-two individuals had a biopsy, of whom 28 had coeliac disease (45%). Of the individuals with-

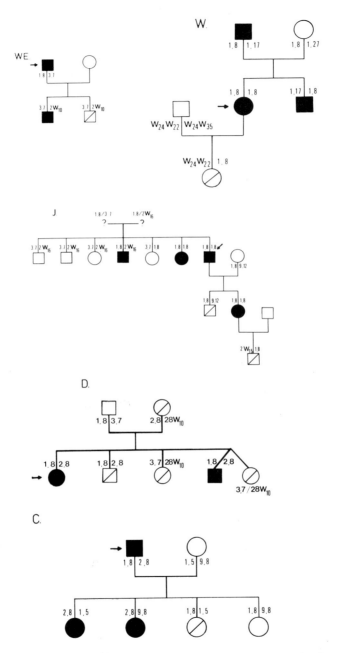

Figure 15.1   Key: ■ ● = coeliac disease; ⊠ ⊘ = normal biopsy; □ ○ = no biopsy done. Pedigrees of the five families with new coeliac patients. HLA typing is described.

Table 15.4   Incidence of HLA-B8 in coeliac patients

	No. of patients	B8 positive patients	%
Dutch family study	28	25	89

out B8 only 3 of the 15 biopsied persons had coeliac disease (20%). Of the individuals who were heterozygous B8, 14 out of the 34 had coeliac disease (41%). Of the 13 homozygous B8 biopsied individuals, all but two had coeliac disease (85%).

Table 15.5   Relation between biopsy proven coeliac disease and HLA-B8

	Non-B8	B8/- (heterozygous)	B8/B8 (homozygous)	Total number of biopsies
Coeliac disease	3	14	11	28
No coeliac disease	12	20	2	34
Total number	15	34	13	62
% Coeliac disease	20%	41%	85%	45%

$$p<0.001$$

The finding that only some of the HLA-B8 positive relatives have coeliac disease (25 out of 47) indicates that it is not only a HLA-linked gene which predisposes for this condition. The locus predisposing for coeliac disease is in linkage disequilibrium with the histocompatibility antigen HLA-B8 and even more with the MLC determinant DW3[10]. It appears that the HLA-linked gene needs only to be present in a single dose to produce coeliac disease. However, our finding that homozygous B8 relatives have a significantly higher risk of having coeliac disease suggests a gene dose effect, possibly involving complementation of the immune response gene, situated on loci closely linked to HLA-B and in linkage disequilibrium with B8.

SERUM FOLATE IN COELIAC PATIENTS AND IN RELATIVES

Folate deficiency is a relatively common phenomenon in coeliac disease[17]. We measured the serum folate concentration in most of the untreated coeliac patients (although in 4 cases we had no pretreatment values). In less than 50% we found a decreased serum folate in the group of patients.

All the 21 relatives who had no coeliac disease had a normal folic acid in serum (Table 15.6). We looked for differences in serum folate in relation to the HLA-B8 genotype in the coeliac patients. Most of the

Table 15.6   Serum folate in biopsied family
members

	Normal folic acid	Low folic acid
Coeliac disease	13	11
No coeliac disease	21	0

homozygous HLA-B8 group had a low serum folate concentration, but because of the small number it is impossible to draw any conclusion.

GLIADIN ANTIBODIES

Since 1975 we have been able to determine the level of gliadin antibodies with the ELISA technique[18,19]. In most untreated coeliac patients the serum antigliadin antibody is elevated. During a gluten-free diet the antibody titre decreases. One of our index patients showed this fall in antibody very well (Figure 15.2).

Because of this effect it was only possible to determine the gliadin antibody titre in a pretreatment condition in 9 of the 28 coeliac patients. These patients used no diet restriction. The gliadin antibodies were high in 7 of the 9 patients (mean: 0.91 E. ± SD 0.39)

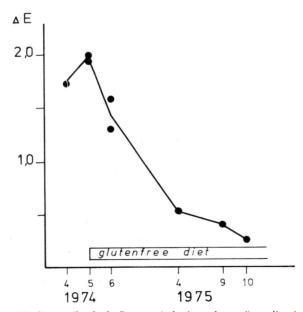

Figure 15.2   Gliadin antibody before and during gluten-free diet in a patient with coeliac disease and dermatitis herpetiformis

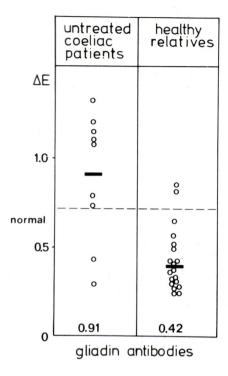

Figure 15.3

We measured the gliadin antibody in 19 biopsy-proven normal family members (mean 0.42 E.± SD 0.19). Two of them had an abnormally high amount of gliadin antibody (0.88 E., 0.83 E.).

CONCLUSIONS

We found in 19 unrelated families with propositi with coeliac disease the same segregation pattern of the disease as has been found in other parts of the world. The incidence of the new cases with coeliac disease is higher than reported elsewhere, possibly due to selection. The incidence of HLA-B8 antigen in the patients with coeliac disease in these families is 89%. The homozygous HLA-B8 individuals in these families have a significantly higher risk of having coeliac disease than the HLA non-B8 or heterozygous HLA-B8 individuals.

References

1. Stokes, P. L., Asquith, P. and Cooke, W. T. (1973). Genetics in coeliac disease. *Clin Gastroenterol.*, **II, No. 3**, pp. 547–556 (London: W. B. Saunders and Co. Ltd.)

2. MacDonald, W. C., Dobbins, W. O. and Rubin, C. E. (1965). Studies of the familial nature of coeliac sprue using biopsy of the small intestine. *N. Engl. J. Med.*, **272**, 448

3. Robinson, D. C., Watson, A. J., Wyatt, E. H., Marks, J. H. and Robberts, D. F. (1971). Incidence of small intestinal mucosal abnormalities and of clinical coeliac disease in the relatives of children with coeliac disease. *Gut*, **12**, 789

4. Mylotte, M. J., Egan-Mitchell, B., Fottrell, P. F., McNicholl, B. and McCarthy, C. F. (1973). Familial coeliac disease. *Quart. J. Med.*, **41**, 527

5. Shipman, R. T., Williams, A. L., Kay, R. and Townley, R. R. W. (1973). A family study of coeliac disease. *Aust. N.Z. J. Med.*, **1975**, 250

6. Rolles, C. J., Kyaw-Myint, T. O. and Sin, W. K. (1974). Family study of coeliac disease. In: *Coeliac Disease*, Hekkens, W. Th. J. M. and Peña, A. S. (eds.) pp. 320–321. (Leiden: Stenfert Kroese)

7. Asquith, P. (1974). Family study in coeliac disease. In: *Coeliac Disease*, Hekkens, W. Th. J. M. and Peña, A. S. (eds.) pp. 322–325. (Leiden: Stenfert Kroese)

8. McCarthy, C. F., Mylotte, M., Stevens, F., Egan-Mitchell, B., Fortrell, P. F. and McNicholl, B. (1974). Family studies on coeliac disease in Ireland. In: *Coeliac Disease*, Hekkens, W. Th. J. M. and Peña, A. S. (eds.) pp. 311–319 (Leiden: Stenfert Kroese)

9. van Rood, J. J., van Hooff, J. P. and Keuning, J. J. (1975). Disease predisposition immune responsiveness and the fine structure of the HL-A supergene. *Transplant. Rev.*, **22**, 75

10. Keuning, J. J., Peña, A. S., van Leeuwen, A. and van Rood, J. J. (1976). HLA-DW3 associated with coeliac disease. *Lancet*, **i**, 506

11. Stokes, P. L., Asquith, P., Holmes, G. T. K., Mackintosh, P. and Cooke, W. T. (1972). Histocompatibility antigens associated with adult coeliac disease. *Lancet*, **ii**, 162

12. Falchuk, Z. M., Rogentine, G. M. and Strober, W. (1972). Predominance of histocompatibility antigen HL-A8 in patients with gluten-sensitive enteropathy. *J. Clin. Invest.*, **15**, 1602

13. McNeish, A. S., Nelson, R. and Mackintosh, P. (1973). HLA 1 and 8 in childhood coeliac disease. *Lancet*, **i**, 668

14. Harms, K., Granditsch, G., Rossipal, E., Ludwig, M., Polymenidis, Z., Scholtz, S. and Albert, E. D. (1974). HLA in patients with coeliac disease and their families. In: *Coeliac Disease*, Hekkens, W. Th. J. M. and Peña, A. S. (eds.) pp. 215–226 (Leiden: Stenfert Kroese)

15. van Hooff, J. P., Peña, A. S., Keuning, J. J., Termijtelen, A., Hekkens, W. Th. J. M., Haex, A. J. Ch. and van Rood, J. J. (1974). SD and LD determinants of the HLA complex in coeliac disease. In: *Coeliac Disease*, Hekkens, W. Th. J. M. and Peña, A. S. (eds.) pp. 233–239 (Leiden: Stenfert Kroese)

16. Solheim, B. G., Baklien, K. and Ek, J. (1974). Association of coeliac disease with HL-A antigens and HLC-antigens. In: *Coeliac Disease*, Hekkens, W. Th. J. M. and Peña, A. S. (eds.) p. 232 (Leiden: Stenfert Kroese)

17. Cluysenaar, O. J. J. (1977). Thesis, Nijmegen University

18. Hekkens, W. Th. J. M. The Toxicity of Gliadin, Review. (In preparation)

19. Editorial. (1976). Elisa: a replacement for radioimmunoassay? *Lancet*, **ii**, 406

Discussion of chapter 15

Jones — Could I ask you about your range for the serum folate because a very high percentage of your coeliac patients had normal folic acid levels.

Rosekrans — The normal level for folic acid in the serum is above 4 mmol/ml so that the abnormal ones had levels below four.

Albert — I would like to ask a statistical question on a critical point: you have said that the B8 homozygotes have a higher relative risk than the B8 heterozygotes, and that this difference is statistically significant. Now, it is very difficult to establish the significance of a difference in association. If you test the relative risk for homozygotes and heterozygotes one may be higher than the other one, but even if the p value for a high relative risk is highly significant it doesn't tell you that the difference between the two elevated relative risks is also significant. It seems with the number of families you have tested that it is unlikely to come up with a statistically significant difference in association.

Rosekrans — The Chi-squared of the three groups is 12 and the measured p is smaller than 0.001. If you look at the three groups separately there is a significant difference between these groups.

Peña — We agree with the comments of Dr Albert. I think what is very interesting here is also in the story of Fiona Stevens, that there are certain populations where this possibly dominant HLA gene is closely linked to B8, and in the Dutch population and in this population that is so, whereas in your part of the world this is not so. I don't think we can draw many conclusions, and in fact we have not calculated relative risk for this data, just because of these criticisms.

Booth — Could I ask a general question of all who have been working on HLA and particularly Dr Albert; are there any examples of linkages of this sort which are associated with specific enzyme defects?

Albert — To my knowledge, there are none. Enzyme deficiencies should be recessive diseases, and this we haven't found. The only disease where there is some indication for recessivity is haemochromatosis, where we do find increased numbers of homozygotes and so forth, but we don't know whether that is an enzyme deficiency. It may very well be, but that would be the only example.

Falchuk — We have recently finished a family study which we are reporting in the Poster session; we were interested in the heterozygotes question as well. Using our techniques of organ culture in a large group of individuals who were heterozygotes, that is, parents and siblings of patients, there is no *in vitro* sensitivity to gluten.

16

Peripheral blood lymphocyte markers in coeliac disease with regard to disease specificity

M. R. HAENEY, H. M. CHAPEL and P. ASQUITH

INTRODUCTION

There is now considerable data suggesting that immunological mechanisms contribute to the pathogenesis of coeliac disease and it has been postulated that the intestinal villous atrophy may be mediated by a local antigen–antibody reaction[1], by activated T-cells[2,3] or by antibody-dependent K-cell mediated cytotoxicity[4].

Indirect evidence for the involvement of these reactions may be provided by the study of lymphocyte subpopulations. A variety of membrane markers have been used for the categorization of lymphocytes into T- or B-cells. Estimations of the concentrations of peripheral blood T-lymphocytes have suggested a reduction in the numbers of circulating T-cells in untreated, but not treated, cases of coeliac disease[5].

The object of studying markers is to define lymphocytes with different functions. We have studied several markers simultaneously; these include markers for B-lymphocytes, T-lymphocytes and a third major population.

The purpose of this investigation was to quantitate the proportional and absolute numbers of these lymphocyte subpopulations in untreated coeliacs using established rosetting techniques to assess the effect of a gluten-free diet on these subpopulations, and to relate any changes in surface markers to the inferred functional activity of that cell population in coeliac disease, particularly with regard to the pathogenesis of the condition.

Table 16.1   Final diagnosis in cases of untreated gastrointestinal disease

Diagnosis	Number of patients
Chronic pancreatitis	3
Contaminated bowel syndrome	3
Tropical sprue	3
Post-infective malabsorption	2
Crohn's disease	3
Ulcerative colitis	2
Tuberculous enteritis	2
Whipple's disease	1
Intestinal lymphangiectasia	1
Total	20

METHODS

Patients studied

Seventy-one subjects, classified into four diagnostic groups, were studied. For the purpose of the study, coeliac disease has been defined as a condition in which there is an abnormal jejunal mucosa with loss of villi, which improves morphologically after treatment with a gluten-free diet.

Group 1 consisted of 15 patients with untreated coeliac disease ingesting a normal diet (coeliac-N.D.). Group 2 was composed of 15 coeliac patients treated with a gluten-free diet for over one year (coeliac-G.F.D.). Group 3 comprised 20 patients with a variety of untreated gastrointestinal conditions (Table 16.1). Group 4 included 21 healthy staff controls of comparable age- and sex-distribution. Routine white cell counts and differentials were done on all subjects.

Lymphocyte separation

Lymphocytes were purified from heparinized (preservative-free heparin, 20 units/ml blood) blood by means of gelatin sedimentation[6], followed by Ficoll–Triosil density gradient centrifugation[7]. A minimum lymphocyte yield of 65% was required before results were regarded as representative. Lymphocytes were washed three times in Hepes-buffered R.P.M.I. 1640 medium (25 mM Hepes salts) and the cell concentration adjusted to 2×10^6/ml after first assessing cell viability by exclusion of trypan blue dye (0.1% in P.B.S.). In all cases, lymphocyte viability exceeded 85%. The resulting cell suspensions contained lymphocytes (88–100%) with some monocyte (0–12%) contamination. Monocytes in the final cell suspension were identified by the ingestion of neutral red (0.1% in sterile distilled water).

Rosetting techniques

E rosettes: Fresh defibrinated sheep red blood cells (E)[8] were diluted to give 330×10^6 red cells per ml and washed once in RPMI-H.

Mouse rosettes: Fresh mouse red cells (M)[9] were diluted to a concentration of 200×10^6 per ml and washed once in RPMI-H.

C3 rosettes: A suspension of dead, fixed yeasts was prepared[10] and washed three times in complement fixation test buffer (C.F.T.). Yeasts (2×10^8) were incubated by continuous rotation with 1 ml of diluted (1:5) human serum at 37 °C for 30 min[11] in order to activate complement (C3). Complement-coated yeasts were washed three times in C.F.T. and adjusted to 1×10^8 per ml.

Fc Hu IgG/Fc Rabbit IgG rosettes: Fresh human rhesus-positive red cells (2.5% suspension) and chicken red cells (1% suspension) were washed and sensitized with heat-inactivated (56 °C, 30 min) human anti-rhesus serum and hyperimmune, heat-inactivated rabbit anti-chicken red cell serum respectively. After incubation at 37 °C for 30 min with continuous rotation, the red cells were washed three times.

Mixed (E+C3+, E+Fc+) rosettes and null (E−C3−, E−Fc−) cells: Combinations of these tests, using sheep red cells with C3 coated yeast[11–13] and sheep red cells with IgG coated human erythrocytes[14,15] were also set up in order to detect cells showing simultaneous binding of E and C3 or of E and Fc and to detect cells failing to bind any of these markers (null cells).

For each marker, equal volumes (0.1 ml) of the lymphocyte suspension and the appropriate indicator cells were then mixed, centrifuged at 200 g for 5 min and left as a pellet overnight at 4 °C. Prior to resuspension one drop of heat-inactivated fetal calf serum was added to each tube to stabilize rosettes. In addition, one drop of trypan blue dye (0.5% in P.B.S.) was added to check lymphocyte viability and to stain the yeasts. Tubes were capped and cells resuspended by gentle continuous rotation at 10 r.p.m. for two minutes. Rosettes were counted in a Fuchs–Rosenthal haemocytometer; 200 lymphocytes were counted and those fixing three or more indicator cells were scored as rosetting cells. The numbers of rosette-forming lymphocytes were expressed both as a percentage of the total lymphocyte population and as absolute number × 10^9/l of blood.

RESULTS

Peripheral blood lymphocyte counts

Figure 16.1 shows lymphocyte counts in the subject groups studied. Although mean counts tended to be lower in the three patient groups compared with healthy controls, no significant differences were found between any of the groups.

Rosetting cells

In untreated coeliacs, the percentages of lymphocytes binding E (Figure 16.2), and E plus C3 (combined test) Figure 16.2) were reduced compared with treated coeliacs and healthy controls. The proportions of lymphocytes failing to bind either E or C3 (E–C3–) and E or Fc (E–Fc–) in the mixed tests, i.e. 'null' cells (Figure 16.3), were increased in coeliacs on a normal diet in comparison with coeliacs ingesting a gluten-free diet and healthy controls. In contrast, the percentages of lymphocytes binding mouse red cells or C3 (Figure 16.2) in untreated coeliacs were similar to those in treated coeliacs and controls.

Lymphocyte subpopulations in coeliacs ingesting a gluten-free diet did not differ significantly from results seen in the healthy control group, with the exception of lymphocytes bearing the Fc (IgG) receptor (Figure 16.3) which were present in greater numbers in treated coeliacs than in controls or untreated coeliacs.

Normal-diet coeliacs showed no significant differences in any of the lymphocyte markers studied when compared with the group of patients with various untreated gastrointestinal conditions.

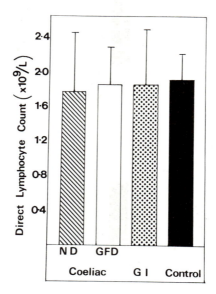

Figure 16.1 Peripheral lymphocyte counts in coeliacs ingesting a normal (ND) or a gluten-free diet (GFD), patients with untreated gastrointestinal disease (GI) and healthy controls

DISCUSSION

Cells which form rosettes with sheep erythrocytes (E rosettes) are considered to be thymus-dependent lymphocytes[8]. The finding of reduced numbers of circulating T-cells in untreated coeliac disease, with normal values in coeliacs on a gluten-free diet, has been previously reported[5]. It may reflect a generalized impairment of lymphocyte production, excessive lymphocyte loss from the gut mucosa or preferential localization of sensitized T-cells to the intestine. Overall lymphocyte production, however, appears unimpaired in that total lymphocyte counts in untreated coeliacs in this and other studies[5,16] have been normal. Indeed, B-cell numbers, as inferred from the proportions of lymphocytes with receptors for mouse red cells[9] or C3[17], are similar in untreated coeliacs, treated coeliacs and healthy controls.

An interesting finding in this study is the depletion of cells binding both sheep erythrocytes and C3 (E+C3+) in untreated coeliacs com-

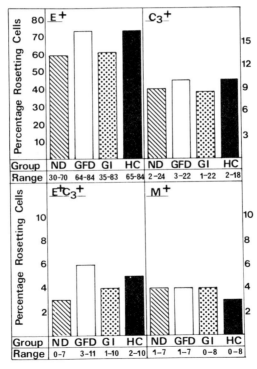

Figure 16.2 Percentages of lymphocytes forming E+, C3+, E+C3+ and M+ rosettes (see text) in coeliacs ingesting a normal (ND) or a gluten-free diet (GFD), patients with various untreated gastrointestinal disease (GI) and healthy controls (HC). Results are shown as group means. Linear scales may differ for each marker

pared with treated coeliacs and healthy controls. The low levels of such cells in normal individuals confirm earlier reports[11,13,14,18]. The combined E- and C3-binding cells may also have receptors for Fc (IgG)[11,14]. There is evidence[11] of increased numbers in untreated cases of T-cell acute lymphoblastic leukaemia and lymphosarcoma. The nature of these mixed rosetting cells, which appear to be a distinct subpopulation, is unknown; they may represent activated T-cells[11]. If this is so, their depletion in normal-diet coeliacs, and return to normal on dietary gluten restriction could imply a loss of activated T-cells from the gut, their increased sequestration in intestinal mucosa or a combination of both mechanisms. Douglas and coworkers[19] have shown an increased enteric loss of radiolabelled autologous lymphocytes in patients with untreated coeliac disease and other intestinal conditions. There is also good evidence that T-cells are sensitized to intraluminal antigens[20] and T-blasts normally migrate preferentially to the gut mucosa[21-24]; this

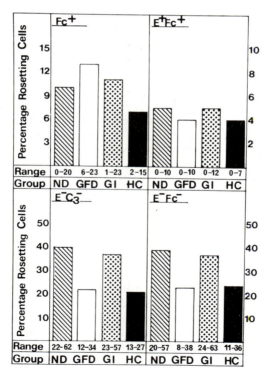

Figure 16.3 Percentages of lymphocytes forming Fc+, E+Fc+, E−C3− and E−Fc− rosettes (see text) in coeliacs ingesting a normal (ND) or a gluten-free diet (GFD), patients with various untreated gastrointestinal disease (GI) and healthy controls (HC). Results are shown as group means. Linear scales may differ between markers

may apply for intraluminal gluten in patients with coeliac disease.

With respect to the other lymphocyte subpopulations studied, there is evidence that human peripheral blood lymphocytes can be divided into two populations of immunoglobulin bearing cells. One population, B-lymphocytes, has both membrane-incorporated immunoglobulin (SmIg) and C3 receptors[25–27]. The second population lacks both SmIg and C3 receptors but possesses Fc receptors capable of binding membrane-labile cytophilic IgG found in serum[25,27]. This population, provisionally named L-lymphocytes[25], differs from T-cells[25] and is non-adherent and non-phagocytic. Unlike B-cells, only L-lymphocytes are effective killers in antibody-dependent lymphocyte cytotoxicity (K-cell test)[28]. Although L-lymphocytes may have K-cell activity, the terms are not synonymous; L-lymphocytes are defined by surface characteristics and K-cells by cytolytic activity. Patients with treated coeliac disease have greater numbers of cells bearing Fc receptors than either normal-diet coeliacs or healthy controls. Possible explanations include the return to the circulation in treated patients of increased numbers of L (?K)-cells sequestered in the small bowel in response to antigenic challenge. Alternatively, the finding may reflect an increased production of these cells to compensate for gastrointestinal loss; the increase in Fc binding cells is only seen when the gut loss is reduced by treatment.

Cells bearing neither T- nor B-cell markers are termed null cells; this study has shown that normal-diet coeliacs have increased numbers of such cells, while numbers are normal in coeliacs following gluten restriction. The nature of null cells is unknown.

The findings in untreated coeliacs are not specific for the condition, similar but less marked changes being seen in the group of subjects with various gastrointestinal diseases. This is in contrast to the reported finding[5] of normal T-cells in patients with malabsorption from non-coeliac conditions but compatible with the observation of increased enteric loss of lymphocytes in a number of unrelated intestinal disorders[19]. Because the changes in lymphocyte subpopulations in normal-diet coeliacs are non-specific, any involvement of lymphocytes in the pathogenesis of villous atrophy cannot be inferred. From the available data, it is not possible to decide whether the predominant mechanism causing this redistribution of subpopulations is a loss of lymphocytes from the gut or increased sequestration of specific sensitized cells in the intestine.

ACKNOWLEDGMENTS

The majority of this work was performed while M.R.H. was in receipt of an MRC research fellowship.

References

1. Booth, C. C., Peters, T. J. and Doe, W. F. (1977). Immunopathology of coeliac disease. In: *Immunology of the Gut. Ciba Foundation Symposium 46 (new series)* pp. 329–346. (Amsterdam: Elsevier, Excerpta Medica, North-Holland)

2. Asquith, P. (1974). Cell-mediated immunity in coeliac disease. In: *Coeliac Disease. Proceedings of the Second International Coeliac Symposium,* pp. 242–260. (Leiden: Stenfert Kroese)

3. Ferguson, A. (1974). Lymphocytes in coeliac disease. In: *Coeliac Disease. Proceedings of the Second International Coeliac Symposium,* pp. 265–276. (Leiden: Stenfert Kroese)

4. Ezeoke, A., Ferguson, J., Fakhri, O., Hekkens, W. Th. J. M. and Hobbs, J. R. (1974). Antibodies in the sera of coeliac patients which can co-opt K-cells to attack gluten-labelled targets. In: *Coeliac Disease. Proceedings of the Second International Coeliac Symposium,* pp. 176–186. (Leiden: Stenfert Kroese)

5. O'Donoghue, D. P., Lancaster-Smith, M., Laviniere, P. and Kumar, P. J. (1976). T-cell depletion in untreated adult coeliac disease. *Gut,* **17,** 328

6. Coulson, A. S. and Chambers, D. G. (1964). Separation of viable lymphocytes from human blood. *Lancet,* **i,** 468

7. Harris, R. and Ukaejifo, E. O. (1969). Rapid separation of lymphocytes for tissue-typing. *Lancet,* **ii,** 327

8. Jondal, M., Holm, G. and Wigzell, H. (1972). Surface markers on human T and B lymphocytes. I. A large population of lymphocytes forming non-immune rosettes with sheep red blood cells. *J. Exp. Med.,* **136,** 207

9. Gupta, R., Good, R. A. and Siegal, F. P. (1976). Rosette formation with mouse erythrocytes. II. A marker for human B and non-T lymphocytes. *Clin. Exp. Immunol.,* **25,** 319

10. Lachmann, P. J., Hobart, M. J. and Aston, W. P. (1973). In: D. M. Wier (ed.) Handbook of Experimental Immunology, pp. 5–8. (Oxford: Blackwell Scientific Publications)

11. Chapel, H. M. and Ling, N. R. (1977). Combined T and B lymphocyte marker test in lymphoproliferative disorders. *Br. J. Haematol.,* **35,** 367

12. Mendes, N. F., Miki, S. S. and Peixinho, Z. F. (1974). Combined detection of human T and B lymphocytes by rosette formation with sheep erythrocytes and zymosan–C3 complexes. *J. Immunol.,* **113,** 531

13. Chiao, J. W., Pantic, V. S. and Good, R. A. (1975). Human lymphocytes bearing both receptors for complement components and sheep red cells. *Clin. Immunol. Immunopathol.,* **4,** 545

14. Chia, J. W. and Good, R. A. (1976). Studies of the presence of membrane receptors for complement, IgG and the sheep erythrocyte rosetting capacity on the same human lymphocytes. *Eur. J. Immunol.,* **6,** 157

15. Sandilands, G. P., Gray, K., Cooney, A., Browning, J. D., Grant, R. M., Anderson, J. R., Dagg, J. H. and Lucie, N. (1974). Lymphocytes with T and B cells properties in a lymphoproliferative disorder. *Lancet,* **i,** 903

16. Winter, G. C. B., McCarthy, C. F., Read, A. E. and Yoffey, J. M. (1967). Development of macrophages in phytohaemagglutinin cultures of blood from patients with idiopathic steatorrhoea and with cirrhosis. *Br. J. Exp. Pathol.,* **48,** 66

17. Bianco, C., Patrick, R. and Nussenzweig, V. (1970). A population of lymphocytes bearing a membrane receptor for antigen–antibody–complement complexes. *J. Exp. Med.,* **132,** 702

18. Shevach, E., Edelson, R., Frank, M., Lutzner, M. and Green, I. (1974). A human leukaemia cell with both B and T cell surface receptors. *Proc. Natl. Acad. Sci. USA,* **71,** 863

19. Douglas, A. P., Weetman, A. P. and Haggith, J. W. (1976). The distribution and enteric loss of ^{51}Cr-labelled lymphocytes in normal subjects and in patients with coeliac disease and other disorders of the small intestine. *Digestion*, **14**, 29

20. Müller-Schoop, J. W. and Good, R. A. (1975). Functional studies of Peyer's patches: evidence for their participation in intestinal immune responses. *J. Immunol.*, **114**, 1757

21. Sprent, J. (1976). Fate of H-2 activated T lymphocytes in syngeneic hosts. I. Fate in lymphoid tissues and intestines traced with ^{3}H-thymidine, ^{125}I-deoxyuridine and ^{51} chromium. *Cell. Immunol.*, **21**, 278

22. Rose, M. L., Parrott, D. M. V. and Bruce, R. G. (1976). Migration of lymphoblasts to the small intestine. I. Effect of *Trichinella spiralis* infection on the migration of mesenteric lymphoblasts and mesenteric T lymphoblasts in syngeneic mice. *Immunology*, **31**, 723

23. Rose, M. L., Parrott, D. M. V. and Bruce, R. G. (1976). Migration of lymphoblasts to the small intestine. II. Divergent migration of mesenteric and peripheral immunoblasts to sites of inflammation in the mouse. *Cell. Immunol.*, **27**, 36

24. Ogilvie, B. M. and Parrott, D. M. V. (1977). The immunological consequences of nematode infection. In: *Immunology of the Gut. Ciba Foundation Symposium 46 (new series)* pp. 183–194. (Amsterdam: Elsevier, Excerpta Medica, North-Holland)

25. Horwitz, D. A. and Lobo, P. I. (1975). Characterization of two populations of human lymphocytes bearing easily detectable surface immunoglobulin. *J. Clin. Invest.*, **56**, 1464

26. Ehlenberger, A. G., McWilliams, M., Phillips-Quagliata, J. M. Lamm, M. E. and Nussenzweig, V. (1975). Immunoglobulin-bearing and complement-receptor lymphocytes constitute the same population in human peripheral blood. *J. Clin. Invest.*, **57**, 53

27. Lobo, P. I. and Horwitz, D. A. (1976). An appraisal of Fc receptors on human peripheral blood B and L lymphocytes. *J. Immunol.*, **117**, 939

28. Horwitz, D. A. (1976). Functional characterization of human peripheral blood L lymphocytes. *Fed. Proc.*, **35**, 473

Discussion of chapter 16

Tripp	You have included a number of patients with other gastrointestinal diseases. Were there any differences within the group, in relation to their immunological basis?
Haeney	We have not broken down the patients with the various gastro-intestinal diseases; obviously it is extremely difficult to find an adequate control for coeliac disease both in terms of immuno-logical mechanisms and in terms of villous atrophy. We have therefore just chosen these patients at random because they were equally as well as the untreated coeliacs.
Cluysenaer	It might be nice to correlate your results with enteric protein loss, because in many intestinal diseases there is an elevated protein loss. If you are unable to measure it you may look for a low serum albumin concentration, and perhaps this gives an indication about subgroups in your coeliac patients and patients with other in-testinal diseases.
Haeney	We are in fact looking at most of these patients for protein losing enteropathy, using faecal alpha-1-antitrypsin levels as a measure of this, but the results are not yet available.
Brueton	Would you comment on the changes in immunoglobulins which you see in coeliac disease in relation to your finding of a normal circulating B-cell population?
Haeney	The fact that the B-cell numbers may be normal, as determined by receptors for C3, is simply a test of marker, it is not necessarily a test of function. Therefore, one would, as I said, tentatively infer that while B-cell numbers may be normal immunoglobulin may be increased, be the same or decreased.
Strober	I might try to help the speaker answer the question by pointing out that the group of patients with very severe pan-hypogamma-globulinaemia can have normal numbers of B-cells. There is no necessary correlation between the numbers of surface positive immunoglobulin bearing cells and the actual level of immuno-globulin in serum. I think one should be cautious about calling complement receptor positive cells, activated T-cells I know of two very good studies, in which they did very careful separations of lymphocyte subpopulations and could definitely rule out the presence of complement receptors on T-cells, so I don't know what population it is that is both E rosette positive and complement receptor positive, but I don't think that they are activated T-cells.
Haeney	There is again equally good evidence from other groups, which

164

suggests that cells which E rosette, and nobody had disputed that cells which form E rosettes are not T-cells, also bind to C3. Again in some disease states, particularly in T-cell acute lymphoplastic leukaemia and in patients with lymphosarcoma one may find increased numbers of cells which bind both to E and to C3, and these are not malignant cells; again we do not know what their function is, but these are not the blast cells in acute lymphoplastic leukaemia. Certainly there is a distinct subpopulation of cells which bind to E and to C3, but it is only a very tentative conclusion that these may be activated T-cells.

Rossipal   Could you find any connection between the duration of the disease and the number of depressed T-cells in your adult treated coeliac? Is there a connection between the duration of the disease and the depression of the T-cells which you also find in treated coeliacs?

Haeney   We did not look.

Section IV
Immunology

17

An immunological theory of gluten-sensitive enteropathy

W. STROBER

The immunological theory of gluten-sensitive enteropathy (GSE) has as its basis the concept that this disease is caused by an abnormal immune response to gluten protein. Within the context of this theory one may postulate an afferent or initiating limb abnormality as well as an efferent or effector limb abnormality. In the former, certain processes unique to patients with GSE allow gluten protein to induce proliferation of lymphoid cells specifically programmed to react to gluten protein either by the production of anti-gluten protein antibody, a B-cell activity, or by the production of gluten protein-specific cell-mediated responses, a T-cell activity. In the latter, the induced cells or their products arising in the afferent limb interact with gluten protein in some manner to induce actual tissue injury (cellular cytotoxicity). In the analysis to follow, I will discuss these elements of the immunological theory of GSE in reverse order by considering first the data bearing on the possibility that there are, in patients with GSE, immunological abnormalities comprising an efferent limb defect; later I will return to the more fundamental question of whether or not there are immunological abnormalities in patients with GSE which comprise an afferent or initiating limb defect.

EFFERENT OR EFFECTOR LIMB ABNORMALITIES

The most obvious fact bearing on the role of immunological processes in the efferent limb of the proposed immunopathologic sequence in GSE is the morphology of the gastrointestinal lesion in this disease. In this regard, the fully developed lesion in GSE is characterized by a lamina propria which contains a dense lymphoid infiltrate dominated by plasma cells as well as an epithelial cell layer which contains an increased number of intraepithelial lymphocytes. The plasma cells are, of course, highly differentiated B cells, whereas the intraepithalial lymphocytes are either thymus-dependent cells or T cells *per se*[1,2]. These morphologic observations can be correlated with two functional observations. First, it can be shown that gluten challenge of individuals with treated GSE (GSE in remission) results in enhanced local mucosal immunoglobulin synthesis. This is demonstrable by utilizing fluorescence techniques or, in a more quantitative manner, by measuring the incorporation of labelled amino acid into immunoglobulin in jejunal biopsy specimens obtained from patients prior to and following an oral challenge of gluten proteins[3,4]. Second, it can be shown that exposure of biopsy specimens to gluten protein *in vitro* results in release of lymphokines—lymphoid cell products whose synthesis requires the presence of T cells but may in fact be produced by either T cells or B cells[5]. Thus, we have in place, at the site of tissue injury, a functioning B cell and T cell population capable of immunologically mediated tissue injury.

The precise identification of an actual mechanism of immunologically mediated tissue injury in GSE is not of major importance to the establishment of an immunological theory of this disease. In point of fact, any or all of a variety of immunological processes including complement-mediated cytotoxicity, antibody-dependent cell-mediated cytotoxicity (K-cell cytotoxicity) or direct cellular cytotoxicity (T-cell cytotoxicity) can conceivably be involved and there is no evidence favouring one of these processes over another[6,7]. Of greater importance to an immunological theory, and indeed a major approach to its proof, is the identification of the specificity of the local mucosal immunological reaction and the nature of the target of the possible immunocytotoxicity.

With regard to the first consideration, the specificity of the proposed immunological reaction, there is the fact that anti-gluten protein antibody is quite consistently found in both the serum and intestinal secretions of patients with GSE[8]. However, it is now clear that these anti-gluten protein antibodies are accompanied by other antibodies having specificities for a large number of dietary proteins[9]. This latter finding has led to the view that the occurrence of anti-gluten protein antibodies in GSE is an incidental or secondary phenomenon which is explained by altered intestinal permeability to potentially immunogenic dietary constituents. While this is not the only interpretation of the antibody data (an alternative interpretation is given later on) it certainly seems premature at the moment to draw any definite conclusions concerning the specificity of the local mucosal immunologic reaction from the nature of the antibodies found in the various body fluids. A more promising approach to discovery of the specificity of the local mucosal immunological reaction in GSE is suggested by the work of Falchuk et al.[10]. These authors measured local mucosal anti-gluten protein antibody production in jejunal tissue in vitro using a labelled amino acid incorporation technique in association with gluten–Sepharose affinity columns. In these studies it was found that a sizeable portion of the newly synthesized immunoglobulin resulting from in vivo gluten challenge has specificity for gluten protein. These studies warrant follow-up and lead one back to the idea that anti-gluten antibody production is indeed a major (albeit non-exclusive) preoccupation of the plasma cells at local mucosal sites in GSE.

With regard to the second consideration, the cellular target of immunocytotoxicity, one might initially think that the mature (villous) epithelial cell is a likely candidate, since this cell appears to be the major casualty in the pathological process. This being said, the epithelial cell per se does not seem a sufficient target since there is no convincing evidence that the local mucosal immunological reaction is autoimmune in nature, and in addition, this reaction is exquisitely sensitive to the presence of gluten protein. An alternative concept is that the mature epithelial cell with gluten protein (or a fragment thereof) bound to its surface is the primary target in GSE. This concept would allow the epithelial cell to be retained as the focus of injury and yet gluten protein would assume the role of the target antigen. In addition, this concept helps explain the fact that the tissue injury in GSE seems neatly compartmentalized in that only a single cell type is affected.

Having arrived at an appropriate target on theoretical grounds, what remains is that this target be substantiated on empirical grounds. Unfortunately, relevant experimental data in this regard are scanty and inconclusive: in the one published report in which this issue is addressed specifically, binding of gluten protein to epithelial cells was indeed found, but binding was seen only on crypt cells and not on villous cells[11]. Clearly, additional work must be done before one can either accept or reject the target proposed. This work must include studies with purified gluten protein as well as fragments derived from such proteins, since it is unlikely that intact molecules are the actual binding moiety. In addition, this work must be accomplished with methods capable of detecting low levels of binding, since relatively few molecules may be necessary to form a target of immunological attack.

The difficulties in establishing the specificity of the local mucosal immunological reaction just discussed in GSE lead to the possibility that the mucosal lymphoid cell infiltrate is after all a consequence rather than a cause of the tissue injury. One approach to this issue which, in a sense, transcends the question of the specificity of the local immune reaction involves the establishment and manipulation of an in vitro (organ culture) model of GSE. As we shall see, the results of these studies suggest, but do not as yet prove, that immunological abnormalities are indeed present which could comprise an efferent limb defect in GSE.

In organ culture studies, bits of intact jejunal tissue are maintained *in vitro* for 24–48 h under conditions that approximate the intestinal mucosa *in vivo*[12,13]. During this period, the status of epithelial cells is monitored by morphological observations or by measuring brush border enzyme activity. This latter criterion has particular importance because brush border enzyme activity develops in epithelial cells *pari passu* with the transformation of crypt epithelial cells into villous epithelial cells and thus can be used to measure the level of maturation of epithelial cells in culture. During organ culture of normal tissue an increase in brush border enzyme activity is quite regularly observed; this indicates that the average level of maturation of epithelial cells increases during the period of culture and that under conditions of culture mature epithelial cells are not replaced by an equal number of nascent immature cells. During culture of tissue from active GSE patients an increase in brush border enzyme activity is also observed, although in this case the baseline level is much reduced; thus, epithelial cell maturation in GSE tissue occurs *in vitro* even if it cannot occur *in vivo*.

The similarity between cultural behaviour of normal and GSE tissue ends when these tissues are cultured in the presence of gluten protein. Then it is observed that the presence of gluten protein in the organ culture medium has no effect on brush border enzyme increases in normal tissue, but has a profoundly inhibitory effect on brush border enzyme increases in GSE tissue. In view of what has been said above, this failure of GSE tissue to exhibit enzyme increases in the presence of gluten protein can be taken as an indication of epithelial cell maturation arrest and as such, an indication of GSE tissue injury *in vitro* which is entirely analogous to the process responsible for the failure of epithelial cell development *in vivo*. Another conclusion worthy of emphasis is that the behaviour of GSE tissue in the presence and absence of gluten protein in organ culture indicates that the injury process depends heavily on the presence of gluten protein, and, therefore, the injury process is not autoimmune in nature.

With the above observations and interpretations concerning organ culture of normal and GSE tissue as a background, various manipulations have been performed with the organ culture system to study the nature of the process responsible for cell injury in GSE. In the first place it has been observed that gluten protein inhibition of brush border enzyme increases in GSE tissue is completely abrogated by corticosteroids[14]. Since steroids can profoundly inhibit immunologic effector mechanisms *in vitro*, these data are compatible with the concept that immunological processes are important in GSE. In the second place it has been shown that the response of GSE tissue in organ culture to gluten protein is dependent on the state of activity of the disease in the patients from whom the tissue is taken[12]. That is, gluten protein inhibits brush border enzyme increases in tissue obtained from active patients but fails to inhibit brush border enzyme increases in tissue obtained from inactive patients. Thus, it can be concluded that mucosa obtained from GSE patients is not subject to injury by gluten protein until one induces a susceptibility by prior exposure to the toxic material; in other words, there seems to be the requirement in GSE for the activation of an endogenous mechanism of cytotoxicity before disease is manifest. It does not seem far-fetched to suggest that the endogenous mechanism we are referring to here is, in fact, the immunological system, which will ultimately interact with gluten protein to result in tissue injury.

Finally, in a set of organ culture studies described at this meeting 3 years ago, an experiment was described which showed that the tissue obtained from inactive patients not susceptible to injury by gluten protein *in vitro,* could be made susceptible to injury by co-culturing the tissue obtained from inactive patients with other tissue obtained from active patients[15]. Interpretation of this experiment, then as now, was that a soluble material can be produced by the tissue obtained from the active patient which can then render the tissue obtained from the inactive patient susceptible to gluten protein injury. Within this co-culture experiments lies the possibility of proving the primacy of the immunological factors in the efferent limb of the proposed immunopathological sequence in GSE, for if the soluble material passing between the active and inactive tissue can be shown to be antibody or some other product of the lymphoid system, then it is possible to say that a necessary and sufficient condition for the production of tissue injury in gluten-sensitive enteropathy involves an immunological process.

AFFERENT OR INITIATING LIMB ABNORMALITIES

Having considered the role of immunological factors in the efferent limb of a possible immunological theory, we can turn our attention to the more difficult question of the role of immunological factors in the afferent limb of such a theory. However, before we begin a discussion of this problem, it will be helpful to have in mind certain facts concerning the organization of the lymphoid system in the gastrointestinal tract as well as certain aspects of the response of this system to antigenic challenge.

It is now known that immune responses in the GI tract are initiated primarily, if not exclusively, in the organized lymphoid tissue of the gastrointestinal wall such as the Peyer's patches[16]. Lymphoid cells in these organized tissues interact with antigen entering into the patch through specialized epithelial cells overlying the patch[17]. However, no antibody is synthesized in the patch itself and it appears that cells leave the patch soon after contact with antigen to complete their development elsewhere[18]. In this latter regard, it has been shown in cell migration studies using radioactive labels that Peyer's patch cells, having passed into draining mesenteric nodes, migrate through the lymphatics and blood vessels and return to the gastrointestinal tract, where they become distributed in a diffuse fashion in the lamina propria. A final point is that lymphoid cells in the patch are heavily oriented toward IgA antibody synthesis and it can be shown that ingestion of antigen is followed by antigen-specific IgA cells in the thoracic duct as well as in the lamina propria[19,20].

It might at first be presumed that ingestion of antigens is invariably followed by positive humoral and cellular immune responses within the organized lymphoid aggregates of the gastrointestinal tract. This is not in fact the case and it has been repeatedly observed that ingestion of antigens leads to specific unresponsiveness. This phenomenon was first demonstrated in the studies of Chase who used simple chemical antigens (DNCB), but subsequently other investigators have observed a similar phenomenon using complex protein antigens such as bovine albumin[21,22]. In recent studies it has also been shown that ingestion of antigen leads to reduced or absent capacity to respond in distant organs (such as the spleen) as well as to the formation of circulating suppressor cells and substances[23]. This has led to the belief that unresponsiveness following oral exposure involves the activity of regulatory mechanisms such as helper T cells and suppressor T cells which are known to exist elsewhere in the lymphoid system (see discussion below). It is also possible that the unresponsiveness involves regulatory mechanisms unique to IgA responses. This latter concept is attractive since it would allow for regulation that would have properties unique to the gastrointestinal lymphoid system.

The fact that GI tract immune responses are highly organized and are under the control of regulatory mechanisms as indicated above introduces the idea that certain pathological states may result from abnormal enhancement or suppression of responses of gastrointestinal lymphoid cells to certain dietary antigens. In the particular case of GSE one might propose that patients with this disease mount an inordinate immune response to gluten protein and/or other antigens because of some error in the regulation of gastrointestinal immune responses with respect to gluten antigen. One can then say that the lymphoid cells induced as a result of this error ultimately migrate to the lamina propria where they mediate tissue injury in the efferent limb of the pathological sequence as discussed above.

At the moment, direct evidence in support of the concept just proposed, i.e. that GSE is an abnormality of immune regulation, is not available. Nevertheless, the hypothesis cannot be dismissed inasmuch as rather compelling indirect evidence in its support has recently come into view. I am of course referring to the important discovery that GSE is associated with certain histocompatibility antigens as well as with certain other lymphoid cell surface antigens not associated with the histocompatibility system. It is appropriate, therefore, to consider these associations in greater detail at this point in the discussion.

One may recall that in the initial studies showing an association between HLA antigen and GSE it was found that some 80% of patients bore the HLA-B8 histocompatilibility type[24,25]. In follow-up studies involving approximately 600 patients this frequency of HLA-B8 was amply corroborated and from the combined data it can be concluded that the risk of having GSE is some 8.8 times greater for HLA-B8 positive individuals than HLA-B8 negative individuals[26]. More recently, a second HLA antigen has been associated with GSE, the D-locus antigen HLA-DW3. In the major study of this association, Keuning *et al.* found that 27 of 28 patients carried the HLA-DW3 type and in fact the frequency of DW3 exceeded the frequency of HLA-B8 in the patient group studied[27]. In other studies carried out by Solheim *et al.* and Peña *et al.*, the DW3 antigen was also shown to occur quite frequently in populations of GSE patients, but in these studies the predominance of DW3 was less clear[28,29]. In any case, there can be no doubt that the DW3 antigen is at least as closely associated with GSE as in HLA-B8.

The fact that HLA-B8 and HLA-DW3 are both associated with GSE correlates with the fact HLA-B8 and HLA-DW3 tend to occur together in normal individuals. A non-random association between two separate HLA specificities in members of outbred populations is called linkage disequilibrium and may occur because the gene combinations responsible for the association confer a selective advantage on the individual bearing the combination. Whatever the cause of linkage disequilibrium, it is clear that as a result of this phenomenon, it is possible that HLA-B8 and/or HLA-DW3 are not in themselves important to the causation of GSE and are only associated with this disease because they are linked as with yet another (as yet unidentified) gene in the HLA complex which is the true 'disease gene'.

To understand how a particular HLA gene or gene combination may be associated with an abnormal immune response in GSE one must be aware of the fact that the cell–cell interactions which comprise the immune response involve surface proteins controlled by histocompatibility genes. For example, at the initiation of an immune response antigen is presented to relevant lymphoid cells by macrophages or macrophage factors. Evidence has recently been obtained in mice which indicates that such presentation involves interactions between surface protein (Ia antigens) which are coded by genes in the major histocompatibility complex[30]. In another phase of the immune response it has been found that T cells, having been presented with antigen, either help (facilitate) or suppress (inhibit) immune responses. Such immunoregulation is carried out by distinct helper T-cell and suppressor T-cell populations and, as in the case of macrophage presentation of antigen, depends on interactions involving Ia antigens. In perhaps the most clearcut demonstration of this fact, it has been shown that helper T-cells and suppressor T-cells, produce soluble products which can mediate immunoregulation and that such factors contain Ia antigens of particular types dependent on whether the factor provides help or suppression[31]. The genes controlling Ia antigens map to the same area of the histocompatibility complex as the Ir genes (immune response genes) and it is likely that the latter act through Ia antigens to influence immune responses at the level of macrophages or immunoregulatory cells. In this regard it is possible that certain Ia genotypes may lead to an enhanced or suppressed immune response to any given antigen by affecting macrophage presentation of that antigen or by affecting the balance of helper T-cell and suppressor T-cell activity for that antigen.

These findings can be directly applied to normal and abnormal human immune responses. It is obvious, for instance, that human HLA genes or genes in linkage disequilibrium with HLA genes can correspond to genes in the mouse located in the Ia region of the mouse histocompatibility complex. This is particularly true for D-locus genes (such as HLA-DW3) which are thought to be cognate to Ia genes in the murine system. Following this line of reasoning further it is possible that certain alleles of human HLA genes may be associated with human Ia genes (in effect, Ir genes) which, in turn, act through macrophages to allow responses to certain antigens but not to others; in addition, certain alleles of HLA genes may be associated with human Ia genes which act through immunoregulatory T cells to favour facilitation or suppression of responses to certain antigens. In this way an individual's HLA type may be predictive of the magnitude of his immune response to certain antigens.

Another possibility not necessarily conflicting with the possibilities already mentioned is that certain HLA genes lead to increased (or decreased) responses to whole classes of antigens or even to antigens in general. In this context it is possible that the HLA-B8 and the HLA-DW3 genes or, more likely, genes in linkage disequilibrium with these genes, constitute components in the human histocompatibility complex which favour general immunofacilitation rather than immunosuppression whereas other HLA genes are associated with general immunosuppression rather than immunofacilitation. One might speculate that individuals bearing the facilitating genes would have relatively vigorous responses to many environmental challenges and have, therefore, a selective advantage in dealing with infection. By the same token such individuals may have a greater tendency to develop autoimmune disease because their threshold for response to native or virally-altered antigen is lower.

The concept that HLA-B8 and HLA-DW3 are associated with a general facilitation of immunological responses is, of course, highly speculative at the moment. It has in its favour, however, the fact that HLA-B8 (and in some cases HLA-DW3) is found not only in GSE but in a number of disparate diseases which are marked by a tendency to over-react immunologically and to display autoimmune abnormalities[32]. In addition, it is increasingly likely that individuals with HLA-B8 hyper-respond to various kinds of specific and non-specific immunological stimuli. In this regard, Osoba et al. have indeed found that individuals with HLA-B8 respond more vigorously than individuals without HLA-B8 in mixed leukocyte cultures[33]. In further support of the concept that HLA-B8 and DW3 is associated with immunologic hyper-responsiveness, it might be mentioned that patients with GSE exhibit a multitude of anti-dietary antigen antibodies. As mentioned above, it has been assumed that these antibodies are a consequence of a disturbance in the gastrointestinal mucosal barrier leading to the penetration of dietary antigens; while this may be true to some extent, it is also plausible that the anti-dietary antibodies occur because of a general immunological hyper-responsiveness. A final point germane to these considerations is the response of GSE patients to non-dietary antigens given by the oral route. In the one controlled study available, oral challenge with polio virus was studied and it was found that patients with GSE produced significantly higher responses than normal[34]. This experiment hints at the possibility that the hyper-responsiveness in GSE may only be demonstrable if antigenic challenge is given orally so that possible regulatory mechanisms unique to the GI tract are involved.

We have so far in our discussion presented the idea that certain genes in the histocompatability complex may influence the strength or weakness of immunological responses to antigenic challenge and that patients with GSE may have an association with certain types of histocompatability antigens which are in fact associated with increased responses to (at least) certain antigens. But the story as so stated is not complete. The missing element is an explanation of the specificity of the abnormality in GSE, for even if we accept that GSE patients hyper-respond to some antigens, we must still explain why their response differs from patients with other diseases also associated with HLA-B8 and why GSE depends so exquisitely on exposure to gluten protein. The answer here may lie in the fact that GSE requires the presence of additional genes which can either channel hyper-responsiveness into immune responses specific for gluten protein or are in fact necessary for hyper-responsiveness *per se*.

In point of fact, the existence in GSE of a second gene totally unrelated to histocompatibility genes can be predicted on purely genetic considerations: firstly, particular HLA complex genes (HLA-B8 and DW3) found in most patients with GSE are found in considerable numbers of normal individuals and yet these individuals do not have GSE. Secondly, within families, siblings of patients may bear HLA antigens identical to the patient yet may not have disease[35]. Thirdly, and most convincingly, at least one family has been found in which transmittance of GSE does not follow that of HLA; that is a family in which a grandmother and two grandchildren have GSE and yet the grandmother is totally HLA-non-identical with the grandchildren[36]. The evidence from this family suggests that a second gene unrelated to HLA is being transmitted which is critical to the causation of disease.

In searching for the second gene important to the development of GSE, the sera of mothers of children with GSE have recently been examined for the presence of antibodies to cell surface proteins specific to this disease on the presumption that such antibodies might develop during pregnancy with children destined to develop GSE. This approach has proven successful in that several sera have been found which react with cells from patients with GSE but only a low percentage of normal cells. Curiously, the cell surface specificity reacting with the maternal antisera is found only on B cells and not T cells, a fact which has unquestionable but as yet unknown significance. Of major importance is the knowledge that the GSE associated B-cell antigen does not appear to be controlled by a gene or a set of genes located in the major histocompatibility locus[38]. First of all, it is detected with sera obtained from mothers who are themselves HLA-B8 and HLA-DW3 positive. Secondly, both normal individuals and patients with GSE are discordant for HLA and GSE-associated B-cell antigens. Finally, and most importantly, family studies show that the GSE-associated B-cell antigens and HLA antigens are separately inherited. Thus, the GSE-associated B-cell antigen is a major new marker protein for GSE distinct from the HLA markers.

The function of the GSE-associated B-cell antigen is not yet understood. One possibility is that this gene codes for a binding site on B-cells which can trigger responses to gluten protein. This idea is supported by the finding that both gluten protein and maternal sera recognizing

GSE-associated B-cell antigens can compete for the same site on the cell membrane; this is indicated by the fact that maternal sera recognizing the GSE-associated B-cell antigens is inhibited by preincubation of target cells with gluten protein. As a working hypothesis it is proposed that the gluten protein recognition site of lymphoid cells is composed primarily of the GSE-associated B-cell antigen. This site is somehow associated on the membrane with an HLA antigen and both act in concert to trigger responses to gluten protein. The gluten protein receptors, while clearly not present on all B-cells, are present on too large a fraction of cells to be only on those cells which have on their surface gluten protein specific idiotypic determinants coded for by immunoglobulin variable genes. Thus, it is further proposed that the interaction of gluten protein with cells in GSE results in the activation of many different cell clones and the production of antibodies to a wide variety of antigens. In this way we can explain a general hyper-responsiveness already alluded to, as well as a specific hyper-responsiveness to gluten protein.

SUMMARY

In the preceding discussion GSE is viewed as a genetically determined disease in which separate genes, one in the HLA complex and one not in the HLA complex, co-operate to produce disease. In the afferent limb of the immunopathological sequence the HLA gene is viewed as affecting the general responsiveness of patients to antigenic challenge and indeed this abnormality may also be found in other immunological diseases. In contrast, the non-HLA gene is viewed as producing a product which interacts with gluten protein more specifically, possibly by comprising the main component of a receptor for gluten protein on cell surfaces which channels the immunological hyper-responsiveness into a path that is gluten protein specific. One caveat here is that the receptor for gluten protein is present on cells of many different clones and, as a result the response to gluten protein may be the production of antibodies having specificities for many antigens.

The genetically determined surface specificities in the afferent limb lead to effector cells which then function in the efferent limb to produce epithelial cell cytotoxicity in the intestinal mucosa. In the discussion of this possibility it was mentioned that an important element in the proof of the immunological theory of GSE was the identification of an appropriate target cell and, in this connection, it was suggested that gluten protein bound to epithelial cells becomes such a target. It seems likely that the same genetically determined surface proteins which are found on lymphoid cells, may also be present on epithelial cells and there form a receptor to which gluten protein binds. This element of the theory insures that even if many antibodies are stimulated by gluten protein in the afferent limb, only gluten protein will be injurious in the efferent limb since a cytotoxic target can only be formed with gluten protein.

In all, the immunological theory of GSE is most critically dependent on the identification of surface components which on the one hand compel an abnormal immune response to gluten protein and on the other hand are important in the formation of the target for the induced cells or antibodies. So far we have identified surface proteins particularly associated with GSE; it remains to be proven that these proteins play a part in the causation of immunologic abnormalities.

References

1. Ferguson, A. (1974). Lymphocytes in coeliac disease. In: W. Th. J. M. Hekkens and A. S. Peña (eds.). *Coeliac Disease* p. 265 (Leiden: Stenfert Kroese)
2. Guy-Grand, D., Griscelli, C. and Vassalli, P. (1974). The gut associated lymphoid system; nature and properties of the large dividing cell. *Eur. J. Immunol.*, **4**, 435.
3. Shiner, M. and Ballard, J. (1972). Antigen–antibody reactions in jejunal mucosa in childhood coeliac disease after gluten challenge. *Lancet*, **i**, 1202
4. Loeb, P. M., Strober, W., Falchuk, Z. M. and Laster, L. (1971). Incorporation of leucine–14C into immunoglobulins by jejunal biopsies of patients with coeliac sprue and other gastrointestinal diseases. *J. Clin. Invest.*, **50**, 559
5. Ferguson, A., MacDonald, T. T., McClure, J. P. and Holden, R. J. (1975). Cell-mediated immunity to gliadin within the small intestinal mucosa in coeliac disease. *Lancet*, **i**, 895
6. Ezeoke, A., Ferguson, M., Fakhri, O., Hekkens, W. Th. J. M. and Hobbs, J. R. (1974). Antibodies in the sera of coeliac patients which can co-opt K cells to attack gluten-labelled targets. In: W. Th. J. M. Hekkens and A. S. Peña (eds.). *Coeliac Disease*. p. 176 (Leiden: Stenfert Kroese)
7. Doe, W. F., Henry, K. and Booth, C. C. (1974). Complement in coeliac disease. In: W. Th. J. M. Hekkens and A. S. Peña (eds.). *Coeliac Disease*. p. 189 (Leiden: Stenfert Kroese)
8. Ferguson, A. and Carswell, F. (1972). Precipitins to dietary proteins in serum and upper intestinal secretions of coeliac children. *Br. Med. J.*, **1**, 75
9. Ferguson, A. (1976). Coeliac disease and gastrointestinal food allergy. In: A. Ferguson and R. N. M. MacSween (eds.) *Immunological Aspects of the Liver and Gastrointestinal Tract*. p. 153. (Baltimore: University Park Press)
10. Falchuk, Z. M. and Strober, W. (1974). Gluten sensitive enteropathy: synthesis of anti-gliadin antibody *in vitro*. *Gut*, **15**, 947
11. Rubin, W., Fauci, A. S., Sleisenger, M. H. and Jeffries, G. H. (1965). Immuno-fluorescent studies in adult coeliac disease. *J. Clin. Invest.*, **44**, 475
12. Falchuk, Z. M., Gebhard, R. G., Sessoms, C. and Strober, W. (1974). An in vitro model of gluten sensitive enteropathy. Effect of gliadin on intestinal epithelial cells of patients with gluten-sensitive enteropathy in organ culture. *J. Clin. Invest.*, **53**, 487
13. Jos, J., Lenoir, G., de Ritis, G. and Rey, J. (1974). In vitro culturing of biopsies from children. In: W. Th. J. M. Hekkens and A. S. Peña (eds.). *Coeliac Disease*, p.91 (Leiden: Stenfert Kroese)

14. Katz, A. J., Falchuk, Z. M., Strober, W. and Shwachman, H. (1976). Gluten-sensitive enteropathy inhibition by cortisol of the effect of gluten protein in vitro. *N. Engl. J. Med.*, **295**, 131

15. Falchuk, Z. M., Gebhard, R. L. and Strober, W. (1974). The pathogenesis of gluten-sensitive enteropathy (coeliac sprue): organ culture studies. In: W. Th. J. M. Hekkens and A. S. Peña (eds.) *Coeliac Disease*, p. 107 (Leiden: Stenfert Kroese)

16. Cebra, J. J., Kamat, R., Gearhart, P., Robertson, S. M. and Tseng, J. (1977). The secretory IgA system of the gut. In: *Immunology of the Gut*, Ciba Foundation Symposium, **46**, p. 5 (Amsterdam: Elsevier)

17. Owen, R. L. (1977). Sequential uptake of horseradish peroxidase by lymphoid follicle epithelium of Peyer's patches in the normal unobstructed mouse intestine: An ultrastructural study. *Gastroenterology*, **72**, 440

18. McWilliams, M., Phillips-Quagliata, J. M. and Lamm, M. E. (1975). Characteristics of mesenteric lymph node cells homing to gut-associated lymphoid tissue in syngeneic mice. *J. Immunol.*, **115**, 54

19. Craig, S. W. and Cebra, J. J. (1971). Peyer's patches: an enriched source of precursors for IgA-producing immunocytes in the rabbit. *J. Exp. Med.*, **134**, 188

20. Pierce, N. F. and Gowans, J. L. (1975). Cellular kinetics of the intestinal immune response to cholera toxoid in rats. *J. Exp. Med.*, **142**, 1550

21. Chase, M. W. (1946). Inhibition of experimental drug allergy by prior feeding of the sensitizing agent. *Proc. Soc. Exp. Biol. Med.*, **61**, 257

22. Thomas, H. C. and Parrott, D. M. V. (1974). The induction of tolerance to a soluble protein antigen by oral administration. *Immunology*, **27**, 631

23. André, C., Heremans, J. F., Vaerman, J. P. and Cambraso, C. L. (1975). A mechanism for the induction of immunological tolerance by antigen feeding: Antigen–antibody complexes. *J. Exp. Med.*, **142**, 1509

24. Falchuk, Z. M., Rogentine, G. N. and Strober, W. (1972). Prodominance of histocompatibility antigen HLA–A8 in patients with gluten-sensitive enteropathy. *J. Clin. Invest.*, **51**, 1602

25. Stokes, P. L., Asquith, P., Holmes, G. K. T., Macintosh, P. and Cook, W. T. (1972). Histocompatibility antigen associated with adult coeliac disease. *Lancet*, **ii**, 162

26. Strober, W. (1976). Abnormalities of the HLA systems and gastrointestinal disease. In: J. Dausset and A. Svejgaard (eds.) *HLA and Disease*, p. 168. (Baltimore: Williams and Wilkins)

27. Keuning, J. J., Peña, A. S., van Leeuwen, A., van Hooff, J. P. and van Rood, J. J. (1976). HLA–DW3 association with coeliac disease. *Lancet*, **i**, 506

28. Solheim, B. G., Ek, J., Thune, P. O., Baklein, K., Bratlie, A., Rankin, B., Thoresen, A. B. and Thorsby, E. (1976). HLA antigens in dermatitis herpetiformis and coeliac disease. *Tissue Antigens*, **7**, 57

29. Peña, A. S., Mann, D. L., Hague, N. W., van Leeuwen, A., van Rood, J. J. and Strober, W. (1977). B-cell antigens in gluten-sensitive enteropathy. (Submitted for publication)

30. Erb, P. and Feldmann, M. (1975). The role of macrophages in the generation of T-helper cells. *J. Exp. Med.*, **142**, 460

31. Tada, T., Taniguchi, M. and David, C. S. (1976). Properties of the antigen-specific suppressive T-cell factor in the regulation of the antibody response of the mouse. *J. Exp. Med.*, **144**, 713

32. Svejgaard, A. and Ryder, L. P. (1976). Associations between HLA and disease. In: J. Dausset and A. Svejgaard (eds.) *HLA and Disease*, p. 46 (Baltimore: Williams and Wilkins)

33. Osoba, D. and Falk, J. (1976). HLA genes regulating the magnitude of the mixed leukocyte rection (MLR). *Fed. Proc.*, **35**, 712

34. Mawhinney, H. and Love, A. H. G. (1975). The immunoglobulin class responses to oral polio vaccine in coeliac disease. *Clin. Exp. Immunol.*, **22**, 47
35. van Rood, J. J., van Hooff, J. P. and Keunning, J. J. (1975). Disease predisposition, immune responsiveness and the fine structure of the HLA–A supergene. *Transplant. Rev.*, **22**, 75
36. Falchuk, Z. M., Katz, A. J., Shwachman, H., Rogentine, G. N. and Strober, W. (1977). Evidence for two genes in the pathogenesis of gluten-sensitive enteropathy. (Submitted for publication)
37. Mann, D. L., Katz, S. I., Nelson, D. L., Abelson, L. D. and Strober, W. (1976). Specific B-cell antigens associated with gluten-sensitive enteropathy and dermatitis herpetiformis. *Lancet,* **i,** 110
38. Strober, W. and Peña, A. S. (1977). Unpublished observations

Discussion of chapter 17

Asquith   This morning you said that when you exposed a coeliac mucosa in exacerbation from a patient who was B8-positive to gluten *in vitro* the toxicity was more obvious then than if the biopsy was from a B8-negative patient. Would that imply a different mechanism and how does it fit with your final hypothesis?

Strober   My working hypothesis concerning my point is as follows:– the HLA antigens, either the B locus antigens or the D locus antigens or some other thing in the HLA complex, play a role not only in the afferent limb, as I tried to point out here, not only in the segment of the pathologic process that is initiating disease, such as production of antibody production of cell-mediated immunity but also in providing a target for the antibody sort of toxicity. Recently a great deal of data has become available indicating that, in fact in T-cell mediated cytotoxicity, the target very frequently is altered histocompatibility antigen. A study showing that either virally altered or chemically altered targets require that the killer cells be histocompatibility related to the targets. These studies seem to indicate that part of the target and T-cell mediated cyto-toxicity is histocompatibility-related. It may be that the histocom-patibility antigens play a role in providing a target for the induced cells and this target will differ depending on the HLA status of the patient. Some targets may be more susceptible than others, giving rise to differences in the extent of disease.

Ferguson   I think we should close there now. I'll just make one point, the newly introduced drug levamisole does what you describe as possibly a genetic mechanism. It does enhance immune status but it will be interesting to see if this influences either the mani-festations of coeliac disease or even the incidence if it's more widely used.

Strober   The only other comment I would like to make is that if we now go back and re-examine the data on responses to gluten as far as antibody is concerned and try to look at the normal population we may be able to select out from the normal population, patients who have part of the genetic background for the production of GSE and yet they never developed disease because they lack all the genetic complement involved. So the fact that certain normals will have anti-food antibodies may not be against the concept of the immune response defect but actually for it.

18

Lymphotoxin production by peripheral blood lymphocytes in inactive and reactivated coeliac disease

R. EIFE, A. ENDERS, R. BERTELE, U. LOHRS, G. HUBNER, E. D. ALBERT and H. K. HARMS

INTRODUCTION

In a previous study, patients with untreated coeliac disease (CD) were found to be defective in their peripheral blood lymphocyte lymphotoxin (LT) production (Eife *et al.,* to be published). A lack of LT production by stimulated human peripheral blood lymphocytes is usually seen in patients suffering from thymus-dependent immunodeficiencies (Eife and August, 1972; Eife, 1975). Defective LT production in patients with certain other diseases may, however, be related to some kind of (secondary) 'immune deviation' with a small number of the potentially cytotoxic lymphocytes in the peripheral blood and an increased number of these cells in those tissues which are mainly involved in the active disease (such as the gut in CD). Thus a study of patients with active CD does not distinguish between an immunodeficiency and some kind of immune deviation as the possible underlying cause of the impaired LT production.

To investigate these two possibilities further we have studied the LT production by stimulated peripheral blood lymphocytes from patients with inactive and reactivated CD.

This work was supported by the 'Deutsche Forschungsgemeinschaft' SFB 37 (B7) and Ha 346/2

METHODS

The methods used are essentially those published recently (Eife *et al.*, 1974)

Lymphocyte cultures

Peripheral venous blood was drawn, heparinized and the erythyrocytes sedimented in 0.2 vol 6% dextran. The buffy coat was harvested, washed twice, and resuspended in tissue culture medium RPMI 1640 (GIBCO, Glasgow) supplemented with pooled human serum (10%), penicillin (100 units/ml) and streptomycin 100 μg/ml). Cultures were established by inoculating 2×10^5 mononuclear cells (lymphocytes and monocytes) into 1.5 ml medium in 12×75 mm tubes, adding 0.1 ml of three dilutions of Bacto-Phytohaemagglutinin-P (PHA) (DIFCO, Detroit) 1:40, 1:80, and 1:320) to each of three cultures and incubated at 37 °C in an atmosphere of moist 5% CO_2 and air. After 72 h the tubes were centrifuged and 1 ml of the cell-free culture fluid removed for assay of its LT content (see below). To the remaining culture, 1.0 μCi of [³H]thymidine was added and the tubes allowed to incorporate the isotope for 3 h. The cultures were terminated by washing the cells on to cellulose acetate filters (Sartorius, Göttingen), and then precipitating the DNA with 5% trichloroacetic acid. The radioactivity was measured by liquid scintillation spectrometry. Lymphocyte blast cell transformation was expressed as the difference between the mean counts per minute (cpm) in the PHA-stimulated and control cultures.

Lymphotoxin assay

Ten thousand HeLa cells [line S_3 (FLOW, Bonn)] suspended in 0.1 ml tissue culture medium MEM (GIBCO) supplemented with fetal calf serum (10%), glutamine (0.04 mmol/ml), penicillin and streptomycin, were placed in each well of a flat-bottomed microculture plate (LINBRO, Oxnard) and incubated at 37 °C in moist 5% CO_2 and air. Twenty four hours later, 50 μl of the cell-free culture medium to be assayed for its toxicity was added to each of the wells and the cultures incubated for 48 h. During the last 3 h of incubation, 0.5 μCi of [³H]thymidine was added. The target cell cultures were terminated by quickly inverting the plates to remove the medium and trysinizing the monolayer. The content of each well was then washed on to glass fibre filters by mean of a multiple cell culture harvester (Skatron, Lierbyan). Lymphotoxin activity was expressed as the percent inhibition of target cell DNA synthesis by cell-free culture medium from PHA-stimulated lymphocytes relative to the DNA synthesis in target cell cultures exposed to medium from unstimulated lymphocytes. Lymphotoxin activity expressed as percent inhibition was therefore calculated as:

$$\left[1 - \frac{\text{cpm (target cells + experimental medium)}}{\text{cpm (target cells + control medium)}} \right] \times 100$$

Patients and controls

Eleven patients with inactive CD and a group of 35 normal control individuals were included in this study. All patients were on a gluten-free diet for at least 2 years (mean duration 5 years). Small bowel biopsies studied by both light and electron microscopy showed a normal mucosa in all patients.

The study was designed in such a way that whenever CD lymphocytes were cultured, the lymphocytes from one normal control individual were cultured simultaneously. Thus every CD patient studied could be paired to one individual control (paired control).

The study was performed over $2\frac{1}{2}$ months. During this period a further 24 healthy individuals were studied in our laboratory. These individuals and the 11 paired controls served as a general control group.

Gluten challenge

Immediately after the first *in vitro* lymphocyte function tests were performed the patients were challenged with gluten (20–40 g per day) over a period of 28 days. This was primarily intended to confirm the initial diagnosis. Lymphocyte function studies were repeated on days 14 and 28 of the challenge. A complete clinical and laboratory investigation (including small bowel biopsy) was repeated on day 28. Mucosal disaccharidases were assayed according to the methods published by Dahlquist (1964).

RESULTS

PHA-induced blast cell transformation in inactive CD

In general the blast cell transformation of lymphocytes from patients with inactive CD was significantly lower than that of lymphocytes of control individuals (Figure 18.1A): the mean value (cpm [³H]thymidine uptake per culture) for the group of patients was 11 700, the range 4000 to 23 800; the mean value for the controls was 38 800, the range 8300 to 85 900. In Figure 18.1B the data from each CD patient paired with his control individual (paired control) is presented as the ratio of CD patient to control transformation: in 10 of 11 pairs the CD lymphocytes responded to a smaller extent than their controls, with an average ratio of approximately 0.7.

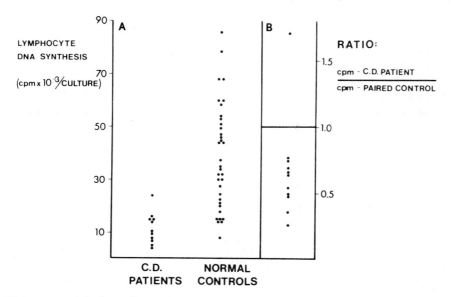

Figure 18.1 (A) Blast cell transformation by CD (gluten-free diet) and normal control peripheral blood lymphocytes. Each dot represents the mean cpm [³H]thymidine uptake per culture. (B) Ratios of blast cell transformation by CD lymphocytes to that of normal lymphocytes for every pair studied

PHA-induced lymphotoxin production in inactive CD

CD lymphocytes produced significantly less LT than did normal lymphocytes (Figure 18.2A): the respective means for the LT activity (expressed as the percent inhibition of target cell DNA synthesis) were 39 and 68%; the range for the CD patients was 15 to 63% and the range for the controls was 45 to 94%. Figure 18.2B shows the paired data for LT production expressed as the ratio CD to control LT: in none of the 11 experiments did CD lymphocytes produce more or equal amounts of control LT; the mean ratio was 0.6, the range 0.3 to 0.9.

However, in about half of the patients the LT production was within the normal range. We have checked all clinical and laboratory findings carefully to look for differences between those patients with an almost normal and those with a severely depressed LT production; the only pathological finding was a mild to moderate suppression of the mucosal lactase in some of the patients (Figure 18.2A): as far as tested, the patients with a depressed LT production showed a suppression of their mucosal lactase activity and the patients with an almost normal LT production showed a normal mucosal lactase activity.

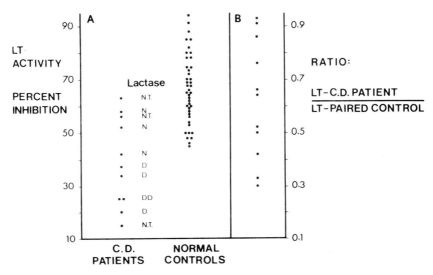

Figure 18.2 (A) LT production by CD (gluten-free diet) and normal control peripheral blood lymphocytes. (B) Ratios of LT production by CD lymphocytes to that of normal lymphocytes for every pair studied. Lactase = Mucosal lactase activity: D = depressed, N = normal, N.T. = not tested

PHA-induced lymphocyte function in reactivated CD

In those patients whose lymphocyte function was reinvestigated during and after gluten challenge, two types of reaction were observed:

(1) In the patients with a very low initial LT production the LT activity increased significantly after 14 days and to an even greater extent after 28 days of challenge (Figure 18.3). The PHA-induced lymphocyte blast cell transformation increased similarly.

(2) In the patients with an initial LT production in the normal range, the LT activity significantly decreased after 14 days and this reduction was more marked after 28 days of gluten challenge (Figure 18.4). Thus, depending on the initial lymphocyte function, the patients showed a totally different reaction pattern *in vitro* upon massive gluten challenge. It should be noted that morphologic studies (small bowel biopsy) confirmed a relapse in all patients. In two patients with an initial intermediate LT production, the LT activity did not change significantly during and after the gluten challenge (data not shown).

LT production in CD families

In some experiments the LT production by PHA-stimulated lympho-

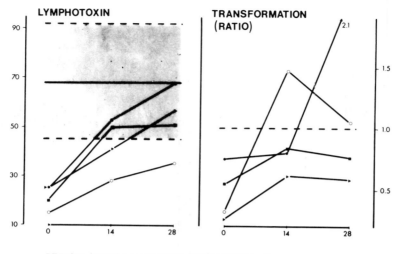

PERIOD (DAYS) OF GLUTEN CHALLENGE (20-40 gms/day)

Figure 18.3 LT production and blast cell transformation in inactive and reactivated CD patients with low initial LT production. LT activity is expressed as per cent inhibition of target cell DNA synthesis. Shaded area: normal range (and mean) LT activity of 35 normal control individuals. Blast cell transformation is expressed as the ratio of cpm [³H]thymidine uptake per culture by CD lymphocytes to that of normal lymphocytes (paired controls)

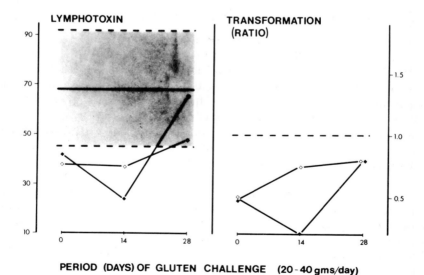

PERIOD (DAYS) OF GLUTEN CHALLENGE (20-40 gms/day)

Figure 18.4 LT production and blast cell transformation in inactive and reactivated CD patients with normal initial LT production. For details see Figure 18.3

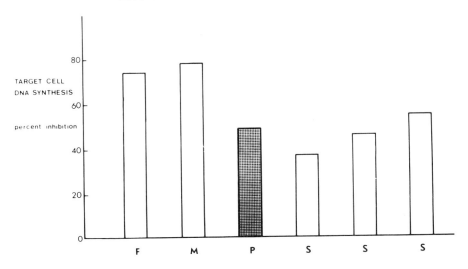

Figure 18.5 Lymphotoxin production in a family with four HLA-identical girls. Lymphotoxin activity is expressed as per cent inhibition of target cell DNA synthesis. F = father, M = mother, P =patient, S = sister

cytes of CD patients and their relatives were investigated. In parallel HLA typing was performed. Figure 18.5 shows the LT activity in a family with four siblings: in comparison to the parents, all four sisters (all being HLA identical) had a reduced LT activity.

DISCUSSION

Recent studies on *in vitro* reactions of peripheral blood lymphocytes in CD patients suggest either a qualitative or a quantitative defect of CD T-lymphocytes (Asquith, 1974). Impairment of cell mediated immunity in CD patients may also be suspected from clinical observations such as an increased risk of lymphoma (Gough *et al.*, 1962; Austad *et al.*, 1967; Harris *et al.*, 1967; Holmes *et al.*, this volume), peripheral lymph node hypoplasia, splenic atrophy (McCarthy *et al.*, 1966), and lack of delayed type hypersensitivity reactions to common antigens (Bullen *et al.*, this volume). It is, however, difficult at present to be sure whether the impairment of the thymus dependent immune system in CD patients is due to a primary or a secondary defect.

The data presented in this study also support the hypothesis that the cellular immune system is impaired in patients with CD. While on a gluten-free diet the patients studied here showed lymphocyte responses to PHA ranging from severely depressed to almost normal values.

These data seem to confirm the hypothesis that the reduced peripheral blood lymphocyte response to PHA is independent of the dietary status of the patient (Asquith, 1974). Upon gluten challenge, however, we found that the responses were reversed: in patients with an initially depressed response the lymphocyte function increased significantly whereas in patients with an initial almost normal response the lymphocyte functions were found to be severely depressed. The reversed responses were, moreover, even more pronounced after 28 days compared with 14 days of gluten challenge and were most clearly observed in the LT activity test.

These observations indicate that (as far as individual patients are concerned) the impairment of CD LT production may indeed depend on the dietary status of the patient. We know of no conclusive explanation, however, for the different reaction pattern of the LT response following gluten challenge in the individual patient.

The different lymphocyte reaction *in vitro* in inactive CD (prior to gluten challenge) may reflect genetic heterogeneity in the disease. Some evidence for such a hypothesis arises from the family study presented in Figure 18.5. In addition, none of our patients showed a LT production above the paired control value, indicating a general depression of LT production which might be genetically determined.

CD patients may, on the other hand, take in minute amounts of gluten even though they are on a 'gluten-free' diet. Such minute quantities may affect the immune system, as seen in our patients after the massive gluten challenge. The suspected gluten intake was not confirmed morphologically in jejunal biopsies. Nevertheless, we observed disorders of mucosal lactase activity in the same patients which had a significant depression of LT production.

If the low mucosal lactase activity is an indicator of a minute gluten intake a secondary defect of the thymus-dependent immune system (represented by the depressed LT activity) has to be discussed.

References

Asquith, P. (1974). Cell mediated immunity in coeliac disease. In: W. Th. J. M. Hekkens and A. S. Peña (eds.). *Coeliac Disease*. pp. 242–260. (Leiden: Stenfert Kroese)

Austad, W. I., Cornes, J. S., Gough, K. R., McCarthy, C. F. and Read, A. E. (1967). Steatorrhoea and malignant lymphoma. The relationship of malignant tumours of lymphoid tissue and coeliac disease. *Am. J. Dig. Dis.*, **12**, 475

Dahlquist, A. (1964). Method for assay of intestinal disaccharidases. *Anal. Biochem.*, **7**, 18

Eife, R. and August, C. (1972). Growth inhibition and cytotoxic factors produced by human peripheral blood leukocytes in vitro. *Pediat. Res.*, **6**, 381

Eife, R., Eife, G., August, C., Kuhre, W. and Staehr-Johansen, K. (1974). Lymphotoxin production and blast cell transformation by cord blood lymphocytes: dissociated lymphocyte function in newborn infants. *Cell. Immunol.*, **14**, 435

Eife, R. (1975). Lymphotoxin-Bildung bei Störungen der Immunität. *Klin. Wocherschr.,* **53,** 929

Gough, K. R., Read, A. E. and Naish, J. M. (1962). Intestinal reticulosis as a complication of idiopathic steatorrhoea. *Gut,* **3,** 223

Harris, O. D., Cooke, W. T., Thompson, H. and Waterhouse, J. A. H. (1967). Malignancy in adult coeliac disease and idiopathic steatorrhoea. *Am. J. Med.,* **42,** 899.

McCarthy, C. F., Fraser, I. D., Evans, K. T. and Read, A. E. (1966). Lymphoreticular dysfunction in idiopathic steatorrhoea. *Gut,* **7,** 140

Discussion to chapter 18

Falchuk	It may or may not affect the interpretation of your data, but I think it might be a bit tricky to use lactase to define whether or not patients are in a strict remission. We and others find quite frequently that lactase is the last of the brush border enzymes to return to normal in patients who are otherwise completely in remission by other criteria.
Eife	I agree, this is indeed a crucial point with regard to the preparation of our data. However, since we could not completely exclude a low gluten intake by out-patients we were cautious in preparing this data as indicating just a delayed return to normal enzyme activity.
Falchuk	There may be a number of different explanations, one of which is that the patients are genetically lactase deficient. I just think that the use of lactase alone may be a problem in terms of defining remission. Professor Rey and his colleagues suggested some years ago that a low level of lactase was a manifestation of accelerated cell transport up the villus.
Eife	Since we have found low lactase activities in about half of our patients, we believe that it is somewhat unlikely that all those patients should be genetically lactase deficient. We therefore are more inclined to suggest an extrinsic factor, such as a low gluten intake.
Rey	We think that it is possible to have apparently normal mucosa with normal villi but increased turnover rates of epithelial cells so if the half-life of the cells is less than 48 hours it is possible there is no lactase at all but normal villi.
Booth	If I could take up that question on lactase. If that hypothesis is true then there should be a general reduction of all brush border enzymes in that situation but there is not. The point that has been made is that lactase is the last one to recover and behaves differently from the other ones and that makes it very unlikely that Rey's hypothesis is true.

19

Antigen–antibody reactions in untreated coeliac mucosa

B. B. SCOTT, D. G. SCOTT and M. S. LOSOWSKY

Although gluten has a central role in the pathogenesis of coeliac disease, it is not known how it exerts its toxic effect. Much evidence suggests that immunological mechanisms are involved. In particular, acute studies of the mucosa following gluten challenge of the treated patient point to antigen–antibody reactions (possibly gluten and gluten antibody) with activation of complement. There is, however, disagreement over the class of antibody involved, two studies having shown mainly IgA and one having shown mainly IgM[3]. Much less attention has been paid to mucosal immunoglobulins and complement in untreated coeliac disease. Of course, it cannot be assumed that the mechanism of acute damage after gluten challenge is the same as the chronic on-going damage in the untreated state. Indeed, Brandtzaeg[4] has postulated that whereas IgA responses are important initially in mucosal tissues, IgG responses are important later. He states that "mucosal IgG responses associated with chronic inflammation probably represent a 'second line of defence' against exogenous and endogenous antigens. . . In the long run a local IgG response may therefore contribute to aggravation and perpetuation of inflammatory disease".

IgG has been noted previously in coeliac mucosa but has been considered non-specific[5]. Involvement of any IgG present in the mucosa in an immune reaction would be suggested by its presence together with complement especially the early components of complement (e.g. C1q which is easily detected). This is because IgG activates the complement cascade via the classical pathway which involves the early components. Thus when IgG is involved in an immune reaction with activation of complement, one would expect to find positive staining for IgG together with C1q and C3. On the other hand, IgA which may also be present, can probably only activate the complement cascade via the alternative pathway which by-passes the early components. Thus when IgA is involved in an immune reaction with activation of complement it is found together with C3 but not C1q.

This study was designed to assess the incidence of immunoglobulins and the C1q and C3 components of complement in untreated coeliac mucosa and compare it with the incidence in treated coeliacs and non-coeliacs.

The subjects studied consisted of seven untreated coeliacs, 11 treated coeliacs, and 16 non-coeliacs. The non-coeliacs were not healthy volunteers but included patients with conditions which might be associated with mucosal immune reactions, e.g. Crohn's disease and cystic fibrosis. Biopsies were taken from just past the duodenojejunal junction and frozen sections stained with fluorescein isothiocyanate-labelled antisera to IgA, IgG, IgM, C1q and C3. The sections were studied blindly by one observer. Only extracellular immunofluorescence was studied and note made of the site (i.e. lamina propria or basement membrane zone) and pattern (i.e. granular or homogeneous). The findings in the lamina propria and basement membrane zone were similar and for convenience only the findings in the basement membrane are presented.

There was a very significantly increased incidence of IgA together with C3 in untreated coeliacs (six out of seven) compared with treated coeliacs (two out of 11; $p = 0.009$) and non-coeliacs (none out of 16 $p = 0.00007$). IgM was only seen in two subjects. IgG was seen in most subjects suggesting it might be without significance. However, it had a granular pattern, suggesting immune complex deposition, in 71% of untreated coeliacs compared with none of the treated coeliacs and 19% of the non-coeliacs. Furthermore, the combination of granular IgG together with C1q was seen in 43% of untreated coeliacs compared with none of the treated coeliacs ($p = 0.04$) or non-coeliacs ($p = 0.02$).

These findings suggest that a local antigen–antibody reaction involving IgA and complement may contribute to the ongoing damage in untreated coeliac disease. In addition, an IgG response may be involved and, since the appearance of IgG has not been seen after acute gluten challenge, it may be a secondary response to the mucosal damage thus contributing to and perpetuating the damage as suggested by Brandt-zaeg.

References

1. Shiner, M. and Ballard, J. (1972). Antigen–antibody reactions in jejunal mucosa in childhood coeliac disease after gluten challenge. *Lancet,* **i,** 1202
2. Lancaster-Smith, M., Packer, S., Kumar, P. J. and Harries, J. T. (1976). Immunological phenomena in the jejunum and serum after re-introduction of dietary gluten in children with treated coeliac disease. *J. Clin. Pathol.,* **29,** 592
3. Doe, W. F., Henry, K. and Booth, C. C. (1974). Complement in coeliac disease. In: W. Th. J. M. Hekkens and A. S. Peña (eds.) *Coeliac Disease,* pp. 189–192. (Leiden: Stenfert Kroese)
4. Brandtzaeg, P. (1973). Structure, synthesis and external transfer of mucosal immunoglobulins. *Ann. Immunol.,* **124C,** 417
5. Shiner, R. J. and Ballard, J. (1973). Mucosal secretory IgA and secretory piece in adult coeliac disease. *Gut,* **14,** 778

Discussion of chapter 19

Douglas	Have you had the opportunity of using this technique to study the mucosa from patients with coeliac disease who are also IgA deficient? What do you think you will find?
Scott	I would not expect to find positive staining for IgA!
Ferguson	Do you think gluten is in the complexes or reticulin or what?
Scott	Obviously, I have no way of telling, but I'd like to think that it was a complex of gluten and gluten antibody.
Ferguson	You have used a number of techniques to study antibodies in the serum of similar patients. Did you do simultaneous serum antibody studies in these because that would be relevant to your hypothesis?
Scott	We did measure serum gluten antibody but found no correlation between serum titres for gluten antibody and the results of mucosal staining.
Strober	Did you specifically absorb your antiserum with purified immunoglobulins to prove their specificity, in other words could you block the IgG staining with IgG but not IgA and IgM?
Scott	We did, yes.

20

A simple immunofluorescence technique for the demonstration of antibodies to wheat

K. P. ETERMAN and T. E. W. FELTKAMP

ABBREVIATIONS

CD	—	Coeliac disease
ELISA	—	Enzyme-linked immunosorbent assay
GFD	—	Gluten-free diet
IFT	—	Immunofluorescence technique
ND	—	Normal diet
RAb	—	Reticulin antibody
RIA	—	Radioimmunoassay

INTRODUCTION

Circulating antibodies to wheat gluten and to other foods are present in the majority of patients with untreated coeliac disease[1,3,10,11,15,18] and tend to disappear when a gluten-free diet is started[1,4]. It seems likely that the antibodies result from increased permeability of the mucosa of the small bowel.

Antibodies to reticulin (RAb) have also been found in a significant number of patients with coeliac disease, dermatitis herpetiformis and Crohn's disease[2,5,13,14,16]. In coeliac disease and dermatitis herpetiformis the antibodies are more common in patients on a normal diet (ND) than in those on a gluten-free diet (GFD)[2,13,17].

The aim of the present study was to develop a simple method for the determination of antibodies to gluten. Such a method might serve as a screening method for coeliac disease. We have already described an immunofluorescence technique performed on cryostat sections of wheat grains which made it possible to detect antibodies to gluten[7]. We now report on some of the results obtained with this technique in patients with coeliac disease and other gastrointestinal diseases, and compare these results with the results of the determination of anti-reticulin antibodies.

Table 20.1 Frequency of antibodies to reticulin (RAb) and gluten (GAb) in patients with coeliac disease

	Number studied	RAb	GAb	RAb and/or GAb
Children ND*	6	2(33%)	6(100%)	6(100%)
Children GFD**	8	0(0%)	7(87%)	7(87%)
Controls	14	0(0%)	0(0%)	0(0%)
Adults ND	36	12(33%)	18(50%)	21(58%)
Adults GFD	59	6(10%)	19(32%)	22(37%)
Controls	95	2(2%)	4(4%)	6(6%)

*ND, normal diet
**GFD, gluten-free diet

FREQUENCY OF ANTIBODIES TO GLUTEN AND RETICULIN

Sera from 95 adults and 14 children with coeliac disease were studied for the presence of antibodies to gluten and reticulin. Antibodies to gluten, demonstrated with the immunofluorescence technique, were found in all the coeliac children on a normal diet and in half of the adults with the untreated disease. In children and adults on a gluten-free diet these frequencies decreased to 87 and 32%, respectively (Table 20.1) (Figures 20.1A and B).

In Crohn's disease, cystic fibrosis, recurrent diarrhoea, dermatitis herpetiformis and ulcerative colitis, the respective frequencies were 52, 42, 37, 18 and 18% (controls 4%) (Table 20.2). Antibodies to reticulin (determined as described by Rizzetto and Doniach[14], with only the R1 and R2 types considered as positive) were found in 33% of coeliac patients on a normal diet. Only 11% of coeliac patients on a gluten-free diet showed these antibodies (Table 20.1).

In patients with dermatitis herpetiformis, 12% had these antibodies, whereas the highest frequency in the other diseases studied (Crohn's disease, ulcerative colitis, cystic fibrosis and recurrent diarrhoea) was 7% (controls 2%) (Table 20.2).

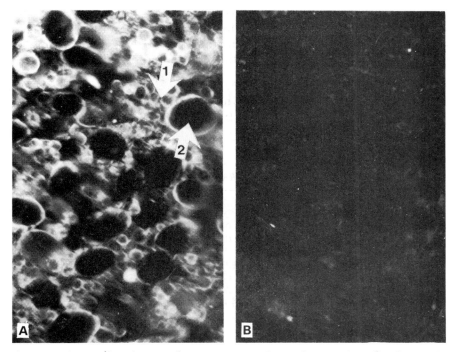

Figure 20.1A. Indirect immunofluorescence technique using a section of a wheat grain as substrate. The section was incubated with serum from a patient with untreated gluten-induced enteropathy followed by FITC-labelled horse anti-human Ig conjugate. Arrow 1: fluorescent granular structure; arrow 2: starch granule, washed out by immunofluorescence procedure (× 274)
B. As (**A**) but instead of a patient serum a normal control was used (× 274)

Table 20.2 Frequency of antibodies to reticulin (RAb) and gluten (GAb) in various diseases.

	Mean age	Number studied	RAb	GAb
Untreated coeliacs (adults)	43	36	12(33%)	18(50%)
Dermatitis herpetiformis	51	34	4(12%)	6(18%)
Crohn's disease	39	50	3(6%)	26(52%)
Ulcerative colitis	40	44	3(7%)	8(18%)
Controls (adults)	44	95	2(2%)	4(4%)
Untreated coeliacs (children)	6	6	2(33%)	6(100%)
Cystic fibrosis	6	17	1(6%)	7(42%)
Recurrent diarrhoea	3	45	1(2%)	17(37%)
Controls (children)	6	60	0(0%)	4(6%)

IMMUNOGLOBULIN CLASSES

The use of an immunofluorescence technique enabled us to determine the immunoglobulin classes of antibody to gluten. The classes were IgA, IgG and IgM, the IgG being most commonly found (Table 20.3). Antibodies to reticulin were of the IgA and IgG classes (Table 20.4). Both antibodies were non-complement fixing.

Table 20.3 Ig class of antibodies to gluten (GAb)

Number studied	Ig class
5 (2 GFD*)	G
1 (1 GFD)	G+A
1	G+M
1	G+A+M
1	A+M
9	

* On gluten-free diet

Table 20.4 Ig class of antibodies to reticulin (RAb)

Number studied	Ig class
6 (2 GFD*)	G
4 (2 GFD)	G+A
4 (1 GFD)	A
14	

* On gluten-free diet

CHARACTERIZATION OF ANTIGEN

Antibodies to wheat were absorbed with gliadin, suggesting that antibodies to gliadin had been determined with the IFT on wheat grains[7]. Further studies in which the results of the IFT on wheat grains were compared with those of the ELISA technique of Engvall and Perlmann[5], in which polystyrene tubes were coated with a gliadin solution, however, showed that a positive but no absolute relation existed between the results of the two tests (Figure 20.2). No significant relation was found between the IFT titres and the extinction values of the Elisa technique[12]. Therefore, we compared the IFT on wheat grains with a radioimmunoassay using [^{125}I]gliadin in the study of coeliac patients and controls. These studies disclosed discrepancies, which suggest that, with the IFT on wheat grains, antibodies may be found not (only) directed to gliadin (Figure 20.3). Furthermore, antibodies to wheat were correlated with coeliac disease significantly better than were antibodies to gliadin (RIA) ($p<0.001$)[9].

DISCUSSION

A simple immunofluorescence technique on cryostat sections of wheat grains enabled us to detect antibodies to wheat, which are very closely connected with coeliac disease. These antibodies were not specific for coeliac disease, a feature they have in common with antibodies to other

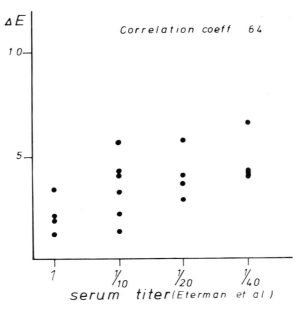

Figure 20.2 Correlation between the serum antigliadin concentration of biopsy-proven coeliacs as determined by the ELISA technique and the anti-wheat titre by the indirect immunofluorescence technique on wheat grains

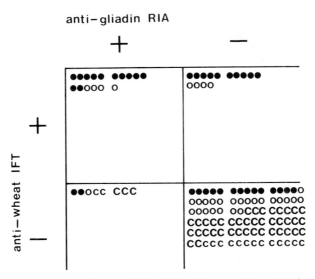

Figure 20.3 Comparison of anti-gliadin RIA with anti-wheat IFT in patients with coeliac disease and healthy controls. ●, untreated coeliac patient; O, coeliac patient on gluten-free diet; C, healthy control (adult); c, healthy control (child)

food antibodies that occur in CD. Antibodies not directed to gliadin accounted for the high number of positive reactions obtained with this technique in patients with coeliac disease. This is further proof of the fact that these antibodies are not of pathogenic significance for CD, but merely another food antibody.

Antibodies may serve as a screening test for the diagnosis of coeliac disease and may also be used in a method for dietary control, although the influence of the half-life of Ig must be kept in mind. The question remains which antigen of the whole wheat grain gives rise to the antibodies found with the IFT on wheat grains.

References

1. Alarcón-Segovia, D., Herskovic, T., Wakim, K. G. and Green, P. A. (1964). Presence of circulating antibodies to gluten and milk fractions in patients with non-tropical sprue. *Am. J. Med.*, **36**, 485

2. Alp, M. H. and Wright, R. (1971). Auto-antibodies to reticulin in patients with idiopathic steatorrhoea, coeliac disease and Crohn's disease and their relation to immunoglobulins and dietary antibodies. *Lancet*, **ii**, 682

3. Berger, E. (1958). Zur allergischen Pathogenese der Cöliakie. *Ann. Paediat. (Beiheft)*, **38**, (New York: S. Karger A. G. and Basel)

4. Carswell, F. and Ferguson, A. (1973). Plasma food antibodies during withdrawal reintroduction of dietary gluten in coeliac disease. *Arch. Dis. Childh.*, **48**, 583

5. Engvall, E. and Perlmann, P. (1971. Enzyme linked immunosorbent assay (ELISA). Quantitative assay immunoglobulin G. *Immunochemistry*, **8**, 871

6. Essen, R. von, Savilahti, E. and Pelkonen, P. (1972). Reticulin antibody in children with malabsorption. *Lancet*, **i**, 1157

7. Eterman, K. P., Hekkens, W. Th. J. M., Peña, A. S., Lems-van Kan, P. H. and Feltkamp, T. E. W. (1977). Wheat grains: a substrate for the determination of gluten antibodies in serum of gluten-sensitive patients. *J. Immunol. Methods*, **14**, 85

8. Eterman, K. P. and Feltkamp, T. E. W. (1977). Antibodies to gluten and reticulin in gastrointestinal diseases. (Submitted for publication)

9. Eterman, K. P. and Aalberse, R. C. (1977). A comparison of antibodies to wheat (IFT) with two antigen-binding assays using ^{125}I gliadin in patients with coeliac disease. (In preparation)

10. Ferguson, A. and Carswell, F. (1972). Precipitins to dietary proteins in serum and upper intestinal secretions of coeliac children. *Br. Med. J.*, **1**, 75

11. Heiner, D. C., Lahey, M. E., Wilson, J. F., Gerrard, J. W., Schwachman, H. and Khaw, K. T. (1962); Precipitins to antigens of wheat and cow's milk in coeliac disease. *J. Pediat.*, **6**, 813

12. Hekkens, W. Th. J. M., Lems-van Kan, P. H., Rosekrans, P. C. M. and Eterman, K. P. (1977). Quantitative determination of gliadin antibodies in serum of patients with coeliac disease. The ELISA technique. (Submitted for publication)

13. Magalhaes, A. F. N., Peters, T. J. and Doe, W. F. (1974). Studies on the nature and significance of connective tissue antibodies in adult coeliac disease and Crohn's disease. *Gut*, **15**, 284

14. Rizzetto, M. and Doniach, D. (1973). Types of 'reticulin' antibodies in human sera by immunofluorescence. *J. Clin. Pathol.*, **26**, 841

15. Rossipal, E. (1970). Precipitins to aqueous extracts of flour in coeliac disease. *Lancet*, **i**, 251

16. Seah, P. P., Fry, L., Rossiter, M. A., Hoffbrand, A. V. and Holborow, E. J. (1971). Anti-reticulin antibodies in childhood coeliac disease. *Lancet*, **ii**, 681

17. Seah, P. P., Fry, L., Holborow, E. J., Rossiter, M. A., Doe, W. F., Magalhaes, A. F. and Hoffbrand, A. V. (1973). Anti-reticulin antibody: Incidence and diagnostic significance. *Gut*, **14**, 311

18. Taylor, K. B., Truelove, S. C., Thomson, D. L. and Wright, R. (1961). An immunological study of coeliac disease and idiopathic steatorrhoea. *Br. Med. J.*, **2**, 1727

Discussion of chapter 20

Ferguson   Professor C. Anderson mentioned, I think at a meeting in the
            Spring, that we talked so much about gluten intolerance whereas
            we are really describing transient wheat intolerance and it's
            nice that you have reminded us to be precise about exactly what
            antigen we are talking about.

21

Immunofluorescent gliadin antibodies in childhood coeliac disease

M. STERN, K. FISCHER and R. GRÜTTNER

INTRODUCTION

Since Berger's[1] original detection of complement-binding wheat-specific antibodies in sera of coeliac children, data concerning pathogenic significance and clinical use of wheat antibodies have been conflicting. The methods reported have been diverse in sensitivity and specificity. Only a few attempts have been made to classify the immunogenic wheat protein fraction. By microimmunodiffusion Beckwith and Heiner[2] were able to show the most distinct precipitin reaction using a fraction later identified to contain mostly alpha-gliadin. Immunoglobulin class determinations of complement-binding antibodies were done by Mietens[3], who found IgM and some IgG anti-gliadin activity in coeliac sera.

We have tried to establish a gliadin antibody test taking advantage of passive haemagglutination and indirect immunofluorescent technique. By this method we were able to identify immunogenic gliadin proteins and immunoglobulin classes of gliadin antibodies.

METHODS AND MATERIALS

From passive haemagglutination we derived the procedure of coupling gliadin in acetic acid solution (pH 2.9) to human group O red blood cells previously stabilized by pyruvic aldehyde according to the method of Ling[4] (Figure 21.1).

The carbonyl aldehyde groups seem to establish a stable coupling over a wide range of pH. Dry films of coated red cells were incubated with patient's serum dilutions in a moist chamber at room temperature for 30 min, washed three times, and incubated with fluorescein-labelled antisera to human immunoglobulin classes G, A, M, D, and E. Con-pH 2.9

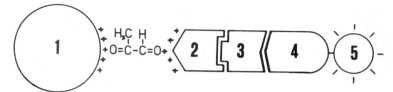

Figure 21.1 Serum gliadin antibodies. Immunofluorescent technique using human red blood cells coupled to gliadin (Cappelle-Desprez) by pyruvic aldehyde in 0.1 M acetic acid. 1, Red blood cell; 2, Gliadin; 3, Anti-gliadin; 4, Anti-human-globulin; 5, Fluorescein isothiocyanate

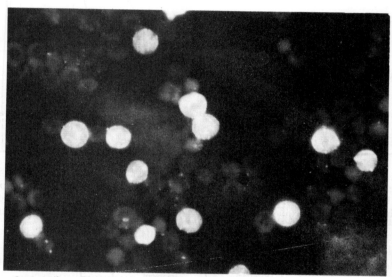

Figure 21.2 Film of 10% gliadin-coated and 90% human albumin-coated human group O red blood cells after incubation with the serum of an untreated coeliac child and with fluorescein-labelled anti-human-IgG. (Fluorescence microscopy, original magnification × 400)

ventional immunofluorescence microscopy was carried out using films of about 10% gliadin-coated mixed up with 90% human albumin-coated red cells for immanent control of specificity. (Figure 21.2).

This control was a condition for semiquantitative evaluation of the test. All antibody activity was shown to be absorbed by preincubation of coeliac sera with a gliadin suspension.

There is a considerable physiochemical and immunogenic heterogeneity of gliadin proteins among different wheat varieties. In order to get a defined starting material we used gliadin prepared from the common European wheat variety Cappelle-Desprez.

By ion exchange chromatography on carboxymethyl cellulose (CMC) eight main fractions were prepared using a sodium acetate buffer pH 3.5 with dimethyl formamide and sequence of sodium chloride gradients according to Patey and Evans[5] (Figure 21.3).

These fractions were identified by means of polyacrylamide disk electrophoresis at pH 2.3, modified after Narayan *et al.*[6] (Figure 21.4).

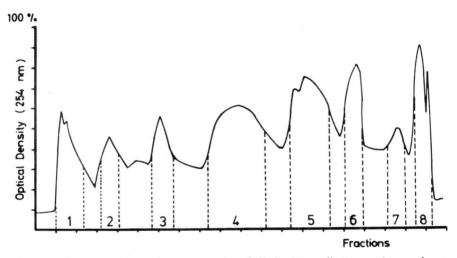

Figure 21.3 Ion exchange chromatography of gliadin (Cappelle-Desprez) on carboxymethyl cellulose (CMC) using a sodium acetate buffer pH 3.5 containing 1 molar dimethyl formamide. Sequence of sodium chloride gradients from 10 to 500 mM. (Patey and Evans[5])

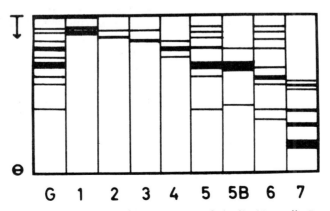

Figure 21.4 Polyacrylamide disk electrophoresis of gliadin (Cappelle-Desprez) at pH 2.3, 5 mA/tube, run 2 hours. (Modified after Narayan *et al.*[6]) G, Gliadin; 1–7, CMC fractions of gliadin 1–7 (Figure 21.3); 5B, Alpha-gliadin after further purification on Sephadex G-100. Migration from top to bottom (cathode)

Glutenin (1) does not penetrate the gel whereas omega- (2), gamma- (3), beta- (4) and crude alpha-gliadin (5) show increasing electrophoretic motility corresponding to their elution sequence on CMC. Wheat albumins and globulin exhibit a spectrum of multiple bands moving in front of gliadin fractions. With the same method we were able to show multiple bands not only confined to the gliadin region using gliadin digests and aqueous wheat flour extracts.

Fifty sera of 45 children were investigated in the coeliac group. The diagnosis was either proven by three jejunal biopsies under different dietary conditions or at least based on the finding of an initial 'flat' mucosa and subsequent clinical remission on a gluten-free diet. Coeliac children on normal diets all showed a 'flat' mucosa including some children on gluten challenge. The 25 coeliac children on gluten-free management all had a normal jejunal mucosa.

Fifty children with various gastrointestinal (GI) disorders (gastro-enteritis, postenteritis malabsorption, cow's milk protein intolerance, cystic fibrosis, ulcerative colitis, Crohn's disease) served as controls as well as 50 normal children and 50 healthy adult blood donors. Coeliac disease had been excluded by biopsy in the majority of GI controls.

RESULTS

All coeliac children had IgG gliadin antibodies in their sera. (Figure 21.5) High titres were almost exclusively present in the coeliac group on normal diets. The IgG antibody titres were diminished on a gluten-free diet of at least three months. These findings were well correlated with the strictness of adherence to the therapy.

Mostly low titres of IgG-anti-gliadin were found in 50% of controls with various GI disorders, in 6% of normal children, and in 4% of healthy blood donors. Although there was a slight overlap between coeliac sera on a gluten-containing diet and the GI control sera, these groups could be distinguished in most cases by IgG antibody titre alone. Distinction is also possible in the coeliac group between different dietary conditions and consequently different jejunal morphology.

Follow-up in a small series of six coeliac patients in the course of gluten-free management showed an initial rise after elimination of the antigenic protein from food and thereafter a slow decline in IgG-anti-gliadin titres (Figure 21.6). There has been no completely negative result even after ten years of gluten-free diet in coeliac children.

Utilizing the purified alpha-, beta-, gamma-, and omega-fractions of gliadin, glutenin, and the pooled wheat albumins and globulins coupled to red cells, we were able to detect IgG antibody activities against alpha-gliadin and against albumins and globulins of wheat (Figure 21.7). There were no immunofluorescent antibodies against

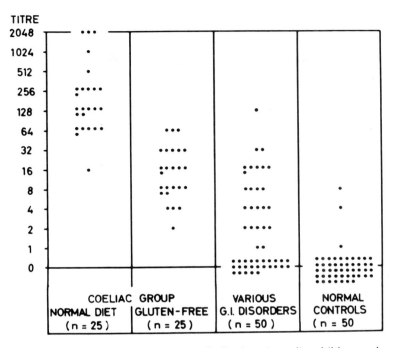

Figure 21.5 Immunofluorescent IgG-anti-gliadin titres in coeliac children and control groups. GI, Gastrointestinal

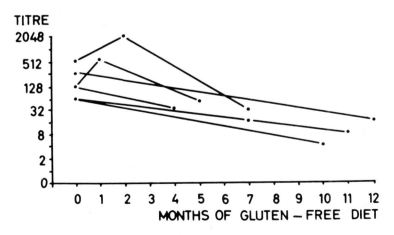

Figure 21.6 IgG-anti-gliadin titres before therapy and in the course of gluten-free management

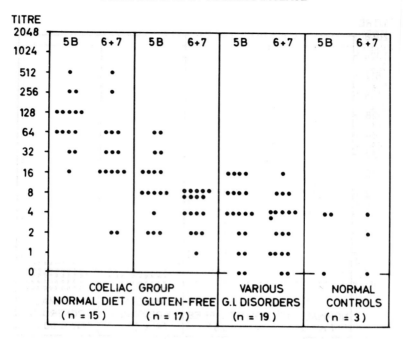

Figure 21.7 IgG antibodies to gliadin fractions in coeliac children and control groups. (Compare Figures 21.3 and 21.4). 5B, alpha-gliadin fraction; 6+7, wheat albumins and globulins, pooled

the remaining wheat protein fractions. Titres of antibodies to the noxious alpha-gliadin fraction did not differ significantly from titres to the harmless water-soluble albumins and globulins. Positive control sera did not show any difference with respect to the antigenic wheat fractions as well. Testing the fraction specificity of antibodies, we could not find any cross-absorption by the fractions used.

IgM-anti-gliadin was found in 96% of coeliac children on a normal diet and in 76% of treated coeliacs (Figure 21.8). IgM antibodies were not as closely correlated with dietary conditions as IgG-anti-gliadin, They could be demonstrated in only 6% of the GI controls and in none of the remaining controls. There were no specific differences in IgM antibodies to the wheat protein fractions used.

IgA-anti-gliadin was found in 20% of coeliac children on a normal diet. IgE antibodies were shown in 8% of the same group. IgD antibodies to gliadin could not be detected at all by immunofluorescence.

Reference data for the same sera were taken by passive haemagglutination using tanned red cells coated with Frazer's Fraction III[7] according to Taylor et al.[8], by microimmunodiffusion using saline extracts of

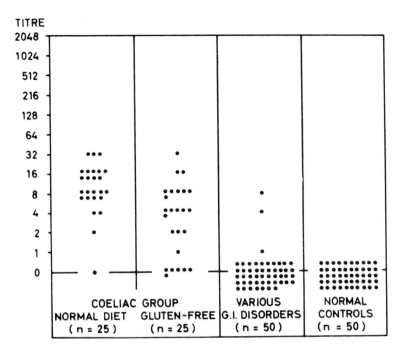

Figure 21.8   Immunofluorescent IgM-anti-gliadin titres in coeliac children and control groups

Table 21.1   Comparison of methods. Wheat protein antibodies

	IF	HA	MID	ID
Coeliac group normal diet	100%	73%	27%	7%
Coeliac group gluten-free	100%	47%	12%	0%
Various GI disorders	50%	38%	9%	0%
Normal controls	6%	18%	3%	0%

GI   Gastrointestinal
IF   Indirect immunofluorescence: IgG-anti-gliadin
HA   Passive haemagglutination (Taylor *et al.*[8])
MID Microimmunodiffusion (Heiner *et al.*[9])
ID   Combined serum electrophoresis and immuno-diffusion (Rossipal[10])

gliadin according to Heiner et al.[9], and by combined serum electro-phoresis and immunodiffusion using an aqueous wheat flour extract according to Rossipal[10] (Table 21.1). The comparability of methods is closely limited by the different starting materials used, in that there are wheat proteins much more saline-soluble than gliadin with its poor solubility in neutral salt solutions. In our series there is a remarkable decline in sensitivity from immunofluorescence over haemagglutination up to immunodiffusion.

DISCUSSION

The immunofluorescent gliadin antibody test using gliadin-coated red cells proved to be superior to the other methods used in our study. By this test we were able to find reliable, though not conclusive, distinc-tions between the groups tested. The sensitive immunofluorescent method allowed us to reinforce the correlations between food antibody titres and dietary conditions in coeliac disease which were demonstrated before in reports[11-13] using different methods.

Our results agree roughly with recent reports on immunofluorescent gliadin antibodies[14,15] with regard to the predominant role of IgG-anti-gliadin antibodies in serum and to the frequency of positive results in coeliac patients. Differences in detail are almost certainly due to minor differences in the techniques.

In our series of 45 coeliac children, serum gliadin antibodies were shown to be mostly IgG and IgM, in some cases IgA, and infrequently IgE immunoglobulins. Antibodies are directed against alpha-gliadin and against wheat albumins and globulins. Because of the discrepancy between noxious and immunogenic properties of wheat proteins in man and because of low titres of gliadin antibodies in conditions other than coeliac disease, we conclude serum gliadin antibodies to be an epi-phenomenon of the mucosal lesion in coeliac disease. There is no direct support for a primary pathogenic role of these antibodies from our investigations.

Although there is no replacement of jejunal biopsy in the diagnosis of coeliac disease by any laboratory test at present, we propose the immunofluorescent gliadin antibody assay to be helpful in pre-estimating children with atypical gastrointestinal complaints and in assessing the strictness of adherence to gluten-free management in coeliac patients.

References

1. Berger, E. (1958). Zur allergischen Pathogenese der Coeliakie. Mit Versuchen über die Spaltung pathogener Antigene durch Fermente. *Ann. Paediatr.,* **67** (Suppl.), 1
2. Beckwith, A. C. and Heiner , D. C. (1966). An immunological study of wheat gluten proteins and derivatives. *Arch. Biochem. Biophys.,* **117,** 239
3. Mietens, C. (1967). Untersuchungen über Antikörperbildung gegen Gliadin und Milchproteine. II. Der Nachweis von αM durch Ultrazentrifugation und Behandlung mit Mercaptoäthanol. *Z. Kinderheilkd.,* **99,** 130
4. Ling, N. R. (1961). The attachment of proteins to aldehyde-tanned cells. *Br. J. Haematol.,* **7,** 299
5. Patey, A. L. and Evans, D. J. (1973). Large-scale preparation of gliadin proteins. *J. Sci. Food Agric.,* **24,** 1229
6. Narayan, K. A., Vogel, M. and Lawrence, J. H. (1965). Disk electrophoresis of wheat flour proteins with a modified apparatus utilizing gels of rectangular cross-section. *Anal. Biochem.,* **12,** 526
7. Frazer, A. C., Fletcher, R. F., Ross, C. A. C., Shaw, B. Sammons, H. G. and Schneider, R. (1959). Gluten-induced enteropathy. The effect of partially d' ,ted gluten. *Lancet,* **ii,** 252
8. Taylor, K. B., Truelove, S. C., Thomson, D. L. and Wright, R. (1961). An immunological study of coeliac disease and idiopathic steatorrhea. Serological reactions to gluten and milk proteins. *Br. Med. J.,* **2,** 1727
9. Heiner, D. C., Lahey, M. E., Wilson, J. F., Gerrard, J. W., Shwachman, H. and Khaw, K. T. (1962). Precipitins to antigens of wheat and cow's milk in coeliac disease. *J. Pediat.,* **61,** 813
10. Rossipal, E. (1971). Nachweis von präcipitierenden Antikörpern gegen waβrige Mehlextrakte bei Coeliakie. *Z. Kinderheilkd.,* **110,** 188
11. Carswell, F. and Ferguson, A. (1973). Plasma food antibodies during withdrawal and reintroduction of dietary gluten in coeliac disease. *Arch. Dis. Child.,* **48,** 583
12. Baker, P. G., Barry, R. E. and Read, A. E. (1975). Detection of continuing gluten ingestion in treated coeliac patients. *Br. Med. J.,* **i,** 486
13. Kumar, P. J., Ferguson, A., Lancaster-Smith, M. and Clark, M. L. (1976). Food antibodies in patients with dermatitis herpetiformis and adult coeliac disease. Relationship to jejunal morphology. *Scand. J. Gastroenterol.,* **11,** 5
14. Bürgin-Wolff, A., Hernandez, R., Just, M. and Signer, E. (1976). Immunofluorescent antibodies against gliadin: a screening test for coeliac disease. *Helv. Paediat. Acta,* **31,** 375
15. Eterman, K. P., Hekkens, W. Th. J. M., Peña, A. S., Lems-van Kan, P. H. and Feltkamp, T. E. W. (1977). Wheat grains: a substrate for the determination of gluten antibodies in serum of gluten-sensitive patients. *J. Immunol. Methods,* **14,** 85

Discussion of chapter 21

Ellis	In the gastrointestinal group how many did you exclude consistent with coeliac disease?
Stern	Exclusion of coeliac disease was performed by biopsy in about 80% of gastrointestinal controls, that means not in the cases of ulcerative colitis and Crohn's disease but in all cases of post-enteritis, malabsorption, and in cases of unclear diarrhoea.
Ellis	In the ones with the positive titres in this control group, were other diseases excluded?
Stern	There are positive titres in controls, but they are distinct from coeliac titres by height.
Ferguson	Had the ones with positive titres jejunal biopsies?
Stern	In the majority of gastrointestinal controls including all patients with IgG antigliadin titres above 8 biopsies were done, and they were all shown to be normal.
Kasarda	I was curious as you found that there were antibodies developed to your alpha-gliadin fraction but not to your other fractions. Do you have any speculations as to why there is a response only to the alpha-gliadin? It seems to me that people have reported that antibodies can be obtained by way of animals to all the gliadin components. Why do you suppose in the case of human beings you find antibodies only to the alpha-gliadins?
Stern	I don't have any explanation for that. I found myself rabbit antibodies after parenteral immunization with total gliadin directed against alpha-, beta- and gamma- not against omega-gliadin, and against albumins and globulins, but in the human material we did not find these results.
Ferguson	I thought that was an important and clear paper differentiating immunogenicity from pathogenicity and something we need to remember for the next couple of days.

22

Immunoglobulin staining in the skin of patients with gastrointestinal disease: specificity and significance of IgA deposition in dermatitis herpetiformis

I. N. ROSS, R. A. THOMPSON, R. D. MONTGOMERY and **P. ASQUITH**

INTRODUCTION

An association between dermatitis herpetiformis (DH) and a small intestinal mucosal lesion resembling that of coeliac disease was first reported by Marks, Shuster and Watson (1966)[1]. Since that time various authors have reported this mucosal lesion present in 25 to 100% of patients with DH[1-9]. However, even in those patients with DH thought to have a normal jejunal mucosa on an ordinary diet, mucosal abnormalities, such as an increase in intraepithelial cell lymphocytes and lamina propria plasma cells, may be induced by stressing with large gluten loads[10,11]. Patchiness of the mucosal lesion may be an additional cause of the discrepancy between the incidences of flat mucosae in DH[2,4,6,60]. Although there are characteristic distinct for both CD and DH there are also many features, other than small intestinal mucosal lesions, that strengthen the association between these two diseases (Table 22.1).

Table 22.1 Similar features and dissimilar features found in CD and DH

Feature	CD	DH	References
Subtotal villous atrophy	+	+ or −	1–9
Symptomatic malabsorption	+	−	2
Increased intraepithelial lymphocytes	+	+	11
Increased numbers of immunoglobulin containing cells in jejunal mucosa	+	+	7,8
Increased *in vitro* jejunal mucosal IgA synthesis	+	+	4
Increased concentration of IgA in jejunal juice	−	+	12,13
Inhibition of *in vitro* alkaline phosphatase increase of epithelial cells by gluten peptides	+	−	4
Gastric mucosal atrophy	+ or −	+	14–17
Splenic atrophy	+	+	18,19
Anti-reticulin antibodies	+	+	20,61
Increased autoantibodies against thyroid, gastric parietal cells and nuclei	−	+	17, 20, 21
Increased serum antibodies to dietary proteins	+	+	22, 23
Serum gluten antibodies	+	−	23
Immune complex formation	+	+	24–26
Serum IgM decreased	+	+ or −	7, 8, 13, 27, 28
Specific B-cell antigens	+	+	29
Increased incidence of HLA–DW3 and HLA–B8	+	+	4, 6, 30–36, 62
Gluten-free diet beneficial	+	+	57

A characteristic marker for the diagnosis of DH is the presence of IgA deposits in areas of normal or peri-lesional skin, as granular or linear deposits at the dermal–epidermal junction (DEJ)[37–39]. Although cutaneous IgA deposition may be seen in some other skin diseases, it is not usually found in skin from normal individuals[40]. In view of the fact that DH may appear some years after the diagnosis of CD[2,41,42] and because of the strong association between the two diseases described above, it seemed pertinent to examine the skin of patients with coeliac disease for the presence of abnormalities such as IgA deposits, that might indicate a predispostion to the development of DH.

PATIENTS AND METHODS

An ellipse of skin 0.5 cm in length was removed from the extensor surface of the proximal area of the forearm in 16 patients with CD, all on a gluten-free diet, 48 patients with other forms of gastrointestinal disease (Table 22.2) and five individuals without gastrointestinal abnor-

Table 22.2   Nature of gastrointestinal abnormality in 48 patients without coeliac disease

Disease	Number
Alpha-chain disease	1
Abdominal pain	1
Crohn's disease	11
Gastric carcinoma	1
Ileocaecal tuberculosis	2
Intestinal lymphangiectasia	2
Intestinal malabsorption	3
'Irritable bowel syndrome'	13
Oral fibrosis	1
Oral granulomata	4
Oral ulceration	3
Post-gastrectomy diarrhoea	1
Thyrotoxic diarrhoea	1
Ulcerative colitis	4

malities. All subjects gave informed consent. Any individuals who gave a history of a previous specific skin disease were excluded from the study.

The biopsy specimen was divided and one part was examined histologically while the other part was snap-frozen. 6 μm sections were examined by direct immunofluorescence for the presence of immunoglobulins and complement (C3) using monospecific anti-IgA, IgG, IgM and C3 conjugated with fluorescein isothiocyanate. Immunofluorescence examination of the skin biopsies was performed by one of us (R.A.T.) on all specimens without prior knowledge of the patients' diagnoses.

Anti-reticulin antibodies were measured in serum by indirect immunofluorescence.

Statistical analysis was performed using the chi-square test and applying Yates' correction.

RESULTS

The nature and distribution of immunoglobulins, and complement in the skin of those patients who were found to have IgA staining in their skin biopsies, are shown in Table 22.3.

Table 22.3 The nature and distribution in the skin of immunoglobulins and complement, found in 9 out of 16 coeliac patients and 5 out of 48 patients with other gastrointestinal disease, all of whom had IgA staining in their skin biopsies

Diagnosis	Papillary	DEJ* 'blobs'	DEJ* granular	Dermal vessels	Dermis
Coeliac disease		IgA IgM			
,,		IgA IgM			IgG
,,		IgM	IgA IgG IgM	IgA IgM C**	
,, + DH		IgM	IgA IgM C		
,,		IgM	IgA		
,,		IgA IgM			
,,	IgA IgG C		IgA IgG C		
,,		IgA IgM			
,,	IgA	IgA IgM	IgA IgM	IgM	IgG
Crohn's disease		IgM	IgM	IgA	IgA
Irritable bowel syndrome	IgG		IgA		
Ileocaecal tubercolosis				IgA	
Alpha-chain disease					IgA
Oral fibrosis	IgA IgM				IgG

* Dermal–epidermal junction
** Complement

IgA in skin

One patient with CD was found to have clinical, histological and immunohistological evidence of DH (occurring 8 years after the diagnosis of CD)[42] and was excluded from the statistical study. Eight out of 15 patients with CD had IgA present in their skin biopsies. This was in the form of granular deposits at the DEJ in 4 patients and as IgA globules or 'blobs' at the DEJ in 5 patients. In addition one patient had staining of the dermal vessels with IgA, while another, who had IgA 'blobs', had an infiltration of the dermis with occasional IgA containing cells. Only one of these 8 patients with IgA deposits complained of a rash which had occurred before starting the gluten-free diet seven years previously.

Five out of the 48 patients with other forms of gastrointestinal disease had IgA deposits in their skin biopsies; however, in only two was this deposition in the DEJ. One of these five patients, with dermal vessel deposition of IgA was found to have cryofibrinogenaemia coexistent with his ileocaecal tuberculosis, while another patient who had alpha-heavy chain disease, had generalized increased staining of the dermis with IgA.

The incidence of IgA staining in the skin of patients with CD was significantly greater ($p<0.05$) than that seen in the gastrointestinal control group.

IgA was not seen in the skin of the five individuals without gastrointestinal disease.

IgG in skin

Although IgG was present in 6 out of 15 patients with CD and in only 7 out of 48 patients without CD, this difference was not statistically significant.

IgM in skin

IgM staining usually as a granular deposition, but with the occasional IgM 'blob' at the DEJ was present in 73% of CD patients, 69% of the patients with other forms of gastrointestinal disease and 60% (3 out of 5) of the individuals without gastrointestinal disease.

Complement in skin

Complement was present in 3 out of 15 patients with CD, but in none of the other 53 patients studied. In one patient it was present at the DEJ, while in the other two including one individual without any visible IgA staining it was present in the dermal vessels.

Histological examination

Apart from the patient with DH, none of the other individuals with IgA in their skin had any significant histological abnormality.

Anti-reticulin antibodies

There was no correlation between the deposition of IgA in the skin and the presence of serum anti-reticulin antibodies.

DISCUSSION

This study has shown that in a group of patients with CD, there was a significantly higher ($p<0.05$) number of patients with IgA deposition in their skin, when compared to individuals without CD. Furthermore the IgA deposits in CD appeared to be confined to the region of the DEJ unlike the majority of the latter group.

There has only been one other study reporting the immunofluorescence appearance of skin in CD[18], which described the presence of IgA globules or 'blobs' in 11 out of 22 patients with CD; only one patient showed papillary deposits of IgA and was concluded to be suffering from DH. The same authors also noted IgA 'blobs' in 2 out of 6 control, non-coeliac disease, patients and concluded that these 'blobs' of immunoglobulins represented a non-specific extravasation of IgA into the skin. However, IgA is rarely reported in other studies of skin immunofluorescence. In one study specifically designed to determine the immunofluorescent appearance of normal skin[40], no IgA deposits were found in 23 healthy individuals. In contrast these same authors found a granular deposit of IgM in the DEJ of 5 out of 23 biopsies examined and the IgG in 3 out of 23. They suggest that the common finding of IgM deposition in skin, as found in the study reported here, may represent the residual products of immunological defence that have become trapped in the peripheral capillaries. An alternative explanation is that the IgM deposits represent immuno-conglutinins formed against complement components in the skin[40,51].

An abnormal histological appearance and perhaps immunofluorescent appearance of the skin might be expected in a small number of patients with CD as various dermatological conditions may be found in association with CD[43–50,63]. However, none of the CD patients studied here had any recognizable skin disease.

Although the immunofluorescent appearances of these CD patients are definite, they are minimal and are not typical of the characteristic IgA deposition found in DH. They may, nonetheless, reflect involvement of the skin in a similar pathogenic process to that causing the intestinal lesion. The absence of IgA in some of these patients with CD may either be due to a sampling error, which may occur even in DH[39] or to the presence of selective IgA deficiency, found in one patient of the present series.

It has been postulated that the deposition of IgA in the skin in DH results from increased permeability of the damaged intestinal mucosa to IgA immune complexes which pass into the circulation and lodge in the dermal vessels due to their size[52]. However, the cutaneous IgA deposition of DH does not appear to be secretory IgA[53,54]. Alternatively, there could be a cross-reaction between the indicating antigen in CD and the skin structure, as it has been suggested that anti-reticulin antibodies present in patients with DH may be absorbed out by gluten and gluten fraction III[18].

If the findings of IgA depostion in the skin of patients with CD described here have any relevance to the CD/DH relationship, then reasons why these individuals do not have the more classical clinical, histological and immunofluorescent appearances of DH may be: (1) a latent period before the appearance of DH[2,18,19,41,55], or (2) the control of any clinical symptoms by a gluten-free diet[56–58].

Finally, the occurrence of IgA in a very small number of non-coeliac gastrointestinal controls is difficult to explain, except for the patient with alpha-heavy chain disease where the marked appearance of diffuse IgA in the dermis may have resulted from the diffusion of the low molecular weight alpha-heavy chain (38 000 daltons)[59] from the circulation.

ACKNOWLEDGEMENT

We would like to thank Dr R. G. F. Parker for reporting the routine histology of the skin biopsies.

References

1. Marks, J., Shuster, S. and Watson, A. J. (1966). Small bowel changes in dermatitis herpetiformis. *Lancet*, **ii**, 1280
2. Brow, J. R., Parker, F., Weinstein, W. M. and Rubin, C. E. (1971). The small intestinal mucosa in dermatitis herpetiformis. Severity of and distribution of the small intestinal lesion and associated malabsorption. *Gastroenterology*, **60**, 355
3. Fry, L., Seah, P. P., Harper., P. G., Hoffbrand, A. V. and McMinn, R. M. H. (1974). The small intestine in dermatitis herpetiformis. *J. Clin. Pathol.*, **27**, 817
4. Gebhard, R. L., Falchuk, Z. M., Katz, S. I., Sessoms, C., Rogentine, G. N. and Strober, W. (1974). Dermatitis herpetiformis. Immunologic concomitants of small intestinal disease and relationship to histocompatibility antigen HL–A8. *J. Clin. Invest.*, **54**, 98
5. Ruppin, H., Weidner, F., Domschke, S., Domschke, W., Classen M. and Hornstein, O. P. (1975). Dermatitis herpetiformis and small intestinal lesion—no strict association in German patients. *Acta Hepatogastroenterol.*, **22**, 105
6. Scott, B. B., Young, S., Rajah, S. M., Marks, J. and Losowsky, M. S. (1976). Coeliac disease and dermatitis herpetiformis: further studies of their relationship. *Gut*, **17**, 759
7. Baklien, K., Brandtzaeg, P. and Fausa, O. (1977). Immunoglobulins in jejunal mucosa and serum from patients with adult coeliac disease. *Scand. J. Gastroenterol.*, **12**, 149
8. Baklien, K., Fausa, O., Thune, P. O. and Gjone, E. (1977). Immunoglobulins in jejunal mucosa and serum from patients with dermatitis herpetiformis. *Scand. J. Gastroenterol.*, **12**, 161
9. Katz, S. I., Hertz, K. C., Rogentine, G. N. and Strober, W. (1977). HLA–B8 and dermatitis herpetiformis in patients with IgA deposits in the skin. *Arch. Dermatol.*, **113**, 155
10. Weinstein, W. M. (1974). Latent coeliac sprue. *Gastroenterology*, **66**, 489
11. Lancaster-Smith, M., Kumar, P. J. and Dawson, A. M. (1975). The cellular infiltrate of the jejunum in adult coeliac disease and dermatitis herpetiformis following the reintroduction of dietary gluten. *Gut*, **16**, 683
12. McClelland, D. B. L., Banretson, R. St. C., Parkin, D. M., Warwick, R. R. G., Heading, R. C. and Shearman, D. J. C. (1972). Small intestine immunoglobulin levels in dermatitis herpetiformis. *Lancet*, **ii**, 1108

13. Lancaster-Smith, M., Kumar, P., Marks, R., Clark, M. L. and Dawson, A. M. (1974). Jejunal mucosal immunoglobulin-containing cells and jejunal fluid immunoglobulins in adult coeliac disease and dermatitis herpetiformis. *Gut*, **15**, 371

14. Hansky, J. and Shiner, M. (1963). Gastric studies in idiopathic steatorrhoea. *Gastroenterology*, **45**, 49

15. O'Donoghue, D. P., Lancaster-Smith, M., Johnson, G. D. and Kumar, P. J. (1976). Gastric lesion in dermatitis herpetiformis. *Gut*, **17**, 185

16. Fausa, O. (1974). Reduction of gastric acid secretion and gastritis in dermatitis herpetiformis. In: *Coeliac Disease. Proceedings of the Second International Coeliac Symposium*. Hekkens, W. Th. J. M. and Peña, A. S. (eds.) p. 373. (Leiden: Stenfert Kroese)

17. Lancaster-Smith, M., Kumar, P. and Johnson, G. (1974). Atrophic gastritis and dermatitis herpetiformis. *Lancet*, **ii**, 777

18. Seah, P. P., Stewart, J. S., Fry, L., Chapman, B. L., Hoffbrand, A. V. and Holborow, E. J. (1972). Immunoglobulins in the skin in dermatitis herpetiformis and coeliac disease. *Lancet*, **i**, 611

19. Marsh, G. W. and Stewart, J. S. (1970). Splenic function in adult coeliac disease. *Br. J. Haematol.*, **19**, 445

20. Seah, P. P., Fry, L., Hoffbrand, A. V. and Holborow, E. J. (1971). Tissue antibodies in dermatitis herpetiformis and adult coeliac disease. *Lancet*, **i**, 834

21. Fraser, N. G. (1970). Autoantibodies in dermatitis herpetiformis. *Br. J. Dermatol.*, **83**, 609

22. Kumar, P. J., Ferguson, A., Lancaster-Smith, M. and Clark, M. L. (1976). Food antibodies in patients with dermatitis herpetiformis—relationship to jejunal morphology. *Scand. J. Gastroenterol.*, **11**, 5

23. Scott, B. B. and Losowsky, M. S. (1976). Proceedings: gluten antibodies (GA) in coeliac disease (CD) and dermatitis herpetiformis (DH). *Gut*, **17**, 398

24. Mowbray, J. F. Holborow, E. J., Hoffbrand, A. V., Seah, P. P. and Fry, L. (1973). Circulating immune complexes in dermatitis herpetiformis. *Lancet*, **i**, 400

25. Mohammed, I., Holborow, E. J., Fry, L., Thompson, B. R., Hoffbrand, A. V. and Stewart, J. S. (1976). Multiple immune complexes and hypocomplementaemia in dermatitis herpetiformis and coeliac disease. *Lancet*, **ii**, 487

26. Teisberg, P., Baklein, K., Fauso, O. and Thune, P. O. (1976). Mediator mechanisms of humoral immunity in patients with dermatitis herpetiformis and enteropathy. *Scand. J. Gastroenterol.*, **11**, Suppl. 38, 21

27. Fry, L., Keir, P., McMinn, R. M. H., Cowan, J. D. and Hoffbrand, A. V. (1967). Small-intestinal structure and function and haematological changes in dermatitis herpetiformis. *Lancet*, **ii**, 729

28. Fraser, N. G., Dick, H. M. and Crichton, W. B. (1969). Immunoglobulins in dermatitis herpetiformis and various other skin conditions. *Br. J. Dermatol.*, **81**, 89

29. Mann, D. L., Katz, S. I., Nelson, D. L., Abelson, L. D. and Strober, W. (1976). Specific B-cell antigens associated with gluten sensitive enteropathy and dermatitis herpetiformis. *Lancet*, **i**, 110

30. Renuala, T., Salo, O. P., Tiilikainen, A. and Matilla, M. J. (1976). Histocompatibility antigens and dermatitis herpetiformis with special reference to jejunal abnormalities and acetylator phenotype. *Br. J. Dermatol.*, **94**, 139

31. Gebhard, R. L., Katz, S. I., Marks, J., Shuster, S., Rogentine, G. N., Trapani, R. J. and Strober, W. (1973). HL–A antigen type and small intestinal disease in dermatitis herpetiformis. *Lancet*, **ii**, 760

32. Falchuk, Z. M., Rogentine, G. N. and Strober, W. (1972). Predominance of histocompatibility antigen HL–A8 in patients with gluten-sensitive enteropathy. *J. Clin. Invest.*, **51**, 1602

33. Katz, S. I., Falchuk, Z. M., Dahl, M. V., Rogentine, G. N. and Strober, W. (1972). HL–A8: agenetic link between dermatitis herpetiformis and gluten-sensitive enteropathy. *J. Clin. Invest.*, **51**, 2977

34. Keuning, J. J., Peña, A. S., van Leeuwen, A., van Hoof, J. P. and van Rood, J. J. (1976) HLA–DW3 associated with coeliac disease. *Lancet*, **i**, 506

35. Thomsen, M., Platz, P., Marks, J. M., Ryder, L. P., Shuster, S., Svejgaard, A. and Young, S. H. (1976). Association of LD–8a and LD–12a with dermatitis herpetiformis. *Tissue Antigens*, **7**, 60

36. Solheim, B. G., Ek, J., Thune, P. O., Baklein, K., Bratlie, A., Rankin, B., Thoresen, A. B. and Thorsby, E. (1976). *Tissue Antigens*, **7**, 57

37. van der Meer, J. B. (1969). Granular deposits of immunoglobulins in the skin of patients with dermatitis herpetiformis, an immunofluorescent study. *Br. J. Dermatol.*, **81**, 493

38. Chorzelski, T. P., Beutner, E. H., Jablonska, S., Blaszczyk, M. and Triftshouser, C. (1971). Immunofluorescent studies in the diagnosis of dermatitis herpetiformis and its differentiation from bullous pemphisoid. *J. Invest. Dermatol.*, **56**, 373

39. Seah, P. P. and Fry. L. (1975). Immunoglobulins in the skin in dermatitis herpetiformis and their relevance in diagnosis. *Br. J. Dermatol.*, **92**, 157

40. Baart de la Faille-Kuyper, E. H., van der Meer, J. B. and Baart de la Faille, H. (1974). An immunohistochemical study of the skin of healthy individuals. *Acta Derm. Venereol.*, **54**, 271

41. Weinstein, W. M., Brow, J. R., Parker, F. and Rubin, C. E. (1971). The small intestinal mucosa in dermatitis herpetiformis. Relationship of the small intestinal lesion to gluten. *Gastroenterology*, **60**, 362

42. Ross, I. N. and Asquith, P. (Unpublished observation)

43. Presbury, D. G. C. and Griffiths, W. A. D. (1975). Coeliac disease with primary cutaneous amyloidosis. *Br. J. Dermatol.*, **92**, 109

44. Bedenoch, J. (1960). Steatorrhoea in the adult. *Br. Med. J.*, **2**, 879

45. Wells, G. C. (1962). Skin disorders in relation to malabsorption. *Br. Med.J.*, **2**, 937

46. Green, F. H. Y. and Carty, J. E. (1976). Coeliac disease and autoimmunity. *Lancet*, **i**, 964

47. Pittman, F. E. and Holub, D. A. (1965). Sjogren's syndrome and adult coeliac disease. *Gastroenterology*, **48**, 869

48. Lancaster-Smith, M. J. and Strickland, I. D. (1971). Autoantibodies in adult coeliac disease. *Lancet*, **i**, 1244

49. Siutala, M., Julkunen, H., Toivonen, S., Pelkonen, R., Saxen, E. and Pitkanen, E. (1965). Digestive tract in collagen diseases. *Acta Med. Scand.*, **178**, 13

50. Ferguson, R., Basu, M. J., Asquith, P. and Cooke, W. T. (1975). Recurrent aphthous ulceration and its association with coeliac disease. *Gut*, **16**, 393

51. Lachman, P. J. (1967). Conglutinin and immunoconglutinin. *Adv. Immunol.*, **6**, 522

52. Cochrane, C. G. and Koffler, D. (1973). Immune complex disease in experimental animals and man. *Adv. Immunol.*, **16**, 185

53. Seah, P. P., Fry, L., Mazaheri, M. R., Mowbray, J. F., Hoffbrand, A. V. and Holborow, E. J. (1973). Alternate-pathway complement fixation by IgA in the skin in dermatitis herpetiformis. *Lancet*, **ii**, 175

54. Provost, T. T. and Tomasi, T. B. (1974). Evidence for the activation of complement via the alternate pathway in skin diseases. Dermatitis herpetiformis. *Clin. Immunol. Immunopathol.*, **3**, 178

55. Fraser, N. G., Ferguson, A. and Murray, D. (1968). Dermatitis herpetiformis in two patients with idiopathic steatorrhoea (adult coeliac disease). *Br. Med. J.*, **4**, 30

56. Fry, L., Seah, P. P., Riches, D. J. and Hoffbrand, A. V. (1973). Clearance of skin lesions in dermatitis herpetiformis after gluten withdrawal. *Lancet*, **i**, 288

57. Heading, R. C., Patersen, W. D., McClelland, D. B. L., Barnetson, R. St. C. and Murray, M. S. M. (1976). Clinical response of dermatitis skin lesions to a gluten-free diet. *Br. J. Dermatol.*, **94**, 509

58. Marks, R. and Whittle, M. W. (1969). Results of treatment of dermatitis herpetiformis with a gluten-free diet after one year. *Br. Med. J.*, **4**, 772

59. Ross, I. N. and Asquith, P. (1977). (Unpublished observations)

60. Scott, B. B. and Losowsky, M. S. (1976). Patchiness and duodenal–jejunal variation of the mucosal abnormality in coeliac disease and dermatitis herpetiformis. *Gut,* **17**, 984

61. Lancaster-Smith, M., Kumar, P., Clark, M. L., Marks, R. and Johnson, G. D. (1975). Antireticulin antibodies in dermatitis herpetiformis and adult coeliac disease. Their relationship to a gluten-free diet and jejunal histology. *Br. J. Dermatol.*, **92**, 37

62. Seah, P. P., Fry, L., Kearny, J. W., Campbell, E., Mowbray, J. F., Stewart, J. S. and Hoffbrand, A. V. (1976). A comparison of histocompatibility antigens in dermatitis herpetiformis and adult coeliac disease. *Br. J. Dermatol.*, **94**, 131

63. Bennett, T. I., Hunter, D. and Vaughn, J. M. (1932). Idiopathic steatorrhoea (Gee's disease): a nutritional disturbance associated with tetany, osteomalacia and anaemia. *Q. J. Med.,* New Series, **1**, 603

Discussion of chapter 22

Marks	I should like to say how much I agree with Dr Asquith about the non-specificity of the IgA test for DH, and words to that effect will appear in the September issue of Clinical and Experimental Dermatology. We have looked at rather a different group of patients from Dr Asquith—namely 141 patients with dermatoses other than DH and in four of these we have granular IgA deposits in the dermal papillae identical with those found in DH. One of the patients had contact dermatitis, one atopic eczema, one urticaria pigmentosa and one a practolol reaction. In addition we have looked back at the last 55 patients with DH who had the diagnosis made by 'steam' methods, that is the before skin IgA was used as a diagnostic aid, and are looking at the IgA in them and there are two of the 55 who in all other grounds have DH, and on several occasions we have been unable to demonstrate IgA. So, looking at the test in two ways we have shown that it is not 100% specific and we should be very wary of saying to people without dermatological expertise that they can diagnose DH merely by demonstrating IgA in the appropriate pattern in clinically uninvolved skin. It is not as easy as that and the test does have to to be taken in conjunction with clinical, histological and other relevant findings.
Strober	There is another pattern of distribution of IgA in the skin of DH patients, namely, a smooth or uniform fluorescence. Did any of the coeliac disease patients demonstrate this form of fluorescence?
Asquith	No; our problem is in respect of forming a large group of patients with DH, for comparison with our non-DH coeliacs. We have not got very many DH patients.
Booth	How do you explain the absence of an IgM response in view of the repeated papers in which has been shown an increased IgM cell population in the lamina propria of the untreated patient and Dr Strober's results in relation to challenge *in vitro*?
Asquith	I don't have an adequate explanation but presumably the IgM that is produced by these cells is not involved in an immune complex in the mucosa. What it is doing I don't know!
Falchuk	In relation to that point, I would like to point out that we have studied a number of patients with IgA deficiency and gluten-sensitive disease and in these patients there is a very high value for local IgM production. The antibody may be related to the disease process.

23

Inhibition of leucocyte migration by α-gliadin in patients with gastrointestinal disease: its specificity with respect to α-gliadin and coeliac disease

M. R. HAENEY and P. ASQUITH

INTRODUCTION

When lymphocytes are stimulated *in vitro* by mitogens or specific antigens, a variety of biologically active mediators, termed lymphokines[1], are released. The production of such mediators may serve as a means of communication between sensitized lymphocytes, macrophages and other cells involved in the immune response. They may also serve as biological amplifiers, recruiting and perhaps activating other inflammatory cells at the reaction site.

Antigen-induced inhibition of cell migration was originally described by Rich and Lewis[2]. Sensitized lymphocytes incubated with specific antigen produce a macrophage migration inhibition factor (MIF) which inhibits migration of peritoneal exudate cells obtained from normal guinea pigs[3]. An adaption of this technique utilizes human buffy coat leucocytes as indicator cells[4], their migration being inhibited by a leucocyte inhibitory factor (LIF) which is distinct from MIF by virtue of its size and the type of cell inhibited[5]. Antigen-induced production of MIF and LIF correlates qualitatively with *in vivo* cutaneous cellular hypersensitivity to the same antigen and is independent of concomitant antibody production[6].

Possible cell-mediated immune reactions to gluten fractions in patients with coeliac diseases have been reviewed[7]. Two recent reports[8,9] have suggested that leucocyte migration inhibition (LMI) to gluten occurs in some adult coeliacs. The purpose of the present study is to assess the ability of coeliac leucocytes to respond normally to established antigens. In addition, the frequency of positive LMI tests to α-gliadin in coeliacs and its specificity with respect to α-gliadin and disease state were determined.

Table 23.1   Subjects studied

Diagnostic group	Number in group	Female:male ratio	Age range (years)	Mean age (years)
Coeliac–ND	16	9 : 7	15–62	36.8
Coeliac–GFD	15	11 : 4	16–65	39.0
Gastrointestinal disease—untreated	16	11 : 5	18–70	40.4
Gastrointestinal disease—treated	7	4 : 3	20–57	40.4
Healthy controls	31	20 : 11	18–70	38.9

MATERIALS AND METHODS

Patients studied (Table 23.1)

Eighty-five subjects, classified into five diagnostic groups, have been studied. Group 1 consists of 16 untreated coeliacs ingesting a normal diet (Coeliac–ND). For the purpose of this paper, coeliac disease has been defined as a condition in which there is an abnormal jejunal mucosa with loss of villi, which improves morphologically after treatment with a gluten-free diet. Group 2 comprises 15 coeliacs treated with a gluten-free diet for over one year (Coeliac–GFD). Group 3 is composed of 16 subjects with untreated gastrointestinal diseases, namely Crohn's disease (4), ulcerative colitis (3), a contaminated bowel syndrome secondary to jejunal diverticulosis (3), tropical sprue (2) and single examples of systemic sclerosis, gastro-oesophageal candidiasis, Whipple's disease and chronic pancreatic insufficiency. Group 4 consists of seven patients from Group 3 restudied following apparently successful treatment of their gastrointestinal disease; contaminated bowel syndrome (3), tropical sprue (2), Whipple's disease (1) and gastro-oesophageal candidiasis (1). No patient was receiving steroids. Group 5 was composed of 31 healthy staff controls. They were age- and sex-matched with coeliacs (Table 23.1) and tested in parallel.

Method

Leucocyte migration from capillary tubes[4] was performed in sterile disposable polystyrene trays (Sterilin Ltd., Richmond, England). Particular care was taken to standardize the technique[10]. Leucocytes were obtained by gelatin sedimentation[11] (1 g, 37 °C 30 min) of heparinized (preservative-free heparin, 20 units/ml blood) peripheral venous blood. The leucocyte-rich supernatant was washed three times (150 g, 10 min) in Eagle's minimum essential medium (Eagle's MEM). Leucocytes were counted, the viability assessed by trypan blue exclusion (0.5% in PBS) and leucocytes resuspended to a concentration of 7×10^7/ml in Eagle's medium supplemented with 10% heat inactivated (56 °C, 30 min) fetal calf serum (FCS). Leucocyte viability exceeded 90% in all experiments. Sterilized (dry heat 150 °C, 2 h) 10 μl capillaries (Bilbate Ltd., Daventry, England) were filled with the cell suspension, plugged at one end with paraffin wax and spun in padded test tubes (150 g, 5 min). Packed capillaries were scored at the cell–fluid interface and cut capillaries mounted in pairs, one pair to each well. Wells were immediately filled with medium alone (three wells) or antigen-containing medium (three wells for each antigen dilution) and sealed with sterile coverslips. Completed migration plates were incubated at 37 °C and results initially read at 4, 8, 18 and 24 h but in the latter part of the study at 18 hours only. Migrating fans of cells were magnified by projection microscopy, traced onto paper, and the area measured by planimetry. Results were expressed as a migration index (MI), derived as follows:

$$MI = \frac{\text{Mean (of 6) migration area in antigen-containing medium}}{\text{Mean (of 6) migration area in medium alone}}$$

The viability of migrating cells was reassessed following incubation to exclude non-specific toxicity of antigen. Even in inhibited cultures, leucocyte viability always exceeded 80%.

Antigens

α-Gliadin was a kind gift from Dr R. Schneider. The same batch was used throughout the study. The gliadin subfraction was eluted from a carboxymethylcellulose column with 0.09 M sodium chloride in a dimethyl formamide-containing buffer. This fraction has been shown to be toxic if fed to coeliac patients in remission[12]. The gliadin fraction was solubilized by enzymic hydrolysis[13], freeze-dried, resuspended in phosphate-buffered saline at a concentration of 50 mg/ml, sterilized by millipore filtration and stored in aliquots at −20 °C. Single aliquots

Table 23.2 Effect of α-gliadin concentration on the viability of leucocytes from three normal subjects

α-Gliadin concentration (mg/ml)	Viability (%)			
	1	2	3	Mean
0	92	99	95	95
1	91	99	100	97
2	94	97	88	93
4	85	88	81	85
8	59	52	73	61
16	33	39	41	38
32	42	16	31	30

were thawed as necessary and diluted in Eagle's medium containing 10% heat inactivated FCS to the appropriate final concentrations. Preliminary studies (Table 23.2) in three normal subjects showed α-gliadin to be toxic (viability< 80%) at concentrations of 8 mg/ml. The highest non-toxic dose (4 mg/ml) was therefore subsequently used in all subjects studied and a dose–response relationship obtained using concentrations of 4 mg/ml, 1 mg/ml, 250 μg/ml and 62.5 μg/ml.

α-Lactalbumin (BDH Chemicals Ltd., Poole, England) was subject to similar sterile procedures as those described for α-gliadin and was used at final concentrations of 2 mg/ml, 1 mg/ml and 500 μg/ml after preliminary assessment of its toxicity using leucocyte preparations from normal donors.

Bacille Calmette-Guérin (BCG: Glaxo Laboratories, England) was supplied in ampoules containing 0.3 mg of freeze-dried bacilli and dissolved in culture medium immediately before use to a final concentration of 25, 12.5 and 6.25 μg/ml[14].

Purified protein derivative (PPD) of human *Mycobacterium tuberculosis* was kindly provided by the Central Veterinary Laboratory, Weybridge. PPD was reconstituted as required to a concentration of 2 mg/ml in sterile distilled water, millipore filtered, and further dilutions made in Eagle's medium + 10% FCS to give final culture concentrations of 200, 100 and 50 μg/ml[15,16].

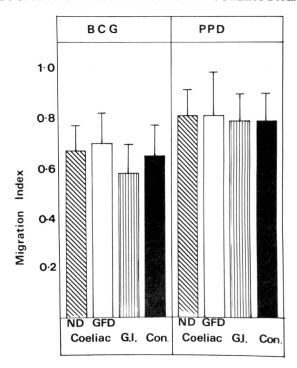

Figure 23.1 Leucocyte migration inhibition (mean±SD) by BCG and PPD in untreated (ND) and treated (GFD) coeliacs, patients with untreated gastrointestinal disease (GI) and healthy controls (Con.)

RESULTS

LMI in coeliacs—assessment of response capacity

Response to BCG

Figure 23.1 shows LMI results for each subject group (mean ± SD). Results in normal diet and gluten-free diet coeliacs are not significantly different from the two control populations.

Response to PPD

There is no significant difference between any of the groups in their LMI responses to PPD (Figure 23.1), although the mean migration indices are higher than those obtained for particulate antigen (BCG).

Leucocyte migration responses to α-gliadin

Length of incubation period

Although 18–21 h incubation is usually regarded as the optimum time

Table 23.3 Optimum culture time for α-gliadin in ten coeliacs (8 GFD, 2 ND)

Culture period (hours)	Number showing lowest M.I. after this time	Number showing significant inhibition after this time
4	0	0
8	2	0
18	7	5
24	1	1

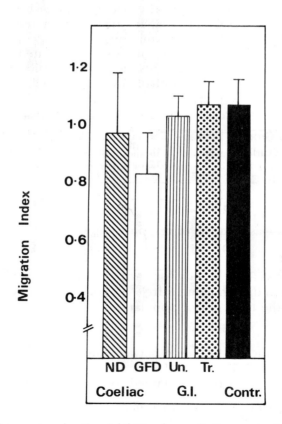

Figure 23.2 Leucocyte migration inhibition by α-gliadin: comparison of responses (mean$\pm$SD) in untreated coeliacs, untreated (Un.) and treated (Tr.) gastrointestinal patients and healthy controls (Contr.)

at which inhibition is likely to occur, each new antigen must be assessed individually[10]. For α-gliadin, results of LMI were read at 4, 8, 18 and 24 h for a group of ten coeliacs (Table 23.3). Results show that significant migration inhibition (5 individuals) was only observed after 18 hours' culture. Inhibition in one individual was also seen at 24 h. Using α-gliadin there was no evidence of an 'escape' from inhibition, i.e. evidence of inhibition during the first 6–8 h of culture which disappeared after 18 h. This 'escape' phenomenon has been demonstrated both for PPD[17] and BCG[18] in Mantoux-positive individuals. In the present study, escape from inhibition was occasionally seen for PPD[19].

Comparison of means

Figure 23.2 shows the migration indices (mean±SD) after 18 hours' culture in the presence of α-gliadin (4 mg/ml) in each subject group. Maximum inhibition is seen in coeliacs ingesting a gluten-free diet, and is significantly greater than in normal diet coeliacs ($p = 0.05$), healthy controls ($p < 0.001$) and subjects with other untreated ($p < 0.001$) or treated ($p < 0.005$) gastrointestinal diseases. Mean inhibition in normal diet coeliacs is greater than in control populations, but not significantly so.

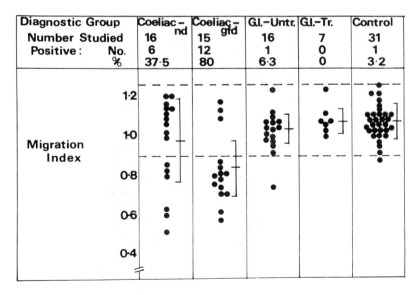

Diagnostic Group		Coeliac – nd	Coeliac – gfd	G.I.–Untr.	G.I.–Tr.	Control
Number Studied		16	15	16	7	31
Positive :	No.	6	12	1	0	1
	%	37·5	80	6·3	0	3·2

Figure 23.3 Leucocyte migration inhibition by α-gliadin: individual results in untreated (nd) and treated (gfd) coeliacs, untreated (Untr.) and treated (Tr.) gastrointestinal patients and healthy controls. Vertical barred lines represent Mean±SD. Horizontal lines indicate normal range (see text)

The normal range (mean ± 2 SD) for the test in 31 healthy controls is 0.89–1.25, while the corresponding ranges for the untreated and treated control groups are very similar at 0.89–1.17 and 0.91–1.23 respectively. These results suggest a slight enhancing effect of α-gliadin on the migration of leucocytes from some non-coeliac individuals. Individual migration indices of less than 0.89 can therefore be taken as showing hypersensitivity to α-gliadin.

Individual results

Figure 23.3 depicts individual migration indices to α-gliadin (4 mg/ml, 18 hours' incubation). Eighty per cent of treated (GFD) coeliacs and 37.5% of untreated (ND) coeliacs show migration inhibition to α-gliadin, compared with only 3.7% of a non-coeliac population.

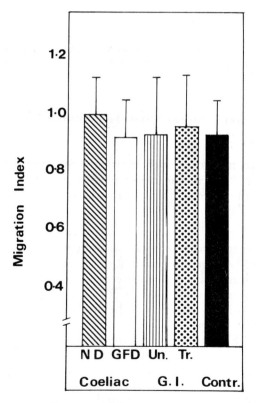

Figure 23.4 Leucocyte migration inhibition by α-lactalbumin: comparison of responses (mean±SD) in untreated (ND) and treated (GFD) coeliacs, untreated (Un.) and treated (Tr.) gastrointestinal patients and healthy controls (Contr.)

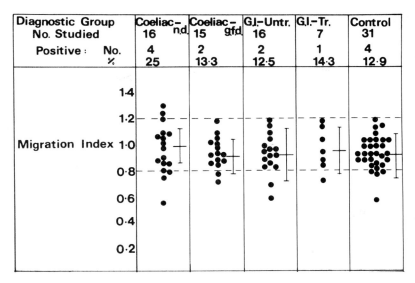

Diagnostic Group No. Studied	Coeliac– nd	Coeliac– gfd	G.I.–Untr.	G.I.–Tr.	Control
	16	15	16	7	31
Positive : No.	4	2	2	1	4
%	25	13·3	12·5	14·3	12·9

Figure 23.5 Leucocyte migration inhibition by α-lactalbumin: individual results in untreated (nd) and treated (gfd) coeliacs, untreated (Untr.) and treated (Tr.) gastrointestinal patients and healthy controls. Vertical barred lines represent mean±SD. Horizontal lines indicate normal range (see text)

Leucocyte migration responses to α-lactalbumin

Comparison of means

Figure 23.4 shows migration indices (mean±SD) for each subject group after 18 hours' culture in the presence of 2 mg/ml of α-lactalbumin. No significant difference in group means can be demonstrated.

Individual results

Figure 23.5 shows individual migration indices to α-lactalbumin (2 mg/ ml; 18 h culture). All groups have some individuals showing definite leucocyte migration inhibition; means are thus less than 1.00 and standard deviations greater than usual. Because no attempt has been made to assess *in vivo* milk sensitivity in the individuals studied (unlike the coeliac population where *in vivo* gluten sensitivity has been demonstrated) it is not known which of these individuals showing LMI to α-lactalbumin are in fact milk-sensitive. Hence the range for LMI to α-lactalbumin in non-sensitized subjects cannot be accurately determined and has been arbitrarily taken as 0.8–1.20. The incidence of LMI to α-lactalbumin is similar in treated coeliacs, treated and untreated gastrointestinal patients and the healthy control population. Inhibition is more frequent in untreated coeliacs, but not significantly so.

DISCUSSION

Before the possible inhibition of coeliac leucocytes to α-gliadin can be assessed, it is first necessary to decide whether their leucocytes are capable of being inhibited by any antigen. BCG and PPD were chosen because most people give positive results in this well-established system[14-16].

This study shows that patients with treated and untreated coeliac disease are capable of showing a normal degree of leucocyte migration inhibition to BCG and PPD and therefore their leucocytes have a normal response capacity in this test. The greater inhibition seen with BCG than with PPD confirms existing reports of the superiority of particulate antigen over soluble antigen[14].

Leucocyte migration inhibition in the presence of α-gliadin occurs in 80% of the treated group, 37.5% of untreated patients and only 3.7% of non-coeliacs and hence is virtually specific for coeliac disease. This pattern is similar to that briefly reported by Bullen and Losowsky[8] using gluten fraction III. They found significant impairment of leucocyte migration in treated, but not in untreated coeliacs, compared with controls, approximately 40% of their treated patients showing inhibition. Douwes[9], using a modification[20] of the LMI test, also showed migration inhibition in the presence of a gluten fraction in a group of 12 coeliacs of unspecified dietary status, while patients with a variety of other gastrointestinal diseases showed no such inhibition. In both studies[8,9], experimental details have not been published.

It is unlikely that the more frequent inhibition in treated coeliacs reflects a non-specific generalized improvement in immune reactivity compared with the untreated populatiom since responsiveness to PPD and BCG is similar in both groups. Although patients with untreated gastrointestinal disease would seem a reasonable control group for untreated coeliac subjects, because most positive results occur in treated coeliacs, a further control group of patients with treated gastrointestinal disease was also studied. Patients with both untreated and treated gastrointestinal conditions do not show any difference in reactivity compared with the healthy control population; thus gastrointestinal disease or treatment of the diseased intestine cannot be held reponsible for the hypersensitivity to α-gliadin shown by those with coeliac disease.

The observed differences, with respect to α-gliadin, between coeliacs and other subjects could reflect non-specific intestinal permeability to many dietary antigens, secondary to villous atrophy. However, this is unlikely in view of the absence of any difference in mean LMI to α-lactalbumin in the five groups studied, the incidence of positive results to α-lactalbumin being similar in coeliacs, patients with gastrointestinal disease and healthy controls.

Observations of immune reactivity to α-gliadin in the peripheral blood of coeliacs provide only an indirect pointer to the possible local jejunal response to that antigen *in vivo*. Nevertheless, this study does support the previous demonstration of LIF release from coeliac jejunal biopsies cultured *in vitro* in the presence of α-gliadin[21]. However, leucocyte migration inhibition to α-gliadin may be due to factors other than LIF generated by activation of T lymphocytes, including non-specific toxicity and specific or irrelevant antigen–antibody complexes[22]. Even where LIF is present, cell-mediated immunity cannot necessarily be inferred since LIF may be released spontaneously by non-lymphoid cell lines[23] or by B-cells in response to specific antigenic stimulation[24]. Despite these alternative explanations, LMI to antigenic challenge shows a qualitative correlation with *in vivo* cell-mediated immunity in the host[6,25]. Our results show that LMI to α-gliadin appears virtually specific for coeliac disease and occurs less frequently in untreated than in treated coeliacs, implying migration of activated T lymphocytes to the gut in normal diet coeliacs in response to immunogenic challenge by intraluminal α-gliadin. There is good evidence that T cells are sensitized to intraluminal antigen. After oral immunization of guinea pigs with live clostridia or BCG, preparations of T cells from Peyer's patches respond by proliferation to *in vitro* stimulation with killed organism[26]. After antigen-induced proliferation, dividing T cells appear to leave the intestinal mucosa and travel via the mesenteric and thoracic duct routes to peripheral blood. T immunoblasts derived from mesenteric lymph nodes[27,28] and activated T cells taken from thoracic duct lymph[29] home to the gut. In situations where the gut is inflamed, increased numbers of T mesenteric blasts migrate to the gut[27]. Peripheral blasts which go to sites of inflamed skin can be diverted to inflamed but not to normal gut[28].

The present study provides indirect evidence that similar mechanisms may be involved in the pathogenesis of coeliac disease: mesenteric T cells activated by intraluminal gliadin home preferentially to the intestine and peripheral blasts may also be diverted to the area. Local cell-mediated immune reactions to gliadin may then be partly responsible for subsequent mucosal damage.

ACKNOWLEDGEMENTS

This work was performed while M.R.H. was in receipt of a research fellowship from the M.R.C. Their financial support is gratefully acknowledged.

References

1. Dumonde, D. C., Wolstencroft, R. A., Panayi, G. S., Matthew, M., Morley, J. and Howson, W. T. (1969). 'Lymphokines': Non-antibody mediators of cellular immunity generated by lymphocyte activation. *Nature (London)*, **224**, 38

2. Rich, A. R. and Lewis, M. R. (1932). The nature of allergy in tuberculosis as revealed by tissue culture studies. *Bull. Johns Hopkins Hosp.*, **50**, 115

3. Bloom, B. R. (1971). In vitro approaches to the mechanisms of cell-mediated immune reactions. *Adv. Immunol.*, **13**, 101

4. Bendixen, G. and Søborg, M. (1970). Comments on the leucocyte migration technique as an in vitro method for demonstrating cellular hypersensitivity in man. *J. Immunol.*, **104**, 1551

5. Rocklin, R. E. (1974). Products of activated lymphocytes. Leukocyte inhibitory factor distinct from migration inhibitory factor (MIF) *J. Immunol.*, **112**, 1461

6. David, J. R. and David, R. R. (1972). Cellular hypersensitivity and immunity. Inhibition of macrophage migration and the lymphocyte mediators. *Progr. Allergy*, **16**, 300

7. Asquith, P. and Haeney, M. R. (1977). Coeliac disease. In: P. Asquith (ed.) *Immunity in Gastrointestinal Disease*, (Edinburgh: Churchill Livingstone)

8. Bullen A. W. and Losowsky, M. S. (1976). Cell-mediated immunity (CMI) to gluten fraction III (GFIII) in adult coeliac disease (ACD). *Gut*, **17**, 813

9. Douwes, F. R. (1976). Gluten and lymphocyte sentization in coeliac disease. *Lancet*, **ii**, 1353

10. Maini, R. N., Roffe, L. M., Magrath, I. T. and Dumonde, D. C. (1973). Standardization of the leucocyte migration test. *Int. Arch. Allergy Appl. Immunol.*, **45**, 308

11. Coulson, A. S. and Chambers, D. G. (1964). Separation of viable lymphocytes from human blood. *Lancet*, **i**, 468

12. Schneider, R., Kendall, M. J. and Hawkins, C. F. (1974). Gliadin subfractionation. In: W. Th. J. M. Hekkens and A. S. Peña (eds). *Coeliac Disease. Proceedings of the Second International Coeliac Symposium*, pp.72–73. (Leiden: Stenfert Kroese)

13. Frazer, A. C., Fletcher, R. F., Ross, C. A. C., Shaw, B., Sammons, H. G. and Schneider, R. (1959). Gluten-induced enteropathy. The effect of partially digested gluten. *Lancet*, **ii**, 252

14. Gorski, A. J. (1974). Superiority of corpuscular BCG to soluble PPD antigen in the leucocyte migration assay. *Clin. Exp. Immunol.*, **18**, 149

15. Rosenberg, S. A. and David, J. R. (1970). Inhibition of leukocyte migration: an evaluation of this in vitro assay of delayed hypersensitivity in man to a soluble antigen. *J. Immunol.*, **105**, 1447

16. Rauch, H. C. and King, K. (1973). Human leucocyte migration inhibition as an indicator of cellular hypersensitivity to soluble antigens. *Int. Arch. Allergy Appl. Immunol.*, **44**, 862

17. Clausen, J. E. (1973). Comparison between capillary tube and agarose migration technique in the study of human peripheral blood leukocytes. *Acta Allergologica*, **28**, 145

18. Brostoff, J. (1974). 'Escape' from leucocyte migration inhibition. *J. Immunol. Methods*, **4**, 27

19. Haeney, M. R. (1976). A study of cell-mediated immune responses to α-gliadin in patients with coeliac disease. M. Sc. Thesis, University of Birmingham

20. Clausen, J. E. (1971). Tuberculin-induced migration inhibition of human peripheral leucocytes in agarose medium. *Acta Allergologica*, **26**, 56

21. Ferguson, A., Macdonald, T. T., McClure, J. P. and Holden, R. J. (1975). Cell-mediated immunity to gliadin within the small intestinal mucosa in coeliac disease. *Lancet*, **i**, 895

22. Spitler, L., Huber, H. and Fudenberg, H. H. (1969). Inhibition of capillary migration by antigen–antibody complexes. *J. Immunol.*, **102**, 404
23. Tubergen, D. G., Feldman, J. D., Pollock, E. M. and Lerner, R. A. (1972). Production of macrophage migration inhibition factor by continuous cell lines. *J. Exp. Med.*, **135**, 255
24. Rocklin, R. E., MacDermott, R. P., Chess, L., Schlossman, S. F. and David J.R. (1974). Studies on mediator production by highly purified human T and B lymphocytes. *J. Exp. Med.*, **140**, 1303
25. Guy-Grand, D., Griscelli, C. and Vassalli, P. (1974). The gut-associated lymphoid system: nature and properties of the large dividing cell. *Eur. J. Immunol.*, **4**, 435
26. Müller-Schoop, J. W. and Good, R. A. (1975). Functional studies of Peyer's patches: evidence for their participation in intestinal immune responses. *J. Immunol.*, **114**, 1757
27. Rose, M. L., Parrott, D. M. V. and Bruce, R. G. (1976). Migration of lymphoblasts to the small intestine. I. Effect of *Trichinella spiralis* infection on the migration of mesenteric lymphoblasts and mesenteric T lymphoblasts in syngeneic mice. *Immunology*, **31**, 723
28. Rose, M. L., Parrott, D. M. V. and Bruce, R. G. (1976). Migration of lymphoblasts to the small intestine. II. Divergent migration of mesenteric and peripheral immunoblasts to sites of inflammation in the mouse. *Cell. Immunol.*, **27**, 36
29. Sprent, J. (1976). Fate of H–2 activated T lymphocytes in syngeneic hosts. I. Fate in lymphoid tissues and intestines traced with ^{3}H–thymidine, ^{125}I–deoxyuridine and [51]chromium. *Cell. Immunol.*, **21**, 278

Discussion of chapter 23

Strober   As stated in your abstract, did you find that there was no significant inhibition in the untreated compared to the control group?

Haeney   There were individuals within that group who showed inhibition compared with the 95% confidence limits of the test.

Strober   The other point I want to make is the general one that it has been shown quite nicely by a number of groups that antigen-induced MIF or LIP production can be accomplished by B-cells, albeit that the response may require the presence of a small number of T-cells, so I would just like to refine the interpretation of your report in saying that while this indicates a specific cell-mediated response, it could indeed be a specific B-cell mediated response as well as T-cell mediated response.

Haeney   I would agree with you, that it is theoretically possible that other factors can cause inhibition of leucocyte migration, not just LIP production by B-cells, but preformed antigen–antibody complexes which we have not excluded. Equally LIF can be produced by non-lymphoid cell lines, such as fibroblast cells in culture. Nevertheless, while one can show this *in vitro* experimentally, nobody has yet shown that leucocyte migration inhibition in humans correlates with anything other than cell-mediated immunity to that antigen and it certainly does not correlate with humoral antibody titres.

Holmes   I think your results have confirmed what we found using a different system; we couldn't understand why it seemed to be in patients on GFD that we were getting transformation. Your idea that these cells are probably sequestrated out somehow when the patient is on a normal diet seems to be a good hypothesis. I think also that people using PHA to transform lymphocytes as a non-specific stimulant generally find that coeliac lymphocytes are as good as normal lymphocytes. An occasional paper has described a depression but on the whole I think the results fall into the normal range, so it is interesting that with a different system we found very similar things.

Haeney   I would like to point out that Dr Bullen from Leeds has also shown (in an abstract in *Gut* last year) that using this system with slightly different antigen and a different dose, that again there was more inhibition in the treated coeliacs than in the untreated coeliacs.

Section V
Gluten tolerance

24

Questionnaire of the European Society for Paediatric Gastroenterology and Nutrition on coeliac disease

D. H. SHMERLING

When Professor Weijers died 1973 the European Society for Paediatric Gastroenterology and Nutrition decided to dedicate a round table conference at the Annual Meeting of the Society in Utrecht 1977 to his memory. Dedicated to his merits as paediatrician, as a pioneer of Paediatric Gastroenterology, as the first President of the Society, and to his outstanding human qualities, the Society also carried out an enquiry into the views of its members on some aspects of diagnosis and management of coeliac disease (CD). The questionnaire was intended to seek information on some of the principles and practices of members of the Society concerning coeliac disease in 1977 and I would like to emphasize that this was an information-seeking enquiry and that the results presented simply reflect the answers of the members of the society to the questionnaire. They do not represent any final consensus or policy of the society itself. Through the courtesy of the President and Council of ESPGAN, I am able to present to you some information relative to today's discussion. The results of the questionnaire as a whole will be published elsewhere.

The questionnaire provided information from 53 paediatric departments in Europe on the diagnosis of CD in the untreated patient, experiences with and the results of late gluten challenges in CD, and some additional questions.

DIAGNOSIS OF CD IN THE UNTREATED PATIENT

Forty-six departments will perform intestinal biopsy in every case of suspected CD, whilst six will do so only after having obtained some other laboratory evidence of malabsorption. The most frequently used test is the 1 hour blood xylose test ($n=19$).

LATE CHALLENGES IN CD

Thirty-eight departments will challenge every case after complete remission has been achieved, whilst 15 will not. The methods used vary from 'wheat ad libitum' in most cases to weighed amounts of gliadin (mostly 0.3 g/kg). Practically all will check the issue of such a challenge primarily by intestinal biopsies at variable intervals of time, but some will also use various laboratory tests. The criteria for a positive challenge response are considered by 31 to be 'reappearance of a flat mucosa' but some will accept a 'deterioration of the mucosa' and other clinical and laboratory findings. Twenty-four departments have observed 60 cases of children initially diagnosed as having CD, who did not relapse after at least two years on a gluten-containing diet, out of a total of 1959 patients ($=3.06\%$). Seven departments reported 21 cases in whom a flat mucosa was not found until the challenge had lasted for over two years and in some instances up to seven years.

COLLAGENOUS TRANSFORMATION OF THE MUCOSA

This was reported in nine cases, mostly toddlers, in a variety of clinical conditions not directly related to CD and not responding to a GFD, frequently with fatal outcome. No case of intestinal lymphoma in children under 18 years with CD was reported.

Discussion of chapter 24

Ferguson	It was clear that some centres rarely or never saw late deterioration of the mucosa in previously treated coeliacs. Did you have an impression that there was a geographical relationship to this?
Shmerling	No.
Nusslé	You imply that when a late gluten challenge is positive that you can make a final diagnosis of gluten intolerance. I would not agree with this, and wonder at what stage it is possible to say that permanent gluten intolerance is present. We may have gluten intolerance persisting for three or four years but we cannot on this basis say that gluten intolerance is life-long, because we cannot predict what the state of the mucosa will be in 15 years' time. There is another point which I would regard as important and that is, in the case of children where late relapse has been shown, what was the state of the mucosa after two years on gluten; was the mucosa not already showing some evidence of damage after two years?
Shmerling	May I answer the second question first; John Walker-Smith is at present trying to get detailed information on every case on this point, that is to say, whether we have documented evidence for a normal mucosa at two years and a deterioration occurring afterwards. We are not in a position to give full information on this point as yet. As to your other question, it is unlikely from the information that we have obtained that we will be able to come to firm conclusions on the various points that you raise. This would need a great deal more detailed information on every single case and while I believe that this is work which should be done I am rather concerned as to its validity until such time as clearcut definitions have been agreed, particularly in relation to diagnosis. We must have clearly defined and generally accepted diagnostic criteria if comparisons between different cases and different centres are to be valid.
Asquith	Concerning the very important question of lymphoma. Do you have any additional details about the 24 patients with respect to their period on gluten-free diets, and as to whether they were responders or non-responders?
Shmerling	We asked for this information, but received it from only one centre. We would need to try to get detailed information in every single case if we are to be able to answer these questions.
Booth	Could I ask two questions—one, whether in childhood there exists a situation of a flat mucosa, non-responsive to a gluten-free diet in an individual, who, when treated with a gluten-free diet (and very often with steroids etc.) regresses with severe malabsorp-

tion, malnutrition and dies. This is a condition with which adult gastroenterologists are familiar, but which I haven't seen described in the literature from childhood, and I wondered if your question-naire produced any information relating to this question, and if so, what is the youngest individual who has been seen with that condition. My second question is, whether in any of the studies on gluten challenge which have been done there have been any patients who have become non-responsive to a gluten-free diet following a gluten challenge?

Shmerling   As to your first question, slide 14 included some information on it. There were nine cases and they had mostly flat mucosa, they had severe malabsorption, did not respond to a gluten-free diet, and had different associated conditions, but these cases were not docu-mented in detail. I personally do not know of any case in childhood who did not respond again to a gluten-free diet after a challenge; perhaps somebody in the audience does?

Rey   We also don't know of any incident of a child who failed to respond to a gluten-free diet following a gluten challenge. With regard to Professor Booth's question about cases non-responsive to gluten-free diets, it is probably not possible to answer this question on the basis of our questionnaire, which was concerned primarily with cases that were regarded as having coeliac disease, and by definition this excluded such problems as infants with intractable diarrhoea, who sometimes have very severe lesions of the intestinal mucosa and who may die despite long-term intravenous nutrition.

Shmerling   There was a question which I have not discussed here about the occurrence of flat mucosa in children not responding to a gluten-free diet. We had 18 centres reporting 26 different cases which included immunodeficiency, cow's milk intolerance, vitamin B_{12} malabsorption, intractable diarrhoea, leukaemia, diabetes, mal-rotation, tropical enteropathy, diffuse systemic sclerosis and one case of eczema.

Cooke   Could I raise the question of transient gluten intolerance? I am a little surprized to note in this meeting that there has been hitherto no reference to what is possibly a fundamental observation of Weinstein in dermatitis herpetiformis, on normal biopsies going through to a flat biopsy, which has profound implications backed up to some extent by Fry's work in treating apparently normal DH patients and getting a fall in the mucosal lymphocyte count. What I want to ask is, is it theoretically possible that it is only children with the coeliac trait who will produce transient gluten intolerance? It follows from Weinstein's observations in dermatitis herpetiformis that this is a possibility. Is there any plan to follow up what happens to these transient gluten intolerances? I am not talking of childhood only when their enzymes are building up and all the rest of their immunological features also, but of later life also. We have certainly had cases whose biopsies were normal during their early childhood and who when they later came to an adult clinic have produced a flat biopsy. I think it is terribly important that apparent transient gluten intolerance should be carefully followed to determine what eventually happens.

Shmerling   Thank you very much for this question, which I believe is an important one. This was not included in the questionnaire, so I can't answer it. Certainly every single one of those who have seen so-called transient gluten intolerance will continue to follow these children very carefully, because we still do not understand it fully, and the information that you have given, Dr Cooke, as to the possibility that these cases will eventually relapse is very important.

Harries   I would like to congratulate Dr Shmerling on transcribing what I thought was an extremely complicated questionnaire, and presenting it with so much clarity. You have obviously had a great deal of time to think about the answers to the questions which were posed in this questionnaire, and I wonder whether we can put the ball back in your court, and ask you whether you have a definition of coeliac disease as a result of your reflections on the questionnaire? Another question is directed towards Professor Booth, and it relates to the terminology of non-responsive coeliac disease in adults which I think is pertinent to the definition of coeliac disease. Does Professor Booth mean by this an adult who has previously had documented improvement on a gluten-free diet, who had then returned to a normal diet and who has subsequently not improved on a gluten-free diet? I am not quite clear what the adult gastroenterologists mean by 'non-responsive coeliac disease'.

Shmerling   It is extremely difficult. I do not have any personal definition of coeliac disease, other than what we tried to define previously together with Visakorpi and Wauters. I believe that we should start with some other definitions before the definition of coeliac disease, because if we include in the definition of coeliac disease a 'flat mucosa' I would very much like to have a definition of flat mucosa before defining coeliac disease, and as a matter of fact I don't believe that when two or three of us look at histological slides that we can all agree as to which show a 'flat' mucosa.

Booth   I'd just like to make one thing quite clear, that the term 'unresponsive coeliac disease' is a misnomer and should never be used. I define coeliac disease as an abnormal jejunal mucosa which responds morphologically to a gluten-free diet. For the adult physician the question of a challenge is not actually a problem although it is for a paediatrician. If I accept that diagnosis, then a patient who does not respond to treatment with a gluten-free diet does not have coeliac disease. I am a splitter not a lumper, and therefore I put those cases into a different file, and I classified them as something different and I think in this I am following Cyrus Rubin's advice. Now if that is the case, then non-responsiveness is not a question. A problem for me is whether there is any truth in the suspicion amongst some adult physicians (which has been stimulated by a patient for whom I personally have been responsible) that gluten challenge can induce a non-responsive situation. Now whether or not that has been clearly documented in other adult patients, it hasn't in ours, so it is only suspicion. Whether challenge is inevitably safe in adults is an important clinical question, but let me reiterate that 'non-responsive coeliac disease' is a misnomer and is a term that should not be used.

25

Prolonged gluten tolerance in treated coeliac disease

B. EGAN-MITCHELL, P. F. FOTTRELL and B. McNICHOLL

In 1974[1] we reported the results of a trial of gluten re-feeding in 40 coeliac children who had been on gluten-free diets (GFD) for a mean of 5.8 years. The trial was carried out in the belief that coeliac disease implied permanent gluten intolerance, our aims being to confirm the initial diagnosis and also the presence of persisting gluten intolerance. At that time, 36 children had had mucosal relapse to an active coeliac state in a mean of 15.4 months, leaving four children with mucosa within the range of morphological normality, with slight depression of brush border enzymes. Of the 36 children, 16 had been under the age of two years at the time of initial diagnosis. We now report the subsequent events in these four children, one of whose mucosa has reverted to active coeliac changes, and two of whom have shown possible evidence of partial or intermittent gluten intolerance.

METHODS

Details of methods used have been given elsewhere[1,2] but the controls have been altered slightly by restricting them to 25 children of age groups comparable to those in the study. Details of anthropometry, mucosal grading and site, HLA antigens, haemoglobin, serum iron, serum or red cell folate, IgA, interepithelial lymphocyte counts (IEL) mucosal lactase, sucrase and alkaline phosphatase are given in Table 25.1. Mucosal grading[3] was as follows: 0=normal mucosa, I=slight, II=moderate and III=severe mucosal damage, grades II and III being regarded as consistent with active coeliac disease. IEL counts were per 1000 epithelial cells, mean and SD for controls were 258 ± 67. Controls for IgA were from a local study of population exposure to lead[4] in 28

Table 25.1 Sex, age, height and weight centiles, HLA antigens, haemoglobin, serum iron, serum or red cell folate, IgA, biopsy grade and site, interepithelial lymphocytes, mucosal lactase, sucrase and alkaline phosphatase at remission and during gluten feeding in four coeliac children

Case No. Sex and age	Months on ND	Height centile	Weight centile	HLA antigens	Hb g/dl	Serum iron μmol/l	Serum folate μg/l	RBC folate μg/l	IgA g/l	Mucosal grade	Site	IEL 10² E.C.	Lactase i.u/g protein	Sucrase i.u/g protein	Alk. phos. i.u/mg protein
144	ND	70	87	A1 A3	14.0				1.0	0	Duo.	228	112.0		
♀6yr.	28	80	80	B7 B8						0–I	Duo.	257	19.6	32.3	23.4
	35	80	80		14.4	27.0	2.5		1.85	0–I	Duo.	415	16.5	44.0	16.2
	47	75	80		15.9	17.5		235	1.76	0–I	Duo.	357	13.1	47.7	7.7
	56	80	65		13.7	11.5		49*	1.18	I	Duo.	514	3.1	13.7	5.3
	59	75	70		13.7	20.0		164	2.4	I	Duo.	416	3.0	16.7	7.5
	63	75	65		13.8			94*		II	Duo.	660	2.6	8.9	3.4
	68	75	65							I	Duo.	472	2.5	9.6	3.6
	74	75	75		12.0	13.5			2.12	II–III	Treitz	618	2.5	8.6	7.9
269	ND	50	87	A2 A3	13.0	19.0	11.2		1.0	0	Duo.	147	28.6	62.3	17.4
♀3.2yr.	15	50	87	B7 B8						0	Duo.	173	28.1	57.3	22.4
	19	50	95		13.4	8.0	13.8		1.46	0	Duo.	74	20.8	46.7	13.5
	32	50	75			16.5		284	0.98	0	Jej.	198	59.7	77.2	16.5
	46	50	75		12.8	12.0		205	1.96	0	Duo.	220	78.8	45.7	18.9
	58	50	75		12.8	30.0		184		0	Duo.	388	24.9	42.5	11.9
110	ND	80	80	A1 AW29	13.3	19.0	24.0		2.1	0	Jej.	100	52.0		
♂7yrs.	17	85	85	B8 B12	13.2	8.0	14.7		1.2	0	Duo.	116	22.8	34.4	11.6
	29	85	85							0	Duo.	264	22.7	36.2	20.1
	35	85	85		13.8	32.5	21.0		1.5	0	Duo.	194	20.8	49.4	12.9
	47	85	85		14.3	22.5		1.12	1.12	0	Duo.	320	15.8	36.7	10.0
	61	90	75		14.2	24.0		215		0	Duo.	186	22.1	43.4	11.7
	73	90	75		13.8	27.0		200		0	Duo.	180	0.6	5.5	8.1
58	ND	45	8	A1 A2	14.1					0	Jej.	106			
♀11.5yr.	25		8	B8 BW35	14.1	29.0	13.6		1.2	0–I	Duo.	287	24.2	56.4	17.6
	33	32	20		13.5	8.5	5.3		3.0	I	Duo.	305	11.7	54.3	14.0
	47	40	15							0	Duo.	264	9.7	29.7	15.5
	53	40	20		13.7	17.5	3.3		1.68	0	Jej.	194	14.4	49.1	10.8
	65	40	30		12.5	24.0		250	1.02	0	Jej.	194	69.4	119.6	16.5

Age at time of commencement of normal gluten-containing diet (ND)

Height and weight plotted on centile charts of Tanner and Whitehouse, 1959

IEL=interepithelial lymphocytes per 1000 epithelial cells; Duo=duodenum; Jej.= jejunum; Hb.=haemoglobin; Alk. phos.=alkaline phosphatase

*These values for serum and red cell folate are below the range of normal for the laboratory in question

children 5 to 10 years of age; mean and SD were 1.29 ($\pm$0.53) g/l, and in 23 children aged 10 to 14 years 1.65 ($\pm$0.79) g/l. Disaccharidases were assayed by Dahlqvist's method[5] and alkaline phosphatase by that of Kelly and Hamilton[6]. Control levels for mucosal enzymes were as follows: in duodenum, lactase 37.6 ($\pm$19.3) i.u. per g protein, sucrase 58.0 ($\pm$33.7) i.u./g, alkaline phosphatase 22.2 ($\pm$7.6) i.u. per mg protein; in jejunum, lactase 62.8 ($\pm$21.6) i.u./g, sucrase 86.9 ($\pm$30.1) i.u./g, alkaline phosphatase 28.9 ($\pm$7.4) i.u./mg.

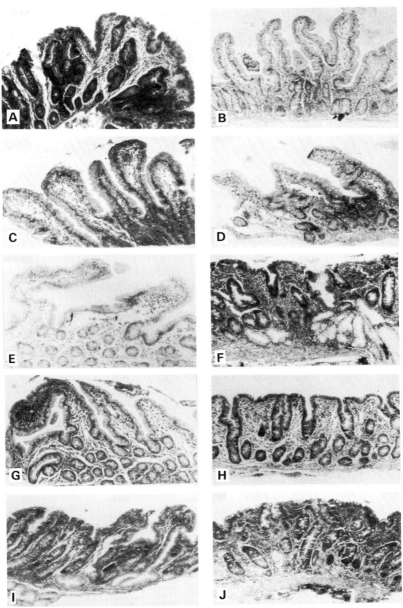

Figure 25.1 A) Duodenal mucosa (D.M.) at initial diagnosis, March, 1966; B) D. M. 57 months later, at time of commencement of ND: C) D. M. after 28 months on ND; D) D.M. after 35 months ND; 20 g gluten daily for two preceding months; E) D.M. after 47 months ND; F) D.M. after 56 months ND; G) D.M. after 59 months ND; H) D.M. after 63 months ND; I) D.M. after 68 months ND, 40 g gluten daily for preceding two months; J) Mucosa at ligament of Treitz, 74 months on ND

RESULTS

Case 144 (Figure 25.1A to 25.1J and Table 25.1) had been diagnosed at the age of 16 months, and had been on a gluten-free diet for 57 months. She probably ate not more than 2 to 5 g gluten daily during the first year on normal diet (ND) but subsequently gradually increased her intake and for two months before the biopsy at 35 months had at our request taken about 20 g gluten daily. This biopsy which did not show definite morphological abnormality, showed trends towards lower mucosal enzyme levels and rising IEL counts, which continued in subsequent biopsies, and from 56 months onwards were consistent with active coeliac disease. The mucosal morphology at 63 months (Figure 25.1) appeared characteristic of coeliac disease (Grade II) and our first reaction was to recommend a return to a gluten-free diet; however, in view of our experience with Case 58 where mild to moderate morphological abnormality associated with a low mucosal lactase at 33 months spontaneously returned to normal (Table 25.1) we decided, with full parental agreement, to prolong the trial. She took approximately 40 g gluten daily for the two months preceding the next biopsy at 68 months, and as this showed some improvement we allowed the trial to continue at a level of gluten intake of her own choice. At 74 months, a multiple biopsy tube was used, three distal duodenal and two proximal jejunal biopsies being taken, (Figure 25.1J) all of which were regarded as characteristic of active coeliac disease, the girl then being counselled to resume her gluten-free diet on a permanent basis.

The three remaining children, Cases 58, 110 and 269 had normal mucosal morphology when last biopsied, 65, 74 and 56 months respectively after starting the gluten trial (Table 25.1). Their initial diagnosis had been made at 68, 15 and 6 months respectively. The mucosal finding in Case 58 at 33 months have already been mentioned, and they were accompanied by a fall of 13 height centiles, a slightly low serum iron of 9 mmol/l and a rise in serum IgA. Subsequent biopsies and her clinical status were normal, but she has not attended for review for two years. Cases 269 and 110 each had a low serum iron on one occasion followed by spontaneous return to normal levels. Case 110 had low mucosal enzymes accompanied by a rise in IEL counts at 47 months, and at 74 months had a marked fall in mucosal enzymes to a level which we are accustomed to finding only in inactive coeliac disease. These four children have appeared to be in normal health throughout the trial, apart from slight fluctuation in height and weight and the occasional mild biochemical abnormalities detailed. Their overall growth has been unaffected and secondary sexual development has occurred normally in those of appropriate age.

DISCUSSION

Case 144 has shown the mucosal changes characteristic of coeliac disease both 63 and 74 months following return to a normal diet and must therefore be regarded as still being intolerant of gluten, presumably for life. It is notable that she ingested gluten, in gradually increasing amounts, for over four years before constantly abnormal morphology persisted, although the mucosal lactase and IEL counts were abnormal from 35 months onwards, sucrase and alkaline phosphatase also being abnormally low in the subsequent biopsies. The slow return to abnormal mucosal changes may be related to the initially low and gradually increasing gluten intake, which may also have allowed some degree of hyposensitization to gluten to have occurred. Adolescent hormonal changes may also have had some protective effect on the mucosa. We believe it probable that cases 58 and 110 will revert to active coeliac disease sooner or later in view of the transient clinical, morphological and enzymological changes in case 58 and the recent fall in enzyme levels in case 110. They might then be regarded as having latent coeliac disease, which could become overt with high level gluten loading, as demonstrated by Weinstein *et al.* in dermatitis herpetiformis[7], or with other stress or illness. It is possible that case 269 may follow a similar course eventually; on the other hand she may be an example of transient gluten intolerance[8] or of flat mucosa due to some other cause. If cases 58 and 110 do revert, then 39 of 40 children diagnosed as CD will have reverted to the coeliac mucosal state (at the least) or to active coeliac disease, on normal diets, indicating persisting and probably permanent gluten intolerance. The course of events in the three girls reported by Schmitz and Rey[9] does however raise the possibility that even in children in whom mucosal relapse has occurred on normal diet, a partial or permanent tolerance may subsequently develop.

Two alternative methods of management are open to us with a child having the generally accepted clinical and mucosal changes of coeliac disease. If we accept that the diagnosis must be confirmed by mucosal relapse produced by gluten re-feeding, we believe that the mucosal changes must include a definite morphological deterioration accompanied by a rise in IEL counts and that demonstration of a fall in mucosal enzymes outside the normal range is also desirable. It is probable that in some children, some years will elapse before definitive changes occur. One must also remember that the morphology of a single mucosal specimen may not be representative. In general, it is our impression that the depression of brush border enzymes is a more consistent as well as earlier indication of gluten intolerance than morphological change.

Alternatively, when the initial diagnosis appears valid, and the other causes of a flat mucosa such as acute enteritis, cow's milk allergy or immune deficiency have been excluded, we can assume that permanent gluten intolerance, albeit of varying degree, will persist in all but an occasional child, 3% according to the ESPGAN questionnaire[10], and consequently counsel life-long gluten abstinence. Regular surveillance, including at least a yearly consultation, would be aimed at ensuring normal growth and nutrition, intestinal biopsy being reserved for those situations where any clinical or biochemical abnormality suggested that the disease might not be under control.

We prefer the latter alternative, since it obviates the stress, discomfort and slight risk of complications of biopsy for a probable 97% of our patients in whom the gluten challenge would be positive. The first alternative would involve our department in 200 further gluten challenges, with at least double that number of biopsies. However, in the case of children where there has been any reasonable doubt about the initial diagnosis, we would regard a gluten challenge, continued until such time as the diagnosis is confirmed or refuted, as mandatory.

This study has demonstrated to us that there is a wide spectrum of response in the treated coeliac child to gluten re-feeding, the occurrence of definite morphological mucosal changes in the upper intestine taking from months to several years to appear. Continued observation of the three children with morphologically normal mucosa, probably for several years, will be necessary to establish if they have persistent intolerance to gluten.

ACKNOWLEDGEMENTS

Our thanks are due to the children and their parents for their whole-hearted cooperation and then to many clinical and laboratory colleagues. We are indebted to Professor J. D. Kennedy for histological reports on the earlier biopsies, Dr H. Grimes for the immunoglobulin assays, Dr F. M. Stevens for the multiple biopsy in Case 144 and S. Baker for lymphocyte counting. The many enzyme assays were made by R. Keane. The Medical Research Council of Ireland supported the enzyme assays and also a Fellowship for B.E-M. Support from the Wellcome Trust and the Western Health Board is gratefully acknowledged.

References

1. McNicholl, B., Egan-Mitchell, B. and Fottrell, P. F. (1974). Varying gluten susceptibility in coeliac disease. In: *Coeliac Disease,* Hekkens and Peña, (eds.) (Leiden: Stenfert Kroese)
2. McNicholl, B., Egan-Mitchell, B., Stevens, F. M., Keane, R., Baker, S., McCarthy, C. F. and Fottrell, P. F. (1976). Mucosal recovery in treated childhood coeliac disease, *J. Paediat.,* **89,** 418

3. McNicholl, B. and Egan, B. (1968). Jejunal biopsy in coeliac disease. *Clin. Paediat.,* **7,** 544

4. Grimes, H. (1975). Biological sampling for monitoring population exposure to lead. *Galway Med. Ann.,* Special Edition, 121

5. Dahlqvist, A. (1968). Assay of intestinal disaccharidases. *Anal. Biochem.,* **22,** 99

6. Kelly, M. H. and Hamilton, J. R. (1970). A microtechnique for the assay of intestinal alkaline phosphatase. *Clin. Biochem.,* **3,** 33

7. Weinstein, W. M., Piercey, J. R. A. and Dossetor, J. B. (1974). Dermatitis herpetiformis and coeliac sprue. In: *Coeliac Disease,* Hekkens and Peña, (eds.) (Leiden: Stenfert Kroese)

8. Walker-Smith, J. (1970). Transient gluten intolerance. *Arch. Dis. Childh.,* **45,** 523

9. Schmitz, J. and Rey, J. (1978). Transient mucosal atrophy in confirmed coeliac disease. *Ibid*

10. Shmerling, D. (1978). Some results of ESPGAN questionnaire. *Ibid*

26

Transient mucosal atrophy in confirmed coeliac disease

J. SCHMITZ, J. JOS and J. REY

INTRODUCTION

According to the ESPGAN criteria, the diagnosis of coeliac disease is based on the following sequence: '1. a structurally abnormal jejunal mucosa on a gluten-containing diet; 2. a clear improvement of villous structure on a gluten-free diet, and 3. deterioration of the mucosa during challenge[17]. This definition implies the permanence of the jejunal mucosa sensitivity to gluten throughout life. Subtotal villous atrophy is thus supposed to persist until and during adulthood in children who eat a gluten-containing diet. This anatomical lesion, and the fear that its persistence could favour malignancy, are in fact among the main reasons why most authors recommend a life-long gluten-free diet once the disease has been recognized. However this view of coeliac disease hardly explains the great variability in the period of time necessary to induce relapse[2], which rarely may not be obtained in cases otherwise indistinguishable from relapsing ones; this view also does not explain the much lower frequency of the disease in adults compared to children[3]. The details of three patients presented here, who had a practically normal mucosa after more than five years on gluten-containing diets, are other facts which question the currently accepted concept of coeliac disease as a permanent stable condition.

PATIENTS

Case 1

Christine B. is a girl born on February the 23rd, 1961, from unrelated healthy parents, measuring respectively 170 cm and 158 cm for the

259

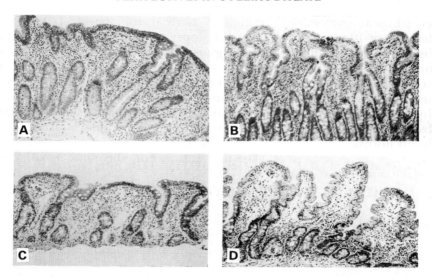

Figure 26.1 Case 1. A, first biopsy, at 1 year and 10 months of age, taken after 3 weeks of a gluten-free diet; B, after 3 months of the same diet; C, after three and a half years of a gluten-containing diet, at 10 years of age; D, after more than 9 years of the same gluten containing diet, at 15 years and 6 months (H.E.×40)

father and the mother. Her first months of life were symptom-free until, after gluten was introduced in her diet at 5 months of age, diarrhoea, failure to thrive, loss of weight, emaciation and a distended abdomen appeared, leading to the first admission to hospital at the age of 8 months. Height was 1.5 standard deviation (SD) below the mean and the clinical picture was typical of coeliac disease. A gluten-free diet was started and she rapidly became more cheerful and began to gain weight. Stools were also more formed. The diet was maintained for 8 months and then stopped to induce a short-term relapse. Two months later at the age of one year and 7 months she was admitted for the second time having lost weight and again passing loose stools. Fat absorption coefficient (FAC) was abnormally low at 82%. After 5 months of normal diet during which the clinical picture became very similar to the initial one, the gluten-free diet was resumed. Three weeks after this the first biopsy revealed a typical subtotal villous atrophy (Figure 26.1A). Simultaneously, however, fat absorption coefficient was already somewhat improved, at 89%, and 3 months later villous atrophy was only partial (Figure 26.1B). The diet, although irregularly followed from the age of 4 years, was maintained until she was 6 years and 4 months old; gluten was then allowed, as periods with it were well-tolerated. In fact she used to eat little bread and her normal diet contained only about 3 g of gluten per day. She continued to grow well and her physical examination remained normal for the next 9 years. However at 10 years of age a control biopsy again showed a flat mucosa (Figure 26.1C), confirming the diagnosis of coeliac disease. Five years later, at 15 years and 6 months of age Christine was readmitted for a short follow-up balance study and a biopsy in September 1976. Her diet had not changed. She measured 162 cm, weighed 51.7 kg; her physical examination was normal as was her nutritional status and fat absorption (FAC=98%). Surprisingly however the jejunal mucosa was almost normal (Figure 26.1D), this normalisation of the mucosa having thus been achieved while Christine was eating the same small but definite amounts of gluten.

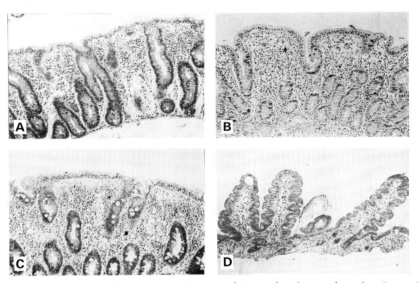

Figure 26.2 Case 2. A, first biopsy at 1 year and 8 months of age, taken after 3 months of normal diet; B, after 1 year of a gluten-free diet; C, after three and a half years of a gluten-containing diet, at 6 years and a half; D, after more than 12 years of the same diet, at 15 years and 6 months. (H.E.×40)

Case 2

Laurence B., a girl, was born on October the 15th, 1960, from unrelated tall parents in good health, measuring 186 cm and 165 cm for the father and the mother respectively. She was still above average height (+1.0 SD) but was failing to gain weight, with diarrhoea and a prominent abdomen for two months, when she was admitted for the first time in the ward at one year of age, gluten having been introduced into her diet at 5 months of age. Fat absorption was low with a FAC of 77%. A gluten-free diet was started, the diagnosis of coeliac disease being the most probable. Her clinical status rapidly improved as she quickly gained weight and after three weeks of this diet the fat absorption coefficient was 89%. After 3 months gluten was reintroduced in her diet; during the next three months she gained less weight and diarrhoea reappeared; the fat absorption coefficient fell to 83% and a biopsy revealed a typical subtotal villous atrophy (Figure 26.2A). The gluten-free diet was then again strictly followed and Laurence's height remained around 2 SD above the mean. At 2 years and two months fat absorption was normal (FAC=96%); however 6 months later the jejunal mucosa still presented partial atrophy (Figure 26.2B). From 3 years to 5 years and 9 months of age Laurence was in a boarding school and the diet was less strictly observed. Since she was in perfect health a normal diet was allowed and after 8 months of it, when she was 6 years and 5 months old, a third biopsy was performed; it showed a flat jejunal mucosa (Figure 26.2C). The normal diet maintained during these years contained around 12 g per day of gluten. In April 1976, Laurence was readmitted for a short follow-up period; for 15 years and 6 months of age she was tall, measuring 171 cm (+1.8 SD) and weighed 52 kg. Her clinical and nutritional status was perfect. So after 12 years and 6 months on a gluten-containing diet, her jejunal mucosa was nearly normal (Figure 26.2D), having thus recovered completely on a diet containing normal amounts of gluten.

Case 3

Isabelle P. is a girl born on January the 26th, 1959, from unrelated healthy parents. Her father was 170 cm and her mother 157 cm tall. She has been receiving gluten for a year when she was first admitted at the age of one year and 5 months, with a history of chronic diarrhoea for 8 months, failure to thrive and profound emaciation. Her height was 1 SD below the mean and she weighed 7.1 kg. Her abdomen was prominent and fat absorption was poor (FAC=66%). Coeliac disease being probable, a gluten-free diet was started. She responded rapidly, gained weight, and after 6 weeks the fat absorption was nearly normal (FAC= 91%). The diet was continued until she was 3 years and 8 months old. She was clinically well at that time, when a gluten challenge was commenced to confirm the diagnosis. Before putting her on a normal diet, the fat absorption was confirmed to be normal (FAC=97%) and a first biopsy was done, showing a normal jejunal mucosa (Figure 26.3A). One year later, her clinical status was still good but her growth was somewhat slower (height = −0.2 SD compared to +0.4SD one year before); the relapse was both biological (FAC=88%) and histological, with a flat mucosa at the second biopsy (Figure 26.3B) although she had eaten little gluten. For the following 8 years, she again strictly observed the

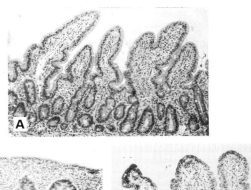

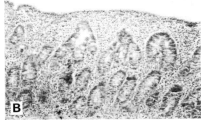
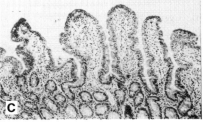

Figure 26.3 Case 3. A, first biopsy at 3 years and 8 months after 2 years and 3 months of a gluten-free diet; B, after 1 year of a diet containing small amounts of gluten; C, at 17 years and 9 months of age, after 5 years of a diet containing similarly little gluten. (H.E.×40)

gluten-free diet. During this period of time she grew normally. At 12 years and 7 months of age, as she was bored by the diet, a normal one was allowed. However she tended to eat little or no bread and her diet contained less than 2 g per day of gluten, mainly in the form of cookies. During the next three years she continued to thrive normally without any clinical symptoms. Between 15 and 17 years of age Isabelle stopped gaining and started losing weight, but it was not clear whether this weight loss was the consequence of a slimming craze (she is a very pretty and self-conscious adolescent) or of the normal diet, and she was readmitted at 17 years and 9 months of age in October 1976 to decide if she had again relapsed. She had reached her final height, 160 cm, was slim (45.6 kg) but otherwise clinically normal. Fat absorption was normal without clearcut signs of relapse as yet (Figure 26.3C).

DISCUSSION

Criteria for the diagnosis of coeliac disease are the subject of continuing discussions. For some this condition should be diagnosed on the basis of a 'flat biopsy in a patient and an unequivocal clinical response to a gluten-free diet'[4]; for the paediatricians gathered in the ESPGAN the specificity of the initial clinical and histological features should be only defined by the deterioration of the mucosa during its challenge by gluten[5]. Although it has been said that in adults the gluten challenge may be hazardous[6], this 'more limiting definition'[7] seems, at least in children, to be justified by the apparent absence of clinical risk during the challenges in this group and the seriousness of a diagnosis which influences the remainder of a patient's life.

The debate is re-opened by the present observations, since, according to the ESPGAN criteria, the diagnosis of coeliac disease can reasonably be made in these girls. Indeed, although histological recovery was only partial in the first two patients who had presented in their first year of life with chronic diarrhoea, malabsorption and failure to thrive responding to a gluten-free diet, the presence of a flat mucosa three and a half years after gluten had been reintroduced in their diet may be considered as equivalent to, and as good a proof of gluten intolerance as, the typical relapse induced in the third case.

It could certainly be argued that the surprisingly normal or nearly normal specimens of jejunal mucosa found after years of gluten-containing diets in these cases of 'confirmed coeliac disease' are not representative of the mucosa as a whole since the biopsies have been performed with one-hole paediatric Crosby capsules at the duodeno-jejunal flexure. If patchy lesions exist in coeliac disease as in dermatitis herpetiformis[8], areas of normal villous architecture may be found in an otherwise flat mucosa. However this has been denied[9,4] and in our experience we have very rarely found a normal mucosa in a child clinically suspected of coeliac disease. If the occurrence of patchy abnormality was frequent in coeliac disease, the histological criteria for diagnosis would have to be reconsidered.

It might also be speculated that the amounts of gluten ingested by cases 1 and 3 when on 'normal' diets were in fact very low and not enough to induce flattening of the mucosa[2,10]. This may be particularly relevant in the third case which, in contrast to the first two, could be regarded as having not yet relapsed; in this latter case, however, it had been noted that Isabelle first relapsed with only small amounts of gluten, probably not very different from those which later on were insufficient to induce a second relapse.

Finally one can question whether the present patients are really affected by coeliac disease, that is to say by a permanent intolerance to gluten, or whether they represent cases of transitory sensitization to dietary proteins, similar to cow's milk allergy, since it is well known that transient gluten intolerance may be observed in this context[1]. However we think that it is more the permanence of the sensitivity of the jejunal mucosa to gluten in coeliac disease which has to be questioned in the light of these observations.

Indeed they raise the crucial point of the true nature of coeliac disease. Is it always induced by gluten in predisposed individuals? Are the anatomical lesions life-long, or do they sometimes disappear during adolescence and reappear in adulthood in only some patients, which would explain the lower incidence of the disease in this age group than in children? Adult coeliacs might thus represent a subgroup among predisposed coeliac patients; or relapse in adulthood might be triggered, as may be the case in infancy, by some factors other than gluten which might then induce histological lesions, depending on individual susceptibility. Anyhow, the frequency of malignancy might have been overestimated if adult coeliacs really represent only a fraction of the whole coeliac population since it has always been evaluated in the adult group. Moreover, it has been demonstrated that, contrary to what has been found in coeliac disease responding to gluten exclusion, the turnover of intestinal epithelial cells is lower than normal in non-responsive coeliac disease in which the incidence of malignancy is particularly high[11]; this raises the question whether abdominal lymphomas are really a complication of adult coeliac disease. It has also been shown that the incidence of malignancy is greater in families where several members are affected by the disease[12] which stresses the importance of genetic factors among others (increased epithelial cell turnover rate, excess of inflammatory cells in the intestinal mucosa, depressed immunologic surveillance) supposed to account for the high frequency of malignancy in coeliac disease[13]. Finally a recent survey has demonstrated that malignancy was independent of the observance of the gluten-free diet[14]. Furthermore one may wonder whether a few years of this diet could have a protective effect against malignancy after as many or more years of mucosal atrophy.

Thus, in our opinion, the question of the permanence of gluten sensitivity as one of the main criteria for coeliac disease and the general custom of systematically leaving coeliac patients on a life-long gluten-free diet once relapse has been obtained, are still debatable. It is our hope that a prospective study of the kind in which we are now involved, comprising patients on gluten-containing diets, who are submitted every five years to short follow-up periods of observation including biopsy, will help to answer these basic questions.

References

1. Visakorpi, J. K. (1974). Definition of coeliac disease in children. In: W. Th. J. M. Hekkens and A. S. Peña (eds.). *Coeliac Disease. Proceedings of the Second International Coeliac Symposium*, pp. 10–16. (Leiden: Stenfert Kroese)
2. McNicholl, B., Egan-Mitchell, B. and Fottrell, P. F. (1974). Varying gluten susceptibility in coeliac disease. In: W. Th. J. M. Hekkens and A. S. Peña (eds). *Coeliac Disease. Proceedings of the Second International Coeliac Symposium*, pp. 413–418. (Leiden: Stenfert Kroese)

3. Bernier, J. J., Bourdeloux, P. and Modigliani, R. (1974). Preliminary data on the incidence of coeliac disease in France. In: W. Th. J. M. Hekkens and A. S. Peña (eds.). *Coeliac Disease. Proceedings of the Second International Coeliac Symposium.* p. 338. (Leiden: Stenfert Kroese)

4. Weinstein, W. M., Shimoda, S. S., Brow, J. R. and Rubin, C. E. (1970). What is celiac sprue? In: C. C. Booth and R. H. Dowling (eds). *Coeliac Disease. Proceedings of an International Conference,* pp. 232–245. (Edinburgh: Churchill Livingstone)

5. Weijers, H. A., Lindquist, B., Anderson, Ch. M., Rey, J., Shmerling, D. H., Visakorpi, J. K., Hadorn, B. and Gruttner, R. (1970). Round table conference on 'Diagnostic Criteria in Coeliac Disease" Proc. ESPGA, Intertaken, 1969. *Acta Paediat. Scand.,* **59,** 461

6. Booth, C. C. (1974). Definition of adult coeliac disease. In: W. Th. J. M. Hekkens and A. S. Peña (eds). *Coeliac Disease. Proceedings of the Second International Coeliac Symposium,* pp. 17–22. (Leiden: Stenfert Kroese)

7. Cooke, W. T. and Asquith, P. (1974). Introduction and Definition. In: W. T. Cooke and P. Asquith (eds). *Clinics in Gastroenterology,* **3,** Coeliac Disease. pp. 3–10. (London: Saunders)

8. Scott, B. B. and Losowsky, M. S. (1976). Patchiness and duodenal-jejunal variation of the mucosal abnormality in coeliac disease and dermatitis herpetiformis. *Gut,* **17,** 984

9. Meeuwisse, G. (1977). Personal communication

10. Jos, J., Rey, J. and Frézal, J. (1969) Effects precoces de la réintroduction du gluten sur la muqueuse intestinale dans la maladie coeliaque en rémission. *Arch. Franç. Péd.,* **26,** 849

11. Barry, R. E. and Read, A. E. (1973). Coeliac disease and malignancy. *Qu. J. Med.,* **42,** 665

12. Barry, R. E., Morris, J. S., Kenwright, S. and Read, A. E. (1971). *Scand. J. Gastroenterol.,* **6,** 205

13. Stokes, P. L. and Holmes, G. K. T. (1974). Malignancy. In: W. T. Cooke and P. Asquith (eds.) *Clinics in Gastroenterology,* **3,** Coeliac Disease. pp. 159–170. (London: Saunders)

14. Holmes, G. K. T., Stokes, P. L., Sorahan, T. M., Prior, P., Waterhouse, J. A. H. and Cooke, W. T. (1976). Coeliac disease, gluten-free diet, and malignancy. *Gut,* **17,** 612

27

Reinvestigation of children previously diagnosed as coeliac disease

J. A. WALKER-SMITH, ANNE KILBY and N. E. FRANCE

INTRODUCTION

The dual concepts that gluten intolerance is permanent in both children and adults with coeliac disease and that spontaneous mucosal recovery does not occur in untreated coeliac disease have both been generally accepted since the observations of Mortimer and her colleagues[1]. Now the observations of Schmitz and his colleagues[2], cast some doubt on this later point.

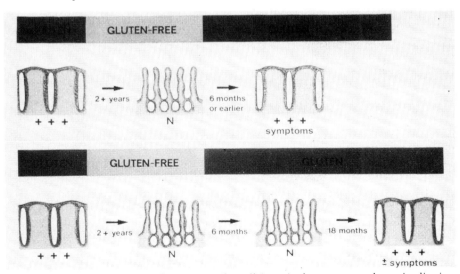

Figure 27.1 Two patterns of response of small intestinal mucosa to gluten in diet in children with coeliac disease

DIAGNOSTIC CRITERIA FOR COELIAC DISEASE

Nevertheless, Figure 27.1 summarizes diagramatically the criteria widely used since 1969, in order to make a final diagnosis of coeliac disease, based upon the demonstration of permanent gluten intolerance[3]. The first requirement is the demonstration of an abnormal mucosa, usually flat, whilst the child is having a gluten-containing diet. Second is the demonstration of a normal mucosa on a gluten-free diet and third the return of an abnormal mucosa on a gluten-containing diet. This diagram also indicates that it may on occasion take some time—at least up to two years and occasionally longer—for the mucosa in some children with coeliac disease to relapse after a return to a gluten-containing diet.

This paper presents the results of reinvestigation of 65 children originally diagnosed as having coeliac disease at Queen Elizabeth Hospital for Children, based upon the concept of gluten challenge producing mucosal relapse in children who have true coeliac disease as shown in Figure 27.1.

TECHNIQUE OF GLUTEN CHALLENGE

Figure 27.2 shows how such a gluten provocation test or challenge was ideally conducted. First, the small intestinal mucosa was shown to be abnormal whilst on a gluten-free diet. Next following a clinical remission on a gluten-free diet, after two years or more the mucosa was shown to be normal or near normal on this gluten-free diet. If it was not, the diagnosis was reconsidered or the accuracy of the gluten-free diet reassessed. The child was then returned to a normal gluten-containing diet.

The amount of gluten in the child's diet was carefully controlled by a dietitian to ensure that the child was, in fact, having an adequate gluten intake for his age. The appropriate gluten intake as grams of wheat protein in children at various age groups has been described[4].

If symptoms recurred on a normal diet, after a week a further biopsy was performed. As a rule a biopsy was not performed earlier as often anxious parents think that any intercurrent symptoms are signs of clinical relapse.

If no symptoms recurred a further biopsy was performed in any event, usually after 3–6 months, although earlier in the study some children were sometimes biopsied earlier. The mucosa was then often abnormal in children who, in fact, had coeliac disease i.e. the diagnosis was confirmed. If the mucosa was still normal observation was continued and when significant symptoms recurred a further biopsy was done after one week. If the mucosa was then abnormal, coeliac disease was confirmed. Failing that, after two years a final biopsy was performed. If it were then normal or near normal we regarded the diag-

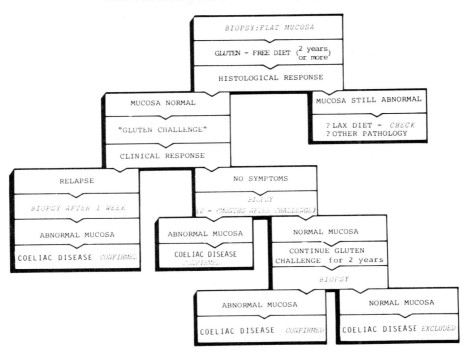

Figure 27.2 Diagnostic criteria and investigation regime for children initially provisionally diagnosed as coeliac disease

nosis of coeliac disease as having been excluded.

In this study it was not possible to follow this ideal sequence in every case, and in our total study of 65 children, we have included both children in whom an original diagnosis was based upon an abnormal biopsy and a clinical response to a gluten-free diet (44 children) and also children where there was clinical and biochemical evidence of coeliac disease and a clinical response to a gluten-free diet but no original biopsy (21 children) (Table 27.1). However, all children in whom the diagnosis of coeliac disease was confirmed, had a mucosal relapse after return to a normal diet and all in whom the challenge was regarded as negative had a normal biopsy after two or more years back on a normal gluten-containing diet.

The criteria for normality in the biopsies of these children is important because morphology of normal small intestinal mucosa in childhood may be different from normal adult morphology.

Mucosal appearances are regarded as normal when under the dissecting microscope there are long thin ridge-like villi, tongue-like villi and leaf-like villi as well as finger-like villi which are uncommon in biopsies from children[5]. On section the villi should be twice as long as the crypts and have a normal intraepithelial lymphocyte count and normal epithelium. Variation in thickness of some villi is a permissible variation of normal. There should be no increase in plasma cells.

If there is some doubtful change we rate the mucosa as ± or near normal. If epithelial abnormality is present, or if shortening or thickening of villi, increase in plasma cells, eosinophils in the lamina propria or elongated crypts are found the mucosa is then regarded as undoubtedly abnormal. A grading system of +, ++, +++ is used, +++ corresponding to a flat mucosa[6].

Table 27.1   Details of gluten challenges

		Initial abnormal biopsy	No initial biopsy
Total number of children challenged	65	44	21
Positive challenges	50	35 { 31 flat / 4 PVA	15
Negative challenges	15	9 { 6 flat / 3 PVA	6

RESULTS OF GLUTEN CHALLENGE (See Table 27.1)

Fifty gluten challenges were positive, whilst 15 were negative. Considering the 44 children who had an initial biopsy, 35 had positive challenge and 9 were negative. Looking specifically at the 37 children in this group who had an initial flat mucosa, 6 did not relapse after two years on a normal diet and are clinically well (i.e. 16%). This is a higher figure than that reported by Shmerling[7] of 3.6% for the members of the European Society for Paediatric Gastroenterology, but is in closer accord with the findings of colleagues in Sweden[8] (8 of 35, or 22%), and in Finland[9] (8 of 83, or 9%).

Since four of the 35 children who had positive gluten challenges had initially had partial villous atrophy, it is clear that this degree of mucosal damage is consistent with a diagnosis of coeliac disease, although found less often than a flat mucosa.

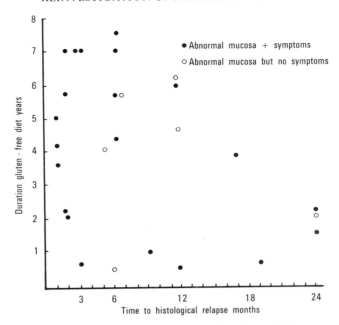

Figure 27.3 Relation between duration of gluten-free diet and time to relapse, after gluten challenge in 27 children with proven coeliac disease

Duration of diet and time to relapse

Twenty seven of these 35 children who had histological relapse were studied for the relationship between the duration of their gluten-free diet and the time to histological relapse. Six of this group were a symptomatic at the time of histological relapse, (Figure 27.3), the remainder being symptomatic. There was no correlation whatever between the duration of their gluten-free diet and the time to histological relapse, nor indeed with those who had clinical symptoms as well.

Delayed relapse

Forty five of the children who had a positive challenge had definite evidence of mucosal relapse at the time of their first post-challenge biopsy, but five did not. Table 27.2 indicates that these five children's first post-challenge biopsies were taken at intervals ranging from 5 weeks to 14 months on a gluten-containing diet. Only one child subsequently became symptomatic and he had a biopsy after 9 months' gluten which was more abnormal than the earlier biopsy. The remainder, despite a grossly abnormal mucosa were symptom-free and were having a routine two year post-challenge biopsy.

Table 27.2 Data concerning five children whose first post-challenge biopsy was not diagnostic

Patient	Sex	Age challenge commenced	Post-challenge biopsy	Time interval on gluten	Final biopsy	Time interval on gluten
B.H.	F.	2 yr. 2 mo.	N.	14 mo.	++/+++	2 yr.
R.J.	M.	3 yr.	N.	5 wks.	+++	2 yr.
J.J.	M.	1½ yr.	N.	5 wks.	+++	2 yr.
S.L.	M.	2 yr.	+	4 mo.	++	9 mo.
J.P.	M.	2 yr. 3 mo.	N.	5 wks.	+++	2 yr.

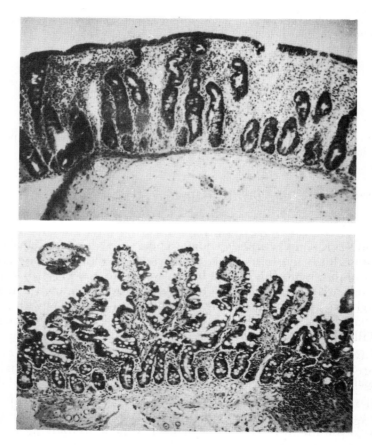

Figure 27.4 Histological appearances of initial biopsy at first presentation (above) from child S.S. aged 3 months and (below) two years two months after return to a normal gluten-containing diet, aged 5 years 3 months

Negative challenges

The nine children who had an initial abnormal biopsy but who despite this had a final biopsy which was normal or near normal after two or more years on a gluten-containing diet, and who do not appear to have coeliac disease, represent an important group. Figure 27.4 demonstrates the histological findings in one of these children.

Seven of these children had serial disaccharidase assay after commencement of challenge. On two occasions disaccharidase activity fell despite normal morphology. This was first reported in such children by McNicholl, Egan-Mitchell and Fottrell[10].

Table 27.3 Histological grading, lactase activity and intraepithelial lymphocyte counts/ 100 epithelial cells (IEL) in serial biopsies from a child S.S. related to age and gluten-containing (G) or gluten-free diet (GF)

Patient	Age	Diet	Histology	Lactase	IEL
S.S.					
	3 mths.	G	++	0.5	81
	3 yr. 1 mo.	GF	N	—	31
	$4\frac{1}{2}$ yr.	G	N	8.1	32
	5 yr. 3 mo.	G	N	2.6	29
	7 yr. 4 mo.	G	±	3.3	48

In only one child has there tended to be a rise in intraepithelial counts (IEL) and this is shown in Table 27.3, related to disaccharidase activity; in view of the rise in IEL his last biopsy was graded as ±. At present he is absolutely well after 3 years 10 months on a normal gluten-containing diet. What is going to happen to this child and the others with a negative challenge? Will the two who had falling disaccharidases and especially the one who also had a rise in his intraepithelial lymphocyte count eventually relapse? Only time will tell.

Original diagnosis in negative challenges

Finally what was wrong with these 9 children originally? (Table 27.4). Their age ranged from 8 weeks to 1 year 5 months at the time of their initial biopsy i.e. all were less than two years of age at that time. Critical review of the early history in three children reveals evidence of a preceding episode of acute enteritis and evidence of other food intolerances e.g. cow's milk protein intolerance, but in the remainder there was no

Table 27.4   Nine children with negative gluten challenges

Patient	Age at initial biopsy	Sex	Histology	Final Diagnosis
D.B.	8 wks.	M.	PVA	Post-enteritis enteropathy
M.M.	10 wks.	M.	Flat	Non-coeliac enteropathy
S.S.	3 mo.	M.	Flat	Non-coeliac enteropathy
T.D.	4 mo.	F.	Flat	Non-coeliac enteropathy
L.S.	4 mo.	F.	PVA	Post-enteritis enteropathy
T.J.	5 mo.	M.	Flat	Post-enteritis enteropathy
T.C.	10 mo.	F.	PVA	Non-coeliac enteropathy
A.K.	1 yr.	M.	Flat	Non-coeliac enteropathy
P.M.	1 yr. 5 mo.	F.	Flat	Non-coeliac enteropathy

such evidence and this group we have designated as non-coeliac enter-opathy.

Within this group there were some children who met the criteria for the initial diagnosis of coeliac disease, as they had a flat mucosa and evidence of malabsorption and responded dramatically to a gluten-free diet. It is impossible now to convince the mothers of some of these children that a gluten-free diet at that time did not account for their clinical improvement. Figure 27.5 shows the weight progress over the years of one of these children. What was wrong with this boy originally? It is probable that he had transient gluten intolerance from which he has recovered (Walker-Smith[11]). Unfortunately, McNeish's strict criteria[12] for transient gluten intolerance in this boy or in the other eight children in our study have not been fulfilled; nonetheless, the original diagnosis of transient gluten intolerance is probable. The cause of such transient intolerance remains a matter for speculation.

The more coeliac disease is investigated, the more difficult it becomes, but the use of serial biopsies related to gluten withdrawal and challenge has been a major advance not only concerning knowledge of this entity but in its practical management in childhood.

ACKNOWLEDGEMENTS

We would like to express our thanks to all those clinicians who referred us patients for diagnosis and reinvestigation, especially Dr O. D. Fisher and Dr M. Stoneman.

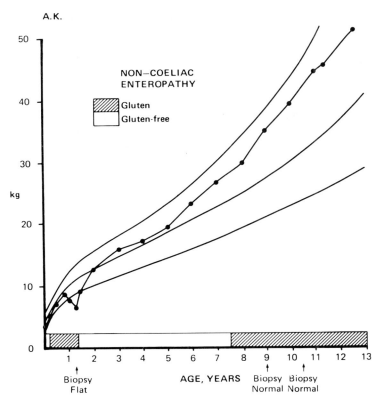

Figure 27.5 Weight chart of child A.K. with non-coeliac enteropathy related to 3rd and 97th percentile. Serial biopsies and dietary changes are indicated

References

1. Mortimer, P. E., Stewart, J. S., Norman, A. P. and Booth, C. C. (1968). Follow-up of coeliac disease. *Br. Med. J.*, **2**, 7
2. Schmitz, J., Jos, J. and Rey, J. (1977). Transient mucosal atrophy in confirmed coeliac disease. *Third International Coeliac Symposium*
3. Meeuwisse, G. W. (1970). Diagnostic criteria in coeliac disease. *Acta Paediat. Scand.*, **59**, 461
4. Francis, D. E. M. (1975). *Diets for Sick Children*. Third Edition, (Oxford and Edinburgh Blackwell Scientific Publications)
5. Walker-Smith, J. A. (1967). Dissecting microscope appearance of small bowel mucosa in children. *Arch. Dis. Childh.*, **42**, 626
6. Harrison, B. M., Kilby, A., Walker-Smith, J. A., France, N. E. and Wood, C. B. S. (1976). Cow's milk protein intolerance: a possible association with gastroenteritis, lactose intolerance and IgA deficiency. *Br. Med. J.*, **1**, 1501
7. Shmerling, D. H. (1977). ESPGAN Questionnaire. *Progress in Coeliac Disease*. McNicholl, McCarthy and Fottrell, (eds.) (Lancaster: M.T.P. Press Ltd.)
8. Lindberg, T. (1977). Personal communication

9. Kuitunen, P., Pelkonen, P., Perkkiö, M., Savilahti, E. and Visakorpi, J. K. (1977). Transient gluten intolerance. *10th Annual Meeting of European Society for Paediatric Gastroenterology and Nutrition.*
10. McNicholl, B., Egan-Mitchell, B. and Fottrell, P. F. (1974). Varying gluten susceptibility in coeliac disease. *Proceedings of Second International Coeliac Symposium.* (Stenfert Kroese: Leiden)
11. Walker-Smith, J. A. (1970). Transient gluten intolerance. *Arch. Dis. Childh.,* **45**, 523
12. McNeish, A. S. (1974). Diagnostic criteria for transient gluten intolerance. Cited in *Disease of the Small Intestine in Childhood,* Walker-Smith, J. A. (Tunbridge Wells: Pitman Medical)

28

Non-coeliac gluten intolerance in infancy

D. NUSSLÉ, C. BOZIC, J. COX, G. DELEZE, M. ROULET
R. FETE and A. MEGEVAND

By definition coeliac disease is a permanent condition associated with gluten intolerance and a flat jejunal mucosa[1]. After normalization of the mucosa on a gluten-free diet, the absence of a histological relapse more than two years after reintroduction of gluten was considered sufficient evidence to exclude the diagnosis of coeliac disease and suggest the diagnosis of transient gluten intolerance. Recent reports have identified a group of children with temporary gluten intolerance and milder intestinal lesions. The majority of these cases had also cow's milk protein intolerance with onset of symptoms in early infancy[2-6]. In the past ten years we have observed two small groups of patients with clinical intolerance to gluten, one without severe villous changes and another with severe villous atrophy, but neither showing mucosal relapse after a challenge with gluten lasting for more than two years.

Of 60 consecutive cases of milk protein intolerance, 11 had a simultaneous intolerance to gluten. Gluten intolerance has been identified with the same criteria as cow's milk intolerance: exclusion of gluten from the diet for several weeks followed by a provocation test. Four of these cases were true coeliacs with severe mucosal atrophy and histological relapse after more than 18 months of gluten-free diet and a short challenge with gluten powder (1–2 months).

Seven cases were considered to have non-coeliac gluten intolerance. In five the initial biopsy showed only mild or absent jejunal changes (*Type 1*). In two, the lesion was severe, indistinguishable from that of coeliac disease, but without relapse after more than two years (two and five years) on a normal gluten-containing diet (*Type 2*). Intraepithelial lymphocyte count[9] as well as mucosal disaccharidases[8] were normal. In this group of seven cases the symptoms associated with gluten intake were, diarrhoea in all cases, vomiting in three, abdominal colic in four, dermatitis in three, rhinitis in four, bronchitis in four, absence of weight gain in two only (these two cases showed severe villous atrophy). Gluten was well-tolerated at the age of 21 to 42 months (mean=34). Before the tolerance to milk in one child (1 year 9 months), at the same age as the milk in three cases (2 to 4 years) and after the milk in two cases (3 years and 3½ years). In one child, cow's milk and gluten were still not tolerated at 5 years of age.

In addition to these seven patients, three cases of type 1 and six patients of type 2, unassociated with cow's milk protein intolerance, were observed.

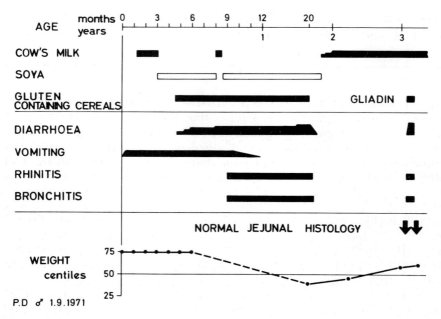

Figure 28.1 Case 1, P. Daniel. Non-coeliac gluten intolerance with allergic manifestations

The first patient (P.D., Figure 28.1) presented with vomiting since birth. He was breast-fed, followed by cow's milk at one month of age. At three months a soya formula was introduced but without effect on vomiting which ceased at the age one year. Gluten was introduced at four months and coincided with the onset of diarrhoea. At nine months of age the mother noted a persistent cough and abundant clear nasal secretions. At 20 months all symptoms disappeared on a gluten-free diet. Cow's milk was reintroduced without difficulty. Diarrhoea as well as the respiratory manifestations reappeared as soon as gliadin (Fluka) at dose of 0.3 g/kg/day was given at the age of three years, and persis-

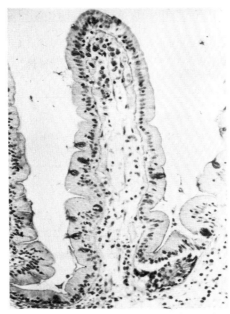

Figure 28.2 Case 1, P. D. Proximal jejunal mucosa after a three week challenge with gliadin. Oedema of the lamina propria Biopsy T 15543/75. PAS 225 ×

ted for the three weeks of its administration.

The jejunal biopsy done at the end of this challenge with gliadin showed only oedema of the lamina propria (Figure 28.2). Several periodic challenges with a gluten-containing diet presented on each occasion the same symptoms of intolerance up to the age of $5\frac{1}{2}$ years. At six years of age a normal diet was well-tolerated.

The second infant (N.A., Figure 28.3) also showed no intolerance to cow's milk. Gluten-containing cereals were introduced at the age of one month. Two weeks later diarrhoea with mucus and blood developed and dermatitis was noted. The patient became asymptomatic on a gluten-free diet. Three subsequent gluten challenges triggered the symptoms on each occasion. At five months, after two weeks of bloody diarrhoea induced by gluten, a jejunal biopsy showed only minimal changes.

Unfortunately, endoscopy and rectal biopsy were not carried out, but there was clinical evidence of haemorrhagic colitis. Intolerance to gluten-containing cereals disappeared at the age of 18 months.

In the third infant (R.V., Figure 28.4) who had received cow's milk from birth, bovine protein intolerance could not be demonstrated. Gluten-containing cereals were introduced at $4\frac{1}{2}$ months. Soon there-after she developed diarrhoea with mucus, anorexia, vomiting, abdo-

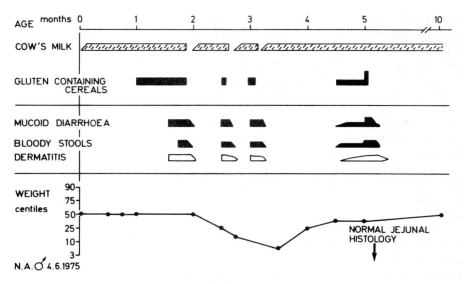

Figure 28.3 Case 2. N. Antoine. Gluten-induced haemorrhagic colitis

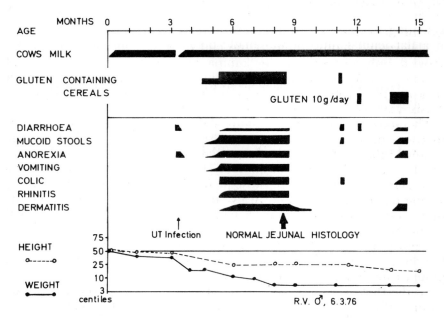

Figure 28.4 Case 3. R. Virginie. Gluten intolerance with symptoms of colitis and allergic manifestations

minal colic, persistent rhinitis and dermatitis. After four months of a gluten-containing diet, the rate of weight gain was diminished, but the jejunal histology was normal. Gluten was then excluded from the diet and all symptoms disappeared. When a challenge with gluten powder was given at 14 months of age, symptoms reappeared.

Six other infants were initially considered as having coeliac disease.

In 59 consecutive children treated for coeliac disease, the effect of reintroduction of a normal gluten-containing diet on the proximal jejunal mucosa after more than 18 months of gluten-free diet was studied.

The criteria for selection of patients were a flat jejunal mucosa before treatment, a good and rapid clinical response to a gluten-free diet, and a normal tolerance to cow's milk, which was not excluded from the diet.

Histological relapse with severe lesions was observed in 47 cases, four months to three years after reintroduction of gluten. In 14 cases the control biopsy was performed only after more than two years of gluten intake and a two year control biopsy is not available. Proximal jejunal histology and mucosal disaccharidases are still normal in six cases after less than two years of gluten challenge (three to 17 months), and in *six cases after more than two years of a normal gluten-containing diet*. Clinical data on these six patients are summarized in Table 28.1. The age of introduction of gluten varied from two to four months. The presenting symptoms were noted soon thereafter. The diagnosis based on a flat jejunal mucosa was made between six and 11 months. In

Table 28.1 Clinical data of the six patients with normal intestinal mucosa $2\frac{1}{2}$–$4\frac{1}{2}$ years after reintroduction of gluten

Patients	M.V.	D.AM	M.M	D.M.	G.CH	S.C.
Age (months) at:						
Introduction of gluten	4	4	2	$2\frac{1}{2}$	3	2
First symptom	5	4	4	$3\frac{1}{2}$	4	$2\frac{1}{2}$
Diagnosis of flat mucosa	9	11	8	6	6	$3\frac{1}{2}$
Early gluten challenge	+	+	ND	+	+	ND
Duration of diets						
Gluten-free (months	21	24	30	60	24	42
Gluten challenge (years)	3 4M	3	2 4M	$4\frac{1}{2}$	3	$2\frac{1}{2}$

Table 28.2 Clinical data in the six infants (II)

	Number of cases	
	A	B
Anorexia	3	3
Vomiting	2	4
Diarrhoea	3	3
Constipation		1
Abdominal distension		4
Colic		1
Poor weight gain	4	6
Dermatitis	1	1
Sudden onset	2	(diarrhoea)
Steatorrhea		3/4
Pathogens in stool culture		0/5
Allergy in first degree relative	2	

A Presenting symptom or sign
B Symptom or sign at time of diagnosis

four cases an early gluten provocation test was performed within the first three months of gluten exclusion and was found to be clearly positive. The remaining two infants were chronically ill and the rapid improvement soon after removal of gluten from the diet was sufficient to incriminate gluten as the substance responsible for the malabsorption. The gluten-free diet was maintained for a period of 21 to 60 months and the duration of the challenge with gluten varied between 2 years 4 months and $4\frac{1}{2}$ years.

Initial clinical findings and those which were present at the time of the biopsy are summarized in Table 28.2. The mode of presentation was variable; as in coeliac disease there was a varying degree and frequency of anorexia, vomiting, diarrhoea, abdominal distension and poor weight gain; colic and dermatitis were observed in some cases. Steatorrhea was present in three of four cases in which faecal lipid was measured. Stool cultures showed no pathogens.

The proximal jejunal biopsies performed in these six children after more than two years of normal gluten-containing diet were normal under both dissecting and light microscopy (Table 28.3, Figures 28.5 and 28.6). Intraepithelial lymphocyte count was low in all cases. Disaccharidase activity of the brush border enzymes was normal except for an isolated low lactase in patient D.M. This finding in the face of the

Table 28.3 Intestinal biopsy in the six patients without relapse more than $2\frac{1}{2}$ years after reintroduction of gluten

	M.V.	D.AM	M.M.	D.M.	G.CH	S.C.
Age (years)	5 10/12	5 8/12	4 9/12	10 2/12	6 2/12	$6\frac{1}{2}$
Dissecting and light microscopy	normal	normal	normal	normal	normal	normal
IE Lymphocytes nb/100 ep. z.	7	11	9	9	6	5
Disaccharidases (UI/g prot)						
Lactase	49	45	29	4	not done	91
Maltase	247	218	266	234		—
Sucrase	81	72	68	85		122
Trehalase	50	22	33	44		48

completely normal histology $4\frac{1}{2}$ years after reintroduction of gluten (Figure 28.5) suggests hypolactasia on a constitutional basis.

DISCUSSION

Sixteen patients who presented with intolerance to gluten and who did not fulfil the criteria of the definition of coeliac disease are described. In all cases the symptoms began in early infancy, seven cases presented an association of gluten intolerance with cow's milk protein allergy.

In the first group (*Type I*), the proximal intestinal mucosa was normal or showed only minimal changes. Diarrhoea containing mucus and with macroscopic blood in one case, suggested colitis, as has been described in cases of milk intolerance[4,10]. The symptoms are similar to those observed in cases of intolerance to cow's milk proteins, with extradigestive allergic manifestations, such as respiratory or cutaneous symptoms.

This type of gluten intolerance can be clearly differentiated from true coeliac disease, and should be considered as a transitory gastrointestinal allergy of infancy.

In the second group (*Type II*), the clinical symptoms as well as the severe lesions of the jejunal mucosa resemble those of coeliac disease, however, two to $4\frac{1}{2}$ years after the reintroduction of gluten;

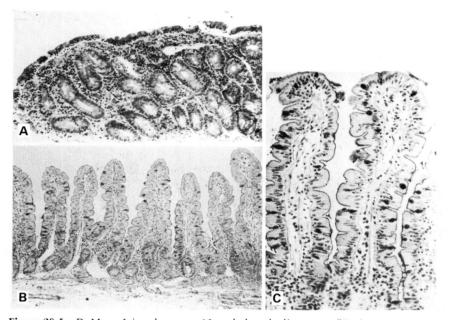

Figure 28.5 D. Marc. Jejunal mucosa 15 cm below the ligament of Treitz.
A) flat mucosa at 6 months of age, with proven gluten intolerance. Biopsy E 1757/68. HE. 44 ×
B) Normal mucosa at 8 years of age, after $2\frac{1}{2}$ years on a gluten-containing diet. Biopsy T 13322/75. PAS 176 ×
C) Normal mucosa at 10 years of age afer $4\frac{1}{2}$ years on a normal gluten intake. Biopsy T 9984/77. PAS 18 ×

the villi as well as the mucosal disaccharidases remained completely normal. In six cases, gluten intolerance was isolated, unassociated with cow's milk intolerance.

One can thus consider two alternatives:

Firstly, we are not dealing with coeliac disease but with a transitory gluten intolerance analogous to other types of food protein intolerance encountered in infancy in which cases one can observe various degrees of histological modifications of the intestinal mucosa, even a completely flat mucosa[4,11]. This entity could thus be considered in a general concept of transitory food protein intolerance in infancy[12,13].

Secondly, that proposed by McNicholl et al.[14], who suggested that in a small number of patients the recommended two years' challenge may not be long enough and that the relapse can be much later, thus it is not possible to specify the time limit.

We do not know of any document in the literature or in other unpublished data which contests the validity of a two year gluten challenge.

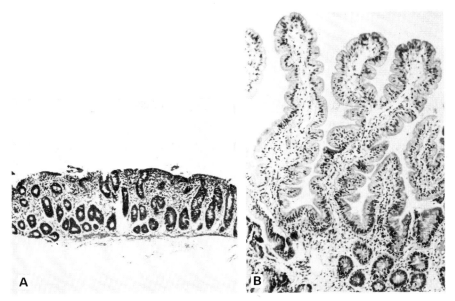

Figure 28.6 M. Valerie. Proximal jejunal mucosa.
A) Typical coeliac lesion at nine months of age, with proven gluten intolerance. Biopsy E 10605/66. HE 21 ×
B) Normal mucosa at the age of 5 years 10 months after a prolonged challenge with gluten of 3 years and 4 months. Biopsy E 16364/71. HE 78 ×

This could only be done by showing a completely normal mucosal histology and normal brush border enzymes after two years of normal gluten-containing diet, and histological relapse later on. In the case described by the above group[15] with histological relapse after more than two years, mucosal enzyme depression was already observed after two years. Nevertheless, considering the considerable variation in susceptibility to wheat gluten in coeliac disease, a definitive conclusion concerning our six cases will require follow-up biopsies, which could eventually force a revision of the accepted definition of coeliac disease.

ACKNOWLEDGEMENTS

The authors are grateful to Dr J. Frei, Head of the central Laboratory of the University Hospital of Lausanne for his valuable help with the disaccharidase assays.

References

1. Meeuwisse, G. W. (1970). Diagnostic criteria on coeliac disease. Round table discussion ESPGAN. *Acta Paediat. Scand.,* **58,** 461

2. Visakorpi, J. K. and Immonen, P. (1967). Intolerance to cow's milk and wheat gluten in the primary malabsorption syndrome in infancy. *Acta Paediat. Scand.,* **56,** 49

3. Kuitunen, P., Visakorpi, J. K., Savilahiti, E. and Pelkonen, P. (1975). Malabsorption syndrome with cow's milk intolerance. *Arch. Dis. Childh.,* **50,** 351

4. Delèze, G. and Nusslé, D. (1975). L'intolérance aux protéines du lait de vache chez l'enfant. *Helv. Paediat. Acta,* **30,** 135

5. Nusslé, D., Delèze, G. and Mégevand, A. (1975). Traitement et évolution des intolérances aux protéines du lait de vache. *XXIVe Congrès de l'Association des Pédiatres de Langue Franĉaise, Vol. 2,* p. 326 (Paris: L'Expansion)

6. Walker-Smith, J. (1970). Transient gluten intolerance. *Arch. Dis. Childh.,* **45,** 523

7. McNeish, A. S., Rolles, C. J. and Arthur, L. J. H. (1976). Criteria for diagnosis of temporary gluten intolerance. *Arch. Dis. Childh.,* **51,** 275

8. Dahlquist, A. (1968). Assay of intestinal disaccharidases. *Anal. Biochem.,* **22,** 99

9. Ferguson, A. and Murray, D. (1971). Quantitation of intraepithelial lymphocytes in human jejunum. *Gut,* **12,** 988

10. Gryboski, J. D., Burkle, F. and Hillman, R. (1966). Milk induced colitis in an infant. *Paediatrics,* **38,** 299

11. Fontane, J. L. and Navarro, J. (1975). Small intestinal biopsy in cow's milk protein allergy in infancy. *Arch. Dis. Childh.,* **50,** 357

12. Rey, J. and Frezal, J. (1974). L'intolérance aux protéines du lait. *Arch. Franc. Pédiat.,* **31,** 933

13. Walker-Smith, J. (1975). Cow's milk protein intolerance. Transient food intolerance of infancy. *Arch. Dis. Childh.,* **50,** 347

14. McNicholl, B., Egan-Mitchell, B. and Fottrell, P. F. (1974). Varying gluten susceptibility in coeliac disease. In: *Coeliac Disease, Proceedings of the Second International Coeliac Symposium.* p. 413 (Leiden: Stenfert Kroese)

15. Egan-Mitchell, B., Fottrell, P. F. and McNicholl, B. (1978). Variability of gluten intolerance in treated childhood coeliac disease. *Ibid*

29

Alterations of the jejunal mucosa after short term instillation of gliadin fractions in children with coeliac disease

M. SINAASAPPEL and W. Th. J. M. HEKKENS

Because of the fact that even today gluten-free diets are sometimes given to patients without an initial histological examination of the jejunal mucosa, the question may later arise as to whether continuation of the diet is necessary.

This question can only be answered by a long-term gluten challenge and histological control of the jejunal mucosa.

Because this is a time-consuming procedure which occasionally causes psychological harm to the patient, we endeavoured to find satisfactory short-term investigation[1,2]. We infused a concentrated gluten solution into the duodenum near the ligament of Treitz. Before and after infusion, mucosal biopsies were taken to investigate the morphology and the enzyme activity.

METHODS

Gluten fractions III and IV were prepared according to Hekkens, which is a modification of Frazer's method, (a purified peptic and tryptic digest of an alcoholic extraction of wheat flour[3]). Ten grams of these fractions were dissolved in water and were infused for four hours into the duodenum, 10 cm above the biopsy site.

The biopsies were taken under fluorescent control with a hydraulic biopsy capsule of small size, specially made for infants and children. Biopsies were taken at time zero, directly after gluten infusion and at four hourly intervals. Early damage to the mucosa was investigated by counting the intraepithelial *lymphocytes* according to the method of Ferguson[4].

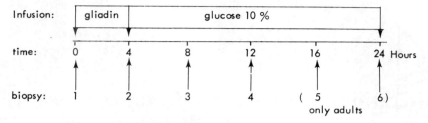

10 gram gliadin fraction III + IV infused during 4 hours, 10 cm above the biopsy site (Treitz) in the duodenum

Biopsies were investigated for morphology and enzyme activity

Figure 29.1   Schedule of the gluten challenge

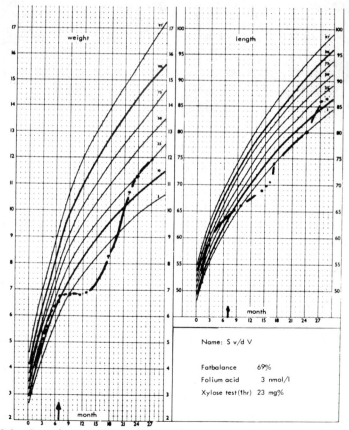

Figure 29.2   Growth chart of a patient with severe coeliac disease. Gluten was introduced at the age of 5 months

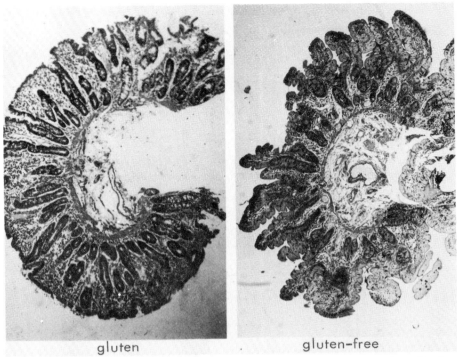

gluten   gluten-free

Figure 29.3 Morphology of the jejunum before and during a gluten-free diet in the same patient as shown in Figure 29.2

The enzyme activity of the mucosa was measured according to Dahlqvist[5]. We estimated lactase, sucrase, maltase, alkaline phosphatase and acid phosphatase activity. The alkaline phosphatase served as a measure of the brush border activity.

In children we stopped at 12 hours, in adults at 24 hours after the start of the procedure (Figure 29.1). Apart from the four children with coeliac disease we investigated four adults with coeliac disease and three control individuals. Only one child was investigated as a control.

The four children had initially shown a total villous atrophy and then a complete recovery after a gluten-free diet. As an example, the growth chart and the histology of one patient are shown in Figures 29.2 and 29.3.

RESULTS

The four children showed a marked depression of the enzyme activities, all of which decreased to below the mean −1 S.D. The most severely affected enzyme was lactase. The time of maximal depression differed

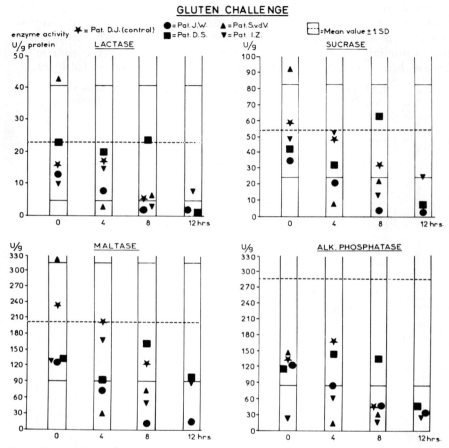

Figure 29.4 Mucosal enzyme activities in four children with coeliac disease and one child without coeliac disease during gluten challenge with 10 g gliadin fractions III and IV

from patient to patient, but was always within 8 h of the gluten infusion. The acid phosphatase level remained stable during the whole procedure. We only once had the opportunity to challenge a non-coeliac child. He also showed some depression of enzyme activity but less than the mean −1 S.D. (Figure 29.4).

The same pattern seen in children was seen in adults. Coeliac patients showed the same strong depression in enzyme activity (Figure 29.5). Control adults also showed some depression when challenged with gluten. One adult was challenged without gluten and did not show any depression of the enzyme activity (Figure 29.6).

Histological evaluation of the biopsies of coeliac patients gave the impression of an increase of the amount of plasma cells in the lamina propria but quantitation has not been done as yet. We counted the intraepithelial lymphocytes as a marker of early damage in coeliac disease, but we could not show an increase in their number (Table 29.1).

Table 29.1 Number of epithelial lymphocytes, expressed as a product of total number of nuclei in the epithelial layer. (normal <40/100)

	Time in hours			
Patient	0	4	8	12
J.Z.	30,2	37	—	33,2
S.v/d.V.	26,6	27,8	30,8	—
D.S.	27,4	22,4	27,6	31
J.W.	38,2	—	—	—

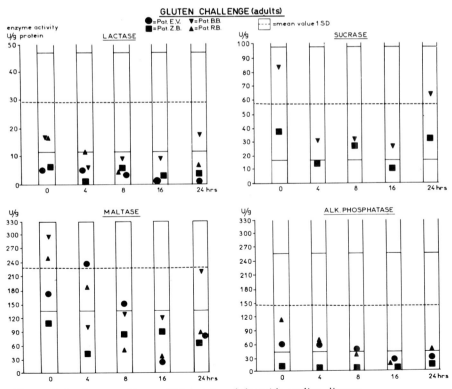

Figure 29.5 Same as Figure 29.4 but in adults with coeliac disease

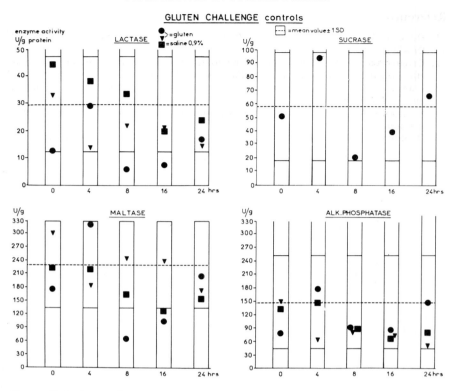

Figure 29.6 Mucosal enzyme activities in two adults without coeliac disease during gluten challenge (10 g) and one adult without coeliac disease in whom only saline infusion was applied

DISCUSSION

In these experiments it is shown that the decrease in the maltase and alkaline phosphatase activity of the mucosa is the most impressive one. Although the decrease in lactase activity is also remarkable, this is less impressive because the value at the start of the experiments is more variable. An explanation could be the more labile character of this enzyme.

CONCLUSION

In a small number of individuals, short-term challenge with gliadin fractions III and IV resulted in a marked depression of brush border enzyme activities in patients with coeliac disease, in contrast to normal controls.

References

1. Hekkens, W. Th. J. M. (1970). In: *Proceedings of the Coeliac Symposium*. Booth and Dowling (eds.), pp. 11–19
2. Dissanayake, D. W. (1974). Identifying toxic fractions of wheat gluten and their effect on the jejunal mucosa in coeliac disease. *Gut*, **15**, 931
3. Frazer, A. C. (1959). Gluten-induced enteropathy: the effect of partially digested gluten, *Lancet*, **ii**, 252
4. Ferguson, A. (1971). Quantitation of intraepithelial lymphocytes in human jejunum. *Gut*, **12**, 988
5. Dahlqvist, A. (1970). Assay of intestinal disaccharidases. *Enz. Biol. Clin.*, **11**, 52

Discussion of chapters 25, 26, 27, 28 and 29

Douglas   I have two particular problems and I wonder whether we may get some resolution of them if there could be some definition and control of what is being done. One problem relates to the histology, and, leaving aside the criteria that were used for abnormality, there is the equally controversial question of whether there is patchy change and therefore when one is making challenges, should one be taking several biopsies rather than just one? The other problem is that of the appropriate amount of gluten to be given, taking into account the age of the patient; there seems to be considerable variation in the studies just reported. I recall that at the second symposium in Leiden there was some discussion regarding the variability of gluten consumption around the world and whether this was related to the variation in incidence. I think we should have an agreed amount of gluten that is given in challenges. It is no good just putting the patient on a normal diet because what is normal for one may contain very much less gluten than an other. I cannot see that anyone is tackling this particular difficulty.

Katz   Seeing that most views expressed have been from Europe, I think I should give a North American view because coeliac disease is still extremely common in Boston, probably because we have a large Irish population. I think the most interesting feature to me is that children under the age of 18 months have an increased susceptibility to develop a flat villous lesion from any cause, whereas a flat villous lesion in adults always seems to be due to coeliac disease, and I think it is just like the giant cells that appear in neonatal hepatitis and doesn't occur in adults with hepatitis due to other causes, and I think that the first important fact is that the initial lesion in coeliac disease in infancy is a diffuse lesion. When you do multiple biopsies it is not usually patchy on initial diagnosis. Secondly, allergic disorders are now becoming more prevalent in the world and also produce a syndrome and a lesion identical to coeliac disease except that this is usually patchy. Thirdly I reinforce Dr Douglas's opinion that it is essential that all patients put on a gluten challenge should have a minimum of at least 10 g of gluten per day, so that when these patients are followed the results of the challenge should clearly be more consistent than in those on a so-called normal diet.

294

Walker-Smith	I'll just briefly comment on patchy enteropathy. We have a poster display in which we tried to indicate that this does exist, and I completely agreed with Dr Katz concerning untreated coeliac disease to the effect that the mucosal lesion is not patchy, whereas mucosa that is being challenged is patchy. I would also agree that in cow's milk protein intolerance and in post-enteritis enteropathy there is little doubt that the enteropathy is patchy.
Watson	Yesterday I think we are reminded about the physiological principle that so much disease is the admixture of seed and soil, and it would seem that in gluten-induced enteropathy the one thing that is relatively constant is that the seed has got something to do with gluten or its fractions, but we must remember that the soil is very variable, and whereas yesterday we were talking about immunological potentiation, other things are important such as the age of the patient. Now in relation to Dr Schmitz's patients, those of us who have seen only adult coeliac patients know very well that they frequently give a history of coeliac disease in childhood or something like it, and what sounded like spontaneous remission in adolescence (in patients who never had the benefit of a gluten-free diet at all because it hadn't become available). I think we should remember that in adolescence the soil changes very radically, and one of the things that is happening is a tremendous upsurge of endocrine activity. Possibly their own endogenous steroids influence the soil (and of course Booth, Peters and Wall showed some years ago that steroids themselves can improve the histological lesion). I would suspect that the adolescent is improving because he is beginning to produce his own augmented quota of steroids which see him through that adolescent period. I think that in the children who have this apparent transient gluten enteropathy other things are happening in the soil. Whether these are allergic or infectious things, gluten is merely the continuing seed working in a different kind of soil environment.
Cluysenaer	I think it is very important when you are speaking about transient gluten intolerance that you realize that the spontaneous course of coeliac sprue is also variable. We also have a poster in the exhibits, and apart from some evidence of the variable course, it also shows that the area of damaged intestinal mucosa is variable. This makes it imperative to state when you are showing biopsies, exactly where they were taken, and this requires that they are always done under fluoroscopic control.
Egan-Mitchell	To partly answer Dr Katz's question, in relation to the age of the patients, of the 37 patients who had mucosal relapse, 17 of them were under the age of $1\frac{1}{2}$ years at the time of diagnosis and five were under one year. In relation to the site of biopsy, we attempt to take the biopsy from the same position, which for some years has been the 3rd or 4th part of the duodenum.
Nusslé	I don't think that you can regard a decreasing lactase activity as only due to gluten toxicity; in our population 10% of children normally have decreasing activity and I don't know what the percentage is in your population, this decrease being on an inherited basis. We find it helpful in differentiating secondary lactase depression from inherited lactase deficiency to take a proximal and a distal jejunal biopsy, the latter about 120 cm

distal to the ligament of Treitz; we then find that in secondary lactase deficiency, whereas the level is low in the proximal jejunum it may be normal in the distal jejunum, whereas in inherited deficiency the level is equally low at both sites.

Editor's Comment In the west of Ireland, inherited lactase deficiency is very unusual, much less that 10%. In the children described by Dr Egan-Mitchell, sucrase and alkaline phosphatase activity became similarly depressed indicating that the cause of the depression was a toxic effect on the brush border.

Bayless I want to ask whether Dr Egan-Mitchell has been troubled with duodenal biopsies, as we have been in adults, especially when people send us endoscopic biopsies. We have trouble with duodenal biopsies because we find the changes much less than in jejunal biopsies.

Egan-Mitchell Usually we do not have any difficulty, and our biopsies would be more distal than endoscopic biopsies.

Cooke I should like to ask the presenters of papers the basis on which they say that there is no heterogeneity in mucosal biopsies. The majority of them have been using a small Crosby capsule: now I can't talk for paediatrics, but I can talk for the adult, and 10 years ago we published material on the heterogeneity of the lesion in coeliac disease with pictures and we have also studied and published more than 30 cases of coeliac disease autopsied within two hours of death, where we examined the whole of the intestine by dissecting microscopy. From these studies we can say that the lesion in coeliac disease is heterogeneous, although admittedly with more damage in the proximal part of the gut than distally with the top $2\frac{1}{2}$ feet usually being severely abnormal.

Rey I am a little puzzled by Dr Egan-Mitchell's statement that two of their patients probably have latent coeliac disease, Dr Walker-Smith having described some of his patients with similar clinical courses as not having coeliac disease. I think it is a most important point to agree on the definition of what is, and what is not coeliac disease, taking into account the duration of the gluten-free diet and also of the time on a normal diet needed to induce a relapse, amongst other things. I also agree with you that if the initial diagnosis is valid, gluten challenge is unnecessary but the problem is to know when the initial diagnosis is valid.

Egan-Mitchell Well, I had rather hoped, Dr Rey, that you would accept that we have shown that the initial diagnosis was correct in 37 of the 40 cases and I was hoping that you wouldn't ask me to set about doing it in another 200 children. I must agree that the definition of coeliac disease, and particularly of latent coeliac disease, is controversial.

Asquith I can accept that it is easy to ensure that the patient is taking the gluten-containing diet during in-patient treatment but I wonder what steps Dr Walker-Smith took to ensure that the patient took a normal diet as an out-patient. It is fine to agree on the total amount to be taken, but do you ensure that it is taken, particularly when patients have shown such a benefit from the gluten-free diet in the first place?

Walker-Smith This was not completely satisfactory but what we aimed to do was to have repeated out-patient visits with our dietitians recording the grammes of wheat protein that the child was having, having regard to the range that Dorothy Francis of Great Ormond Street has laid down for normal gluten intake in English children. We were not giving high doses, say 20 or 40 g of gluten, to very young infants, because I think that is a completely different ball park. We were trying to keep as closely as possible to the amount of wheat protein that children would ordinarily be having in the community. I agree that diets may be variable, but believe that with many out-patients visits to senior and experienced dietitians they are fairly reliable. We abandoned giving whole gluten because some of our parents felt that their children were being poisoned by directly taking gluten powder. We found that the normal diet is usually more acceptable.

Katz   Dr Nusslé, did some of your patients appear to have a form of wheat sensitivity? Did any of them have protein-losing enteropathy or peripheral eosinophilia?

Nusslé   No.

Trier   In regard to the studies of gliadin instillation, quite a number of years ago we did similar studies in Seattle, and found that the results were much more dramatic in terms of response to wheat and gliadin instillation, if one instilled the test substance more distally into the bowel towards the mid-jejunum or at least towards the jejunal-ileal junction and made serial biopsies there. For some reason the proximal bowel seemed more resistant to the instillation than the distal bowel and I wonder if you have had a chance to study the response more distally where you might see more dramatic changes than in the proximal bowel?

Sinaasappel   I did not have the opportunity.

Stroder   Dr Nusslé, have you measured IgE levels in any of your patients?

Nusslé   IgE levels were normal in all cases.

McNicholl   I think it is clear that we must try to achieve some agreed criteria for diagnosis, particularly regarding mucosal morphology. This seems important, especially in children who appear to have transient intolerance, or prolonged tolerance. Could we ask Dr Walker-Smith and Professor Booth to form the nucleus of a small panel to collect and assess material, including photomicrographs, of these controversial patients?

Editor's comment   It was agreed to ask Walker-Smith and Booth to form a panel.

Section VI
Malignancy and ulceration in coeliac disease

30

Malignant lymphoma in coeliac disease

G. K. T. HOLMES, B. T. COOPER and W. T. COOKE

INTRODUCTION

Gough and his colleagues in 1962[1] were the first to suggest that intestinal lymphoma is a complication rather than just an association of coeliac disease. This view was strengthened in a further publication by the Bristol group[2] and shown to be statistically valid by Harris and his co-workers[3] in their survey of 202 patients with coeliac disease or idiopathic steatorrhoea. This series has been reviewed and to date 99 deaths have occurred of which 39 have been due to malignant disease, and in particular 18 due to lymphoma of which 14 involved the gastrointestinal tract.

This group has allowed longitudinal study of a group of coeliac patients who between 1965 and 1977 developed 11 new malignancies of which 4 were lymphomas, 4 gastrointestinal carcinomas and 3 carcinomas of other sites (Table 30.1). Since two patients each had two tumours the total number of malignancies in the series stands at 43. The mean follow-up is now approximately 14 years.

Table 30.1 Review of 202 patients with CD/IS

Malignancies	1965–1977
Lymphoma	4
GIT Carcinoma	4
Other	3
Total	11

Table 30.2 Deaths due to malignancy among 210 patients with coeliac disease

	Expected	Observed	p
All malignancies	5.048	21	<0.001
Reticulum cell sarcoma	0.114	13	<0.001

Since many individuals in this series died before the technique of jejunal biopsy became available a further study of the causes of death has been carried out with special reference to malignancy in all patients with histologically proven coeliac disease seen in the Nutritional and Intestinal Unit up to the end of 1972 and followed to the end of 1974[4]. Among these patients 21 deaths occurred due to malignancy when only 5 would have been expected ($p < 0.001$). There was a great excess of deaths due to reticulum cell sarcoma; 13 were observed when 0.11 were expected ($p<0.001$). (Table 30.2).

Since the prognosis of patients who develop these complications is so very poor (the mean duration of symptoms attributed to lymphoma was 7.6 months and to carcinoma 8.3 months) an attempt was made to ascertain whether the risk of dying from malignancy is lessened by prior treatment with a gluten-free diet. A total of 134 patients who had been treated with a gluten-free diet for at least one year were used in the assessment together with 70 patients who had taken a conventional diet. There was no evidence from this study that gluten withdrawal was in any way protective. Seven deaths were observed in the gluten-free group and eight in the normal diet group, both significantly in excess of the numbers expected (Table 30.3). This was also true for reticulum cell sarcoma considered separately.

Table 30.3 Deaths due to malignancy in coeliac disease in relation to dietary history

	No.	Expected	Observed	p
All malignancies				
GFD	134	1.259	7	<0.001
ND	70	3.787	8	<0.05
Reticulum cell sarcoma				
GFD	134	0.038	4	<0.001
ND	70	0.759	4	<0.001

GFD=gluten-free diet
ND=normal diet

It was perhaps optimistic to expect to demonstrate any such effect in patients who had already been exposed to an oncogenic stimulus for many years, probably since birth. It may be that if a gluten-free diet does offer any protection against malignancy it will only become apparent from an analysis of a group of patients who have been on the diet since childhood.

An alternative approach to try to improve the appalling prognosis would be to identify clues to earlier diagnosis. Thus the clinical and laboratory data from 27 patients with coeliac disease complicated by lymphoma who have attended the unit have been analysed with this in view. In 20 patients coeliac disease was diagnosed by the characteristic jejunal biopsy. The remaining seven patients were seen before the introduction of this technique to our hospital and are classed as having idiopathic steatorrhoea.

AGE AND SEX

There were 15 men and 12 women whose ages at diagnosis of lymphoma ranged from 35 to 82 years (mean 55 years) with a peak incidence in the seventh decade.

LYMPHOMA IN RELATION TO COELIAC DISEASE

The patients fell into two main groups: those 10 in whom coeliac disease and lymphoma were diagnosed within a short time (<one year) of each other, and a group of 16 patients in whom the diagnosis of coeliac disease clearly preceded that of lymphoma. There remained one patient in whom the diagnosis of Hodgkin's disease was made 14 years before that of coeliac disease though in retrospect symptoms suggestive of coeliac disease had been present for many years before the diagnosis of lymphoma.

Half of the patients in whom coeliac disease and lymphoma presented together were aged between 30 and 40 years (Figure 30.1). By contrast, for the group in which the diagnosis of coeliac disease was made prior to that of lymphoma the great majority of tumours occurred over the age of 50 years and almost two-thirds over the age of 60 years. (Figure 30.2).

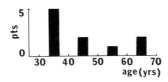

Figure 30.1 Age distribution at presentation (by decade) for 10 patients in whom coeliac disease and lymphoma were diagnosed within a short time of each other

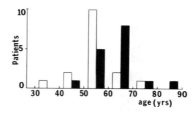

Figure 30.2 Age distribution at presentation (by decade) of coeliac disease (open columns) and lymphoma (filled columns) for 16 patients in whom the diagnosis of coeliac disease clearly preceded that of lymphoma

SYMPTOMS AT PRESENTATION

In general symptoms developed insidiously, but occasionally the presentation was acute such as with peritonitis or pneumonia (Figure 30.3). The commonest symptom was weight loss. It was the major warning sign that things were not satisfactory in an otherwise apparently healthy patient, was insidious and persistent, and usually the first symptom when it appeared. The generalized weakness affecting nearly half the

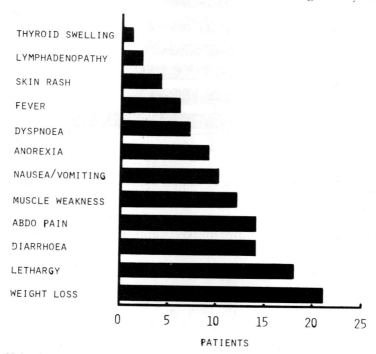

Figure 30.3 Symptoms at presentation in 27 patients with coeliac disease complicated by lymphoma

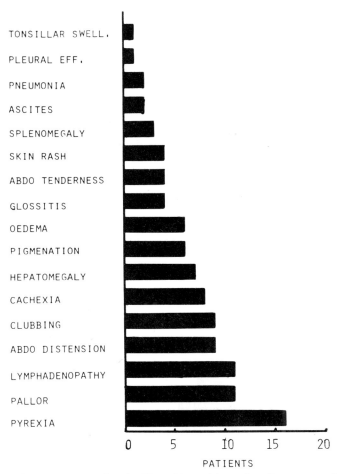

Figure 30.4 Signs at presentation in 27 patients with coeliac disease complicated by lymphoma

patients needs special emphasis. It involved voluntary muscles, becoming progressively more marked, and leading to almost total inability to walk or perform other motor functions but without any objective neurological abnormalities apart from reduced power.

SIGNS AT PRESENTATION

The signs were many and variable (Figure 30.4). The commonest were fever, superficial lymphadenopathy, clubbing and abdominal distension. Apart from skin pigmentation only four patients had skin rashes at presentation and of these only one was due to lympho-matous infiltration of the skin.

Table 30.4 Lymphoma in CD (27 cases). Indices at presentation

	No. measured	Abnormal	No. abnormal	% abnormal
Hb	27	< 12.5 g/100 ml	18	67
MCV	21	> 95 fl	10	48
Retics	13	> 1%	8	62
WBC	27	> 10.000/cu.mm	6	22
WBC	27	< 4.500/cu.mm	8	30
ESR	21	> 13 mm/h	15	71
Folate	16	< 3.1 ng/ml	8	50
Iron	15	< 60 g/100 ml	10	67
Albumin	23	< 35 g/l	16	70
Globulin	23	> 30 g/l	11	48
IgA	9	> 450 mg/100 ml	5	56
Alkaline phosphatase	23	> 13 K.A. units	12	52
Faecal fats	20	> 5 g/24 h	15	75

LABORATORY DATA

No patient had entirely normal blood indices (Table 30.4). Most patients were anaemic. Other commmon abnormalities were a raised ESR, low serum folate, low serum iron, low serum albumin and a raised alkaline phosphatase.

RADIOLOGY

Slightly more than half of the patients (15) had a barium meal and follow-through performed but these were disappointing for only one showed narrowed areas in the jejunum and three lesions in the stomach. Two-thirds showed only a malabsorption pattern, but in this group half of the patients were subsequently shown to have lymphomatous involvement of the small bowel.

CONFIRMATION OF DIAGNOSIS

The diagnosis was confirmed by biopsy in a third and by autopsy in another third of the patients. The remaining third were diagnosed by laparotomy. Of the nine in whom laparotomy was carried out, four were operated upon for diagnostic reasons since lymphoma was suspected from their clinical deterioration for no apparent reason. Three were operated upon for lesions in the stomach or jejunum. The remaining two individuals had perforation of the gastrointestinal tract.

TREATMENT AND SURVIVAL

With two exceptions the clinical course was a steady deterioration with an average survival of $9\frac{1}{2}$ months. Of the two exceptions (not included in this survival figure) one had Hodgkin's disease diagnosed in 1950 which was treated by radiotherapy with excellent results. In 1965 coeliac disease was diagnosed although in retrospect symptoms compatible with coeliac disease had been present for a number of years. The patient was treated with a gluten-free diet which resulted in clinical remission and morphological improvement in the jejunal histology. However, in 1976 he presented with abdominal pain, weight loss and severe haemolytic anaemia, which was attributed to Hodgkin's disease found in the bone marrow at autopsy. The remaining patient, the only survivor, is alive and well after treatment of his thyroid lymphoma.

Of the 18 patients diagnosed during life 13 received some form of treatment, though somewhat haphazard. If the long-term survivor with Hodgkin's disease and the living patient with a thyroid lymphoma are excluded from the reckoning the 11 remaining patients who were treated survived for a mean of 103 days (8–226 days) while the five untreated only survived for an average of 16 days (2–28 days). These figures probably reflect no more than that the untreated patients were severely ill when first diagnosed and that those who were treated were encountered at a slightly earlier stage of the disease.

DISCUSSION

Early diagnosis of lymphoma in patients with coeliac disease is difficult, since clinical features are non-specific and often indistinguishable from coeliac disease itself. In seeking helpful diagnostic features in a series of 27 coeliac patients with lymphoma, two groups have emerged. The first group comprises those in whom coeliac disease and lymphoma presented together. We believe that such patients should be regarded as having coeliac disease complicated by malignancy. They almost always have long histories compatible with coeliac disease, while in the occasional case who does not, the diagnosis is not invalidated, since asymptomatic coeliac patients are described[5]. Of those patients in this group who were treated with a gluten-free diet only one patient showed a transient clinical response; the remainder derived no benefit. Thus patients often in their fourth decade who present with coeliac disease which does not respond to gluten withdrawal should be regarded with great suspicion.

The second group comprises those who symptoms had been well-controlled by a gluten-free diet but whose condition subsequently deteriorated. All too often this reversal is attributed to dietary indiscretion and thus valuable weeks or months may be lost. Signs and symptoms were similar to those encountered in coeliac patients presenting without malignancy, although the presence of muscle weakness, pyrexia and lymphadenopathy encountered in the present series is unusual or only rarely found in uncomplicated coeliac disease[6-8]. Although many abnormalities were noted in the laboratory investigations, no particular pattern emerged and radiology was frequently unhelpful. Unfortunately in the great majority of patients, even in those subjected to laparotomy, lymphoma was widely disseminated at diagnosis, making the outlook for this group extremely poor. It is not known whether lifelong treatment with a gluten-free diet will prevent malignant complications arising, but efforts must be directed towards their diagnosis at a very much earlier stage if the prognosis is to be improved. Finally, there had been a suggestion that, from the plasma cell counts in the lamina propria of the jejunal mucosa, it may be possible to predict which patients are more likely to develop lymphoma[9]. This may identify a group at special risk who would require very careful follow-up. However, the problems of making an early definitive diagnosis of malignancy would probably still be considerable.

References

1. Gough, K. R., Read, A. E. and Naish, J. M. (1962). Intestinal reticulosis as a complication of steatorrhoea. *Gut*, **3**, 232
2. Austad, W. I., Cornes, J. S., Gough, K. R., McCarthy, C. F. and Read, A. E. (1967). Steatorrhoea and malignant lymphoma. The relationship of malignant tumours of lymphoid tissue and coeliac disease. *Am. J. Dig. Dis.*, **12**, 475
3. Harris, O. D., Cooke, W. T., Thompson, H. and Waterhouse, J. A. H. (1967). Malignancy in adult coeliac disease and idiopathic steatorrhoea. *Am. J. Med.*, **42**, 899
4. Holmes, G. K. T., Stokes, P. L., Sorahan, T. M., Prior, P., Waterhouse, J. A. H. and Cooke, W. T. (1976). Coeliac disease, gluten-free diet and malignancy. *Gut*, **17**, 612
5. Stokes, P. L., Ferguson, R., Holmes, G. K. T. and Cooke, W. T. (1976). Familial aspects of coeliac disease. *Qu. J. Med.*, **XLV**, 567
6. Cooke, W. T., Peeney, A. L. P. and Hawkins, C. F. (1953). Symptoms, signs, and diagnostic features of idiopathic steatorrhoea. *Qu. J. Med.*, **XXII**, 59
7. Benson, G. D., Kowlessar, O. B. and Sleisenger, M. H. (1964). Adult coeliac disease with emphasis upon response to the gluten-free diet. *Medicine* (Baltimore), **43**, 1
8. Barry, R. E., Baker, P. and Read, A. E. (1974). The clinical presentation. In: Cooke, W. T. and Asquith, P. (eds.) *Coeliac Disease*, pp. 55–69 (London: Saunders)
9. Ferguson, R., Asquith, P. and Cooke, W. T. (1974). The jejunal cellular infiltrate in coeliac disease complicated by lymphoma. *Gut*, **15**, 458

Discussion of chapter 30

Ferguson   When I went to the Western General Hospital two and a half years ago I shared your impression of an appalling prognosis in patients with lymphoma and coeliac disease, but the previous experience of the Unit was not quite as bad as you have suggested. I think we have had about a dozen coeliacs with lymphomas of whom the majority were submitted to laparotomy and if possible resection, followed by radiotherapy to the abdomen. Three such patients have survived for long periods. Two have recently died, seven and nine years aftrer the initial operation. One man is alive and completely well 11 years after three laparotomies in quick succession for lymphoma. Early surgery, I think, is certainly still advisable. If it is proceeded with it is worth doing a proper staging laparotomy with bone marrow biopsy, liver biopsy and so on to allow formal management of the lymphoma as we would with any other lymphoma. Could I now ask you a question? Is there evidence of reticulum cell sarcoma developing in anyone who has been documented as having return of the jejunal mucosa to be absolutely normal for two, three or more years on a gluten-free diet?

Holmes   Yes, there is a case report actually which was written up in 1969 in *Gut,* of a woman whose intestinal mucosa had become normal on a gluten-free diet when she developed lymphoma, and the biopsy stayed normal.

Stewart   The duration of a gluten-free diet clearly is of great importance, but can you tell us something about the strictness of the diet, because this is remarkably difficult to determine in out-patients.

Holmes   I accept that, that is an intrinsic problem for any gluten-free diet research. We know all of the 134 patients personally and follow them closely. We can never exclude the possibility that they do take gluten. I think the best we can say is that their gluten load is less than when they were on normal diet.

Stevens   We have one man with coeliac disease who has a brother with coeliac disease. A third brother with a normal small intestinal mucosa has a lymphosarcoma of the intestine.

Asquith   You said a third of the diagnoses had been made by biopsy. Were you talking about intestinal biopsy? So you think that a multiple proximal intestinal biopsy, looking for low plasma cell counts and high lymphocyte counts might be justified if lymphoma is suspected?

Holmes   We didn't make any diagnosis on histology of intestinal biopsy. I am speaking about liver biopsy and lymph node biopsy.

Rey If the incidence in lymphoma is related to the intestinal lesion, do you expect an effect from a gluten-free diet after 40 to 50 years of flat mucosa? Did you try to correlate the incidence of lymphoma with genetic markers?

Holmes We did not look at genetic markers. I agree, of our 18 lymphomas, 14 have involved the GI tract, but four didn't, so that more general mechanisms have to be considered in pathogenesis. I accept your point and I think this is one reason we were unable to show any advantage of a gluten-free diet. We had had patients on a gluten-free diet for roughly eight years, whereas they have had a life-long exposure to a normal diet, so it is a bit optimistic to expect any improvement. We may have to wait another 20 years.

Albert I would like to know whether any cases of lymphoma in first-degree relatives of coeliac patients have been observed or are included in your series.

Holmes No, there are no relatives in this. We have had a family study, and we have as far as I know been unable to find any lymphomas in first-degree relatives. One would expect to. We did find an increase in cancer generally.

31

Intestinal ulceration, flat mucosa and malabsorption: report of registry of 33 patients

T. M. BAYLESS, A. BAER, J. H. YARDLEY and T. R. HENDRIX

Since our initial report of intestinal ulceration occurring as an apparent complication of well-documented coeliac disease, we have maintained a registry of similar patients. We have received reports on 33 patients with a flat jejunal mucosa and malabsorption and small bowel ulcerations. Fourteen had either proven or probable coeliac disease. Eight others may have coeliac disease but the pathogenetic role of gluten is less clear. Ten additional patients were refractory to an adequate trial of corticosteroids and/or a gluten-free diet. The term 'non-granulomatous ulcerative jejuno-ileitis' had been used for many of these patients.

Twenty-four of the 33 patients died of complications of the small bowel ulceration. Sixteen died within 7 months of the onset of symptoms referable to the ulcers. Six of the nine who survived had undergone extensive resections of the ulcerated areas. Two patients who had received corticosteroids without surgery survived over five years.

None of the 33 patients developed lymphoma, but six other patients in the registry presented with non-specific intestinal ulcers and were subsequently found to have a definite or probable lymphoma. Atypical lymphoproliferative inflammation was present in the base of the ulcers of three of these patients, which should have helped distinguish them from the non-specific 'wastebasket' diagnosis of non-granulomatous ulcerative jejuno-ileitis.

Our own most recent patient with multiple intestinal ulceration and malabsorption had skin biopsy confirmed dermatitis herpetiformis as well as a patchy small bowel lesion. This patient seems to provide another link between coeliac disease and dermatitis herpetiformis.

References

1. Artinian, B., Lough, J. O. and Palmer, J. D. (1971). Idiopathic ulceration of small bowel with pseudolymphomatous reaction. A clinicopathological study of 6 cases. *Arch. Pathol.*, **91**, 327

2. Bayless, T. M., Kapelowitz, R. F., Shelley, W. M., *et al*: (1967). Intestinal ulceration —a complication of coeliac disease. *New Engl. J. Med.*, **276**, 996

3. Blau, J. S., Stolzenberg, J. and Toffler, R. B. (1971). Small bowel ulcerations—an unusual complication of coeliac disease. *J. Canad. Assoc. Radiol.*, **25**, 77

4. Evans, D. J. and Booth, C. C. (1971). Fatal malabsorption unresponsive to gluten-free diet in the adult. *Gut.* **12**, 858

5. Jeffries, G. H., Steinberg, H. and Sleisenger, M. H. (1968). Chronic ulcerative (non-granulomatous) jejunitis. *Am. J. Med.*, **44**, 47

6. Klaeveman, H. L., Gebhard, R. L., Sessons, C., *et al* (1975). In vitro studies of ulcerative ileojejunitis. *Gastroenterology*, **68**, 572

7. McCarthy, C. F. and Mylotte, M. J. (1972). Coeliac disease – a premalignant disease? *J. Irish Med. Assn.*, **65**, 241

8. Moritz, M., Moran, J. M. and Patterson, J. F. (1971). Chronic ulcerative jejunitis. Report of a case and discussion of classification. *Gastroenterology*, **60**, 96

9. Stuber, J. L., Wiegman, H., Crosby, I., *et al.* (1971). Ulcers of the colon and jejunum in coeliac disease. *Radiology*, **99**, 339

10. Thompson, H. (1974). Necropsy studies on adult coeliac disease. *J. Clin. Pathol.*, **27**, 710

11. Tönder, M., Sörlie, D. and Kearney, M. S. (1976). Adult coeliac disease. A case with ulceration, dermatitis herpetiformis and reticulosarcoma. *Scand. J. Gastroenterol.*, 11:107

12. Whitehead, R. (1968). Primary lymphadenopathy complicating idiopathic steatorrhoea. *Gut*, **9**, 569

Discussion of chapter 31

Booth   I have asked Professor Delmont if he will show us a patient that he has seen at Nice.

Delmont   The patient was a 31-year-old Algerian woman with a history of six years of diarrhoea and weight loss of 10 kilograms. She entered our unit with acute diarrhoea and malabsorptive state and the barium enema showed us a fistula between the right part of the transverse colon and the third portion of the duodenum. The fistula was closed surgically but symptoms recurred two months later and a jejunal biopsy was done which showed an atropic pattern. With a gluten-free diet there was clinical improvement in 10 days, but a biopsy in three months showed no improvement. A further barium enema showed a recurrence of the fistula which was closed surgically again. Two years after the operation she is well. Repeat biopsy has not been possible because of the narrowing in the second part of the duodenum. We do not know how to classify this patient.

McCarthy   Could I ask about associated diseases in those patients with intestinal ulceration. I ask because we have a patient with a flat intestinal mucosa, a 44-year-old woman who responded partly to a gluten-free diet and steroids with some improvement of the mucosa. She died because of bleeding ulcers in the terminal ileum. The histology of these ulcers is still debated as to whether it is malignant or non-malignant. She also had chronic active hepatitis cirrhosis and cutaneous vasculitis.

Bayless   Pericholangitis was found in five patients, two others had excess lymphocytes in the portar triads. Those were mainly these people with the atypical lymphoproliferative disorder. Four had chronic pancreatitis, 12 had enlarged hyperplastic lymph nodes, one had splenic atrophy.

Cluysenaer In a series of 47 patients with coeliac disease, we found four patients with intestinal ulceration and this seems to prove that ulceration is not as rare as usually thought. One of our patients also had a fistula between the duodenum and transverse colon. We were very much impressed that two of these patients only responded to a gluten-free diet after additional corticosteroids and also reduction of the dietary fat intake.

Scott   In the patients who had both ulceration and lymphoma do you think that the ulceration results in the lymphoma or do you think they both result from underlying coeliac disease?

Bayless   Obviously, I don't know the answer to that question. Some of the patients who have well-established coeliac disease develop

313

benign ulcerations for two or three years. I mentioned two had laparotomy and nothing was found and then the lymphoma appeared. What the cause of the ulceration in the non-lymphomatous bowel, was, we don't know.

Clarke   Your overall mortality was 70%. Was there very much variation in the groups? One has impression that ones with ulceration usually die.

Bayless   All figures that I gave for mortality were among those 33 patients, the first two categories that is, as I said, 16 of the 33 died within seven months of the onset of ulcers. Nine survived the complications. Seven patients were followed up over five years and one died at seven years and the other died at 13 years. Two are still alive at 13 and 15 years.

Weiser   May I assume that hypersecretory hormonal cases of a flat mucosa such as hypergastrinaemia have been excluded?

Bayless   The question of Zollinger–Ellison syndrome has been taken into account. Most of these patients have been seen in the last five years and the patients were studied for that. On autopsy there was no evidence of hyperplasia of the stomach and duodenal ulcers were very uncommon. Most of these people had very simple ulcerations, not like peptic ulceration.

32

Aphthous ulceration – the incidence of coeliac disease and gluten sensitivity

P. ASQUITH and M. K. BASU

The incidence of recurrent aphthous ulceration (RAU) in the population is high. Approximately 20% of unselected hospital out-patients and 10% of patients seen in general practice have such ulcers[1]. Their aetiology is unknown, however, there is a long recognised association of RAU with gastrointestinal disease, particularly coeliac disease[2]. This has lead several groups to screen such patients for intestinal lesions including performing jejunal biopsies. The reported incidence of flat biopsies compatible with coeliac disease has varied from 24%, in a study by Ferguson, Basu, Asquith and Cooke 1976[3] to less than 4% in two other series [4,5] Protocols have not usually included tests for absorption or investigation of the patient's immunological status. More importantly, follow-up jejunal biopsies after gluten withdrawal have not been reported. In view of this, and also because of the large variation in the reported incidence of flat biopsies, a further study of patients with RAU has been performed.

PATIENTS AND METHODS

Patients studied

A total of 36 patients (14 male and 22 female, mean age 32.2 years) were studied having been referred with a single complaint of RAU. The patients had to have suffered from RAU for more than 1 year with recurrent (maximum freedom of up to 4 weeks) or continuous lesions. Following initial evaluation (see below) the patients were then followed for a further 3–6 months as out-patients to further confirm the inclusion criteria.

Methods

Laboratory investigations were performed at least twice at intervals of 2–6 weeks. Tests included a full blood count, serum iron, TIBC, serum folate, red cell folate and B_{12}, a biochemical profile, serum IgG, IgA and IgM, C3, C4, and reticulin, antinuclear factor and smooth muscle antibodies. After full explanation and having giving informed consent the patients were then admitted to the Metabolic Unit for the following investigations. Faeces were collected for 3–5 days for fat estimation; a 1 hour blood xylose absorption test and a lactose tolerance test were performed and intestinal fluid aspirated for IgG and IgA estimations. Also performed were jejunal biopsies using a suction multiple biopsy capsule[6]. The mucosa was examined under the dissecting microscope and routinely processed. Sections were classified using criteria of Roy-Choudhury *et al.* 1974[7]. Cell counts were performed of plasma cells and lymphocytes per mm² of lamina propria and the number of epithelial lymphocytes per 200 epithelial cell nuclei were counted[8]. Sections were also stained with fluorescene labelled antisera specific for IgG, IgA and IgM. Jejunal mucosal lactase, sucrase and maltase esimations were also carried out using standard techniques. Because of the occurrence of RAU in Behcet's syndrome and because some patients with this syndrome are unaware of for example rectal ulcers, all patients had a sigmoidoscopy. Three additional patients were found to have rectal ulcers and were therefore excluded from the series. To allow certain comparisons, 12 patients with untreated coeliac disease, 100 healthy controls and 8 patients with irritable colon were also studied.

The results were analysed using Student's t test and the x^2 test with the Yates's correction.

RESULTS

Three of 28 RAU patients had a mosaic appearance on dissecting microscopy and Grade III histological changes. One of these (M.F.) was an Irish girl and one (R.H.) had a grand-daughter with known coeliac disease. One other patient had a family history of coeliac disease in a maternal aunt. He has refused a jejunal biopsy. Whilst on a normal diet none of the three had steatorrhoea, only one (M.F.) had an abnormal blood xylose absorption test. The lactose tolerance test was normal in all three but two (M.F. and R.H.) had low mucosal levels of lactase, sucrase, and maltase. These three patients were treated solely with a gluten-free diet for 3–6 months. The mouth ulcers cleared

Table 32.1 Results of blood tests and jejunal biopsies on a normal diet and after a gluten-free diet in the three patients who showed Grade III changes

Patient		Hb	Fe	IBC	Serum folate	RCF	IgG	IgA	IgM	C3	C4	Jejunal biopsy
M.F.	N.D.	10.2	1.4	71.8	0.8	50	406	659	109	131	26	Grade III
	G.F.D.	10.0	3.3	80.5	2.2	58	850	570	70	238	46	Grade II
	(6 months)											
R.H.	N.D.	16.4	9.8	66.0	2.8	113	1380	820	108	200	90	Grade III
	G.F.D.	15.8	29.0	71.0	—	—	1370	890	120	163	73	Grade II
	(6 months)											
E.B.	N.D.	12.8	17.4	58.2	7.8	106	630	275	32	213	24	Grade III
	G.F.D.	13.6	15.1	53.9	8.6	151	855	595	70	256	45	Grade II
	(3 months)											

within 2–4 weeks and have not recurred. Table 32.1 shows the results of their tests before and after gluten withdrawal. All showed morphological improvement in their jejunal biopsies.

More than one biopsy was obtained in 15 patients; 12 patients had two, two had three, and one had seven biopsies. 42% of the patients showed either a Grade O or Grade I biopsy, 35% showed a combination of Grades I and II, 3% Grades I, II and III, 7% showed Grade II appearances alone, and 10% Grade III alone, namely the three already mentioned. Excluding the three Grade III biopsies, 6 of 26 patients (23%) showed an abnormal 1 hour corrected xylose test. However, abnormal results did not correlate with the grading of the jejunal biopsies. Only one patient had steatorrhoea.

The results of haematological, biochemical and immunological tests in patients with RAU and untreated coeliac disease are shown in Tables 32.2 and 32.3. A substantial number (up to 50%) of patients with RAU had deficiences of folate, red cell folate or of iron. There were few changes with respect to serum levels of IgG, IgA and IgM. However, in patients with RAU 83% had raised C3 and 72% raised C4 levels, and their mean values showed significant increases for both components compared with the mean results in the 100 healthy controls ($p<0.001$). Reticulin antibodies (IgG class), anti-nuclear factor antibodies and smooth muscle antibodies were found in only 4, 4 and 1 patient(s) respectively. Semiquantitative assessment of mucosal immunoglobulin containing cells showed little change; quantitative estimation of immunoglobulins in intestinal fluid aspirate showed mean concentrations of IgG of 16.68 ± 2.88 mg/100 ml and IgA 11.65 ± 4.17 mg/100 ml in 18 patients with RAU, results which did not differ significantly from those

Table 32.2 Results of laboratory investigations (percent abnormal) in patients with aphthous ulcers and coeliac disease

Test	N.R.	Aphthous ulcers (n = 36)	Untreated coeliacs (n = 12)
Hb.	male 12–16 g/dl	7(19%)	7(58%)
	female 14–18 g/dl		
P.C.V.	male 370–470	10(28%)	9(75%)
	female 420–520		
M.C.H.C.	32–36 g/dl	0	8(66%)
R.C.F.	160–600 μg/l	18(50%)	9(75%)
Folate	2.5–18 μg/l	5(14%)	7(58%)
B_{12}	150–800 ng/l	6(17%)	0
Fe	14.3–28.6 μmol/l	15(42%)	7(58%)
T.I.B.C.	45–72 μmol/l	7(19%)	2(17%)
Albumin	34–45 g/l	0	1(8%)
Calcium	2.30–2.60mmol/l	low: 12(33%)	low: 7(63%)
		high: 2(6%)	high: 1(8%)
Alkaline phosphatase	17–75 I.U./l	4(12%)	3(25%)

in patients with untreated coeliac disease (n=9): IgG 20.83±4.38 mg/100 ml, IgA 11.41±2.01 mg/100 ml.

With respect to mucosal cell counts (Table 32.4), significant increases were found in the lamina propria plasma cells in both patients with RAU and untreated coeliac disease ($p<0.001$). Compared to controls, lamina propria lymphocytes were also increased in RAU ($p<0.01$), but not in coeliac disease, whilst epithelial lymphocytes were significantly increased in both patient groups ($p<0.01$). Patients with coeliac disease showed a further significant increase in plasma cells compared to RAU but not for lymphocytes either in the lamina propria or epithelial cell layer.

DISCUSSION

In a group of individuals presenting with mouth ulcers, we have found three patients out of a total of 28 who were biopsied, who satisfy a current definition of coeliac disease[9]. One had several features of coeliac disease, however, the other two did not, and would have been missed had the jejunal bioipsies not been carried out as a result of too much attention being given to the results of the initial screening tests. Nevertheless, one was a grandfather of a known coeliac and could have been picked up as a result of a family survey which included jejunal biopsies. The mucosal abnormalities of the three patients were gluten responsive, so

Table 32.3 Results of serum immunoglobulins, C3, C4 (percent abnormal) and autoantibodies and mucosal immunofluorescence (percent abnormal) in patients with aphthous ulcers and untreated coeliac disease

	N.R.		Aphthous ulcers (n=36)		Untreated coeliacs (n=12)	
IgG	6.00–16.00	g/l	Low	0	Low	1(8%)
			High	3(8%)	High	2(16%)
IgA	1.25–4.80	g/l	Low	1(2%)	Low	0
			High	5(14%)	High	5(41%)
IgM	0.50–20	g/l	Low	3(8%)	Low	2(16%)
			High	4(11%)	High	1(8%)
C3	0.78–1.62	g/l	Low	0	Low	0
			High	30(83%)	High	7(58%)
C4	0.15–0.45	g/l	Low	0	Low	0
			High	26(72%)	High	6(50%)
Reticulin Ab.						
IgG	—			4(11%)		2(16%)
IgA	—			0		1(8%)
A.N.F.	—			4(11%)		—
S.M.A.	—			1(2%)		—
Mucosal IgG	—			1(2%)		2(16%)
,, IgA	—			2(4%)		6(50%)
,, IgM	—			2(4%)		4(33%)

Table 32.4 Mean (± SE) cell counts per mm² of lamina propria and per 200 epithelial cell nuclei in groups of patients studied

	Controls (n=8)	Patients with aphthous ulcers non-coeliac (n=17)	Patients with coeliac disease on normal diet (n=9)
Lamina propria:			
Plasma cells	1082±118	1777±121	4640±506
Lymphocytes	2175±139	2945±203	2573±213
Epithelial lymphocytes	36±4	60±6	75±9

were their mouth lesions. It is tempting to postulate that the mouth lesions of a significant proportion of the other patients are gluten induced, more importantly are dependent on an intestinal mucosal lesion rather than a gut independent direct effect of gluten on the mouth mucosa. Such a hypothesis would be difficult to prove because the lesion is patchy and in any case may be minimally represented by increased cell counts in the jejunal mucosa. In this latter respect our results are similar to those found by Ferguson et al 1976[3]. That the lesion is patchy is illustrated by one patient who had three separate jejunal biopsies producing in all a total of seven pieces of intestinal mucosa. One piece, from the third procedure, showed Grade III changes but Grades I and II were also present in other pieces. This patient has been treated with a gluten-free diet. His mouth ulcers have disappeared and there has been improvement in his clinical and blood status but he has yet to undergo a post-gluten-free jejunal biopsy. Hence at the moment he has not been given a definite diagnosis of coeliac disease. A patchy lesion would explain the different incidence of flat biopsies found in the literature [3,4,5] and this seems the most reasonable explanation. Different inclusion criteria is another possibility. Patients with less severe RAU may have lower incidences of flat biopsies and it is thus essential to have comparable patients for series comparisons.

Abnormal D-xylose tests were found in 23% of our patients but no correlation was found with the results of a single jejunal biopsy. Again this may be due to the patchy nature of the lesion. Results of serum complement, mucosal cell counts, mucosal immunoglobulin containing plasma cells and intestinal immunoglobulin levels resemble those found in untreated coeliacs. With respect to intestinal immunoglobulins, unfortunately a non-coeliac control group was not included but it still seems relevant and worth noting that the intestinal fluid immunoglobulin concentrations in aphthous ulcer patients are just as abnormal as in untreated coeliacs. We propose but have not proven that many of the listed abnormalities in patients with RAU are gluten dependent. To this end 12 patients with Grade 0 or 1 biopsies have been treated with a gluten-free diet. To date eight have shown a reduction in the incidence of their RAU. It is tempting to postulate that the mouth lesions in many of these patients are the mouth equivalents of the skin lesions found in dermatitis herpetiformis, the intestine of the patient being the source of circulating gluten antibody, or immune complexes, or sensitized T-cells which on reaching the mouth induce either a humoral or cell-mediated reaction.

References

1. Sircus, W., Church, R. and Kelleher, S. (1957). Recurrent aphthous ulceration of the mouth. A study of the natural history, aetiology and treatment, *Q. J. Med.*, **26**, 235

2. Cooke, W. T., Peeney, A. L. P. and Hawkins, C. F. (1953). Symptoms, signs and diagnostic features of idiopathic steatorrhoea. *Q. J. Med.*, **22**, 59

3. Ferguson, R., Basu, M. K., Asquith, P. and Cooke, W. T. (1976). Jejunal mucosal abnormalities in patients with recurrent aphthous ulceration. *Br. Med. J.*, **1**, 11

4. Wray, D. Ferguson, M.M., Mason, D.K., Hutcheon, A.W. and Dagg, J.H. (1975). Recurrent aphthae: treatment with vitamin B$_{12}$, folic acid and iron. *Br. Med. J.*, **2**, 490

5. Challacombe, S.J., Barkhan, P. and Lehner, T. (1977). Haematological features and differentiation of recurrent oral ulceration. *Br. J. Oral Surg.*, **15**, 37

6. Roy-Choudhury, D.C., Nicholson, G.M. and Cooke, W.T. (1964). Simple capsule for multiple intestinal biopsy specimens. *Lancet*, **2**, 185

7. Roy-Choudhury, D.C., Cooke, W.T. and Tan, D.T. (1966). Jejunal biopsy: criteria and significance. *Scand. J. Gastroenterol.*, **1**, 57

8. Holmes, G.K.T., Asquith, P., Stokes, P.L. and Cooke, W.T. (1974). Cellular infiltrate of jejunal biopsies in adult coeliac disease in relation to gluten withdrawal. *Gut*, **15**, 278

9. Cooke, W.T. and Asquith, P. (1974). Definition of coeliac disease – In W. T. Cooke and P. Asquith (eds) *Coeliac Disease: Clinics in Gastroenterology* Vol. 3 No., 1, pp 3–10 (London: Saunders)

Discussion of chapter 32

Ferguson	My colleague, Dr James Rose, has studied 25 patients referred to the Edinburgh Dental Hospital with aphthous ulceration. The study was to define whether or not coeliac disease was present in any of the patients. In 23, jejunal morphology including intra-epithelial lymphocyte count was unequivocally normal. Disaccharidase levels were also normal. In one slim tall teenager aged 16, jejunal biopsy was flat, epithelial lymphocyte count high and disaccharidases were low. She has been put on a gluten-free diet. There is no change in her aphthous ulceration and she has not yet had a repeat biopsy. One further patient had minor abnormalities, reduction in villous height, high intraepithelial lymphocyte count and reduction in sucrase level. A repeat biopsy six months later on a normal diet was unequivocally normal. We interpret this as meaning that the changes in his original biopsy were due to intercurrent infection. From this study the incidence of coeliac disease is 4% of patients with aphthous ulceration.
Douglas	If I saw your data correctly there appeared to be a higher IgG than IgA in the intestinal secretions. This appears to be very different from data Paul Crabbé, Jack Hobbs and myself reported in 1970. David Shmerling has drawn attention to the difficulties in measuring immunoglobulins in intestinal juice. Are you sure that you really were measuring all the IgA that was there?
Asquith	Yes, these were monospecific antisera. We have excluded non-specific precipitation. This was a single radial diffusion technique. We have not excluded the fact that some degradation of IgG occurred, but at least samples were collected in appropriate conditions.
Moynihan	Did you look at patients with dermatitis herpetiformis and possible association with aphthous ulceration?
Asquith	No. With respect to the ethics of the study. We deliberately followed the patients for about six months as out-patients to check that they were really suffering severe mouth lesions and they satisfied our inclusion criteria. Many of the patients came once and then the ulcers disappeared and clearly such intensive investigation would be unjustified in those patients.
Booth	I may have missed it, but did you tell us the results of the rectal studies?
Asquith	The rectal studies were done deliberately because of the possibility of rectal ulcers. Three patients were excluded because they had rectal ulcers—Behcet's syndrome in other words.
Nusslé	Have you done viral studies?
Asquith	No.

33

Refractory sprue

J. H. M. v. TONGEREN, O. J. J. CLUYSENAER and
P. H. M. SCHILLINGS

INTRODUCTION

The majority of patients who suffer from malabsorption associated with
a flat jejunal mucosa respond to treatment with a gluten-free diet.
Some of them, however, only respond to a combination of a gluten-free
diet and corticosteroids. In the course of time most of these patients
become gluten-sensitive again. A few patients respond not at all and run
an almost pernicious course resulting in death from gross malnutrition
or from complications.

This paper presents two patients with severe malabsorption. a flat
jejunal mucosa and fatal outcome.

CASE HISTORIES

Patient 1 (reg. no. 2209212D), female, was born in 1921. Prior to 1963
she had noticed several periods of weight loss without a demonstrable
reason. She recovered spontaneously from such episodes and always
returned to her normal body weight. In 1963 she complained of fatigue,
dizziness and weight loss. A diagnosis of adrenal cortical insufficiency
was considered and treatment with cortisone, 65 mg daily, resulted in
marked improvement and 18 kg weight gain. In November 1965 she
noticed pain in the left buttock and her weight fell to 39 kg. X-ray
examination of the left sacroiliac joint showed a slight irregularity and a
surgical biopsy specimen from this region was suggestive of a reticulum
cell sarcoma. After irradiation of the joint the pain disappeared and
radiological features were normalized. Her body weight increased to
57 kg. In 1966 she first complained of watery stools with bowel movements up to 20 times daily. This resulted in a decrease in body weight
to 45 kg. The patient felt weak and vomited frequently. Serum K, Mg

and Ca levels were very low (1.7, 0.5 and 1.2 mmol/l, respectively) and the patient was admitted to our hospital in October 1966. Her body weight was then 39 kg.

No pigmentation was observed in the mouth or on the palms of the hands. Physical examination of the abdomen revealed no abnormalities. Bowel action was 3–5 times daily. The amount of faeces largely depended on the food intake and varied from 500 to 3000 g/day. Faeces contained no blood or pathological bacteria.

Haemoglobin was 7 mmol/l (11.2 g/dl), serum folate 0.9 ng/ml but bone marrow was not clearly megaloblastic. Fat absorption was 55%. Serum albumin was reduced to 27 g/l. Cortisone therapy was gradually stopped. Three weeks later the plasma cortisol level was normal (250 μg/l). After intravenous administration of 120 U ACTH the plasma cortisol rose to 950 μg/l, thus indicating normally functioning adrenal cortices.

Lymphangiography of the lumbar and para-aortic lymph nodes and the thoracic duct was normal. A jejunal biopsy showed a flat mucosa. Gluten was withheld from the diet but no effect on the diarrhoea was observed. The diarrhoea was relieved only by complete exclusion of oral food. The patient was treated with intravenous glucose, supplemented with minerals, whilst vitamin supplements including B-group, B_{12}, C,A,D,K and folic acid were administered parenterally. To increase the serum protein level plasma infusions were given. Later, corticosteroids were introduced in an effort to improve both the histological abnormality of the small bowel mucosa and absorption, but all these measures had little effect. Oral feeding continued to cause diarrhoea, so minerals, glucose and vitamins eventually had to be given through a vena cava catheter. A few weeks later the patient developed *E. coli* sepis which was successfully treated with ampicillin and streptomycin. However, she developed rapidly progressive jaundice and the liver enlarged markedly. A liver biopsy revealed extreme steatosis, many bile plugs and intercellular bile pigment. The portal areas were enlarged and there was a moderate accumulation of lymphocytes and granulocytes, especially eosinophils. The patient slowly deteriorated. The temperature remained high but repeated bacteriological examinations of the blood were negative. She died on 3rd January 1967. Autopsy was performed within a few hours. The entire small bowel mucosa was flat and reduced in thickness, showing relatively few crypts of Lieberkühn. Paneth cells were absent. The bowel wall was extremely thin too (Figure 33.1A). There was no subepithelial collagen. The colon was normal. Examination of the mesenteric blood vessels and lymph nodes revealed no abnormalities. The liver showed an extreme fatty change and weighed 2460 g. Metastases of a reticulum cell sarcoma in the liver were not found and there was no large duct obstruction. The spleen weighed

90 g. The pancreas was normal and tumours were not observed in this organ. No signs of malignancy were found in the left sacroiliac joint.

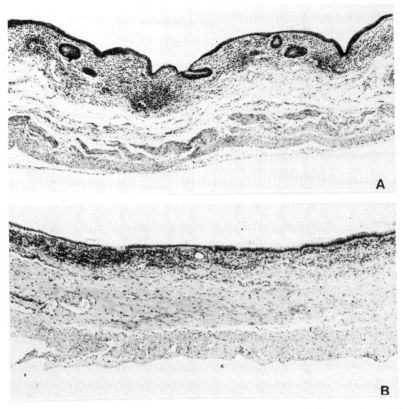

Figure 33.1   Post-mortem specimens of the small intestinal wall from patient 1(A) and 2(B) with refractory sprue. The thinness of the intestinal wall and paucity of mucosal crypts are apparent. (Reproduced from Cluysenaer and van Tongeren, 'Malabsorption in Coeliac Sprue', Martinus Nijhoff Medical Division, The Hague, 1977; with permission of authors and publisher).

Patient 2 (reg. no. 1012191K) began to pass frequent pulpy stools at age 54 and lost 6 kg body weight. He also felt tired and listless. When questioned he stated that as a child he had sometimes suffered from meteorism, diarrhoea, anaemia and retardation of growth. The abdominal symptoms which had now developed were so severe that hospitalization was necessary. The patient was vomiting and produced large amounts of watery faeces (1–5 kg per day). The body weight had decreased to 50 kg (height 1.68 m). Biochemical tests revealed a normal haemoglobin concentration but a markedly decreased serum folate level (less than 1 ng/ml). The serum albumin concentration was markedly decreased (19 g/l), due to an increased enteric protein loss (500 ml plasma per day). There was moderate steatorrhoea (absorption coefficient 68%), decreased excretion of D-xylose (2 g in 5 h) and vitamin B_{12} (0.6% in 48 hours). The number of microorganisms in the proximal jejunum was not increased. The 'breath' test ($[^{14}C]$glycocholic acid) for bile acid deconjugation showed an increased peak value (5.25 × 10^{-5} of the administered dose), probably due to reduced absorption of bile acids in the ileum. Cholestyramine had no effect on the diarrhoea. Gluten withdrawal was prescribed in view of a flat jejunal mucosa with marked inflammatory changes and superficial erosions, but had no more effect than 3 weeks of an elementary diet or parenteral administration of fluids, plasma, minerals and vitamins. The progressive deterioration of the patient's condition was accelerated by disturbed liver function, jaundice and sepsis. The patient died cachectic, seven months after the onset of diarrhoea. At the post-mortem, performed within 2 h of death, a palpably thin small intestine was resected. A small amount of serous fluid was found in the abdominal cavity. The liver showed extensive steatosis and signs of cholangitis. The pancreas was normal apart from slight atrophy of the exocrine glands. The spleen was atrophic. The mesenteric blood vessels seemed normal. The abdominal lymph nodes were markedly enlarged: microscopy revealed a chronic inflammatory infiltrate with an increase of connective tissue. No signs of a specific inflammatory or malignant process were found. The mucosa of the small intestine was flat over its entire length, and lined by cubical to high-cylindrical enterocytes. The lamina propria contained an inflammatory infiltrate consisting of granulocytes as well as plasma cells and lymphocytes. In this patient the number of mucosal crypts was also extremely reduced with moderate mitotic activity (Figure 33.1B). Paneth cells were absent. No subepithelial collagen deposits were seen.

COMMENT

Refractory sprue, although relatively rare, is not unique judging from the number of published case histories[1-19]. It seems that the patients in question may well belong to a heterogeneous group having in common severe malabsorption, a flat small bowel mucosa and failure to respond to any kind of treatment. The names given to this condition such as non-responsive coeliac disease, intestinal mucosal atrophy, fatal malabsorption syndrome, fatal (non-tropical) sprue, collagenous sprue and ulcerative jejunoileitis, express either the fatal outcome or characteristics of the small bowel wall at autopsy. In the published cases stress is laid on five lesions: ulceration of the small bowel

wall with, in some cases, perforation, obstruction or severe haemor-
rhage, widespread collagen deposition beneath the epithelium, foci of
intestinal lymphoma, the absence of Paneth cells in the crypts, and an
extremely thin-walled small intestine with true atrophy of the small
mucosa.

Small bowel ulceration in coeliac sprue is not rare[1,2,4,5,9,11,13]. The
localization and morphology of these ulcers can vary significantly,
being either superficial or very deep. Although there are many cases
of ulceration in the small intestine, the rather high frequency of
intestinal ulceration in coeliac patients suggests a relationship with
coeliac sprue. Although a high rate of complications is a striking
characteristic of these patients, healing of the ulcers may occur[20,21].

Widespread subepithelial collagen deposition was stressed by Weinstein et al.[14] to carry a particularly bad prognosis. It is true that a
number of therapy-resistant cases of severe malabsorption and a flat
intestinal mucosa have large amounts of collagen beneath the epithelium[3,9,16]. A distinctly recognizable amount of collagen, however,
may be found in no fewer than one-third of the intestinal biopsies of
untreated coeliac patients[3,22,23]. Collagen can disappear with 2–6
months after gluten withdrawal. Most patients respond well to gluten
withdrawal with or without temporary corticosteroid treatment[17,21,24].
For these reasons it seems to us not a primary phenomenon but the
result of the pathological process in the intestinal mucosa.

Abdominal lymphoma is in general not associated with a flat mucous
membrane of the small intestine but cases have been described which
exhibit this combination[17]. It is likely that malignant lymphoma may
occur as a complication of coeliac sprue, although it has been suggested
that a flat mucosa can occur in response to a pre-existing lymphoma
or prelymphoma[12].

Paneth cell function has been related to secretion of a protein–
carbohydrate complex necessary for the luminal nutrition of the crypt
cells. Absence or marked reduction of Paneth cells in the crypts of
Lieberkühn is not uncommon in patients with severe and extensive
intestinal mucosal lesions who do not respond to a gluten-free diet[6].
Not all cases of refractory sprue however, are associated with Paneth
cell deficiency[9]. It seems that Paneth cell deficiency is not the primary
cause of the morphological lesions but more likely an expression of
the basic abnormality.

The extremely thin-walled and atrophic small intestine, as was found
in our two patients, has been reported by others in similar cases of
refractory sprue[6,14]. In the two cases presented we were struck by the
extreme atrophy of the intestinal wall over the entire length. Histological examination of the intestinal mucosa revealed features of an
exhausted regeneration. Only a reduced number or very few crypts,

in which a moderate number of mitotic figures, were discernible. Others have reported similar findings[3,6,11,14,19]. That a decreased production of enterocytes can be present in such patients was demonstrated by Barry *et al.*[17] by DNA determination in perfusion fluid from intestinal loops. The epithelial cell turnover in coeliac sprue has been shown to be raised using this method[17,25]. This difference in epithelial cell kinetics distinguishes this type of refractory sprue from uncomplicated coeliac sprue. However, the lesion in these two patients is not only characterized by true atrophy of the epithelium and decreased mucosal thickness but also by partial disappearance of the submucosa and muscular coat. The flat mucosa in these two patients, resembling that in coeliac sprue, and the paucity of mucosal crypts seem to be the end-result of true crypt atrophy. Analogous to comparing the turnover pattern of the intestinal epithelium in coeliac patients with haemolytic anaemia[26,27], one might compare the pattern in refractory sprue with aplastic anaemia.

Although this disease process produces a flat mucosa it is questionable if it has anything to do with coeliac sprue. Neither of our two patients nor the rare cases described in literature give enough evidence in support of that connection. Unless equivocal evidence has been produced we consider these two disorders as different.

References

1. Himes, H. W., Gabriel, J. B. and Adlersberg, D. (1957). Previously undescribed clinical and post-mortem observations in non-tropical sprue: possible role of prolonged corticosteroid therapy. *Gastroenterology*, **32**, 60
2. Kelley, M. L. and Terry, R. (1958). Clinical and histological observations in fatal non-tropical sprue. *Am. J. Med.*, **25**, 460
3. Hourihane, Do'B. (1963). The histology of intestinal biopsies. *Proc. Roy. Soc. Med.*, **56**, 1073
4. Shiner, M. (1963). Effect of a gluten-free diet in 17 patients with idiopathic steatorrhoea. *Am. J. Dig. Dis.*, **8**, 969
5. Smitskamp, H. and Kuipers, F. C. (1975) Steatorrhoea and ulcerative jejuno-ileitis. *Acta Med. Scand.*, **177**, 37
6. Pink, I. J. and Creamer, B. (1967). Response to a gluten-free diet of patients with the coeliac syndrome. *Lancet*, **i**, 300
7. Stewart, J. S., Pollock, D. J., Hoffbrand, A. V. *et al.* (1967). A study of proximal and distal intesinal structure and absorptive function in idiopathic steatorrhea. *Qu. J. Med.*, **36**, 425
8. Cooke, W. T. (1968). Adult celiac disease. In: G. B. Jerzy Glass (ed.) *Progress in Gastroenterology, Vol. I*, pp. 299–338. (New York: Grune & Stratton)
9. Clinicopathological Conference. (1968). A case of adult coeliac disease resistant to treatment. *Br. Med. J.*, **2**, 678
10. Jeffries, G. H., Steinberg, H. and Sleisenger, M. H. (1968). Chronic ulcerative (nongranulomatous) jejunitis. *Am. J. Med.*, **44**, 47
11. Barry, R. E., Morris, J. S. and Read, A. E. (1970). A case of small intestinal mucosal atrophy. *Gut*, **11**, 743

12. Hourihane, Do'B. and Weir, D. G. (1970). Malignant coeliac syndrome. *Gastroenterology*, **59**, 130
13. Clinicopathological Conference. (1970). A case of malabsorption, intestinal mucosal atrophy and ulceration, cirrhosis and emphysema. *Br. Med. J.*, **3**, 207
14. Weinstein, W. M., Saunders, D. R., Tijtgat, G. N. and Rubin, C. E. (1970). Collagenous sprue—an unrecognized type of malabsorption. *New Engl. J. Med.*, **283**, 1297
15. Clinicopathological Conference. (1972). Non-responsive coeliac disease. *Br. Med. J.*, **3**, 624
16. Doe, W. F., Evans, D., Hobbs, J. R. and Booth, C. C. (1972). Coeliac disease, vasculitis and cryoglobulinaemia. *Gut*, **13**, 112
17. Barry, R. E. and Read, A. E. (1973). Coeliac disease and malignancy. *Qu. J. Med.*, **42**, 665
18. Marche, C., Bocquet, L., Mignon, M. and Preel, J. L. (1974) Syndrome de malabsorption avec cavitation ganglionnaire mésentérique et atrophie splénique. *Sem. Hôp. Paris*, **50**, 879
19. Modigliani, R., Matuchansky, C., Galian, A. *et al.* (1975). Maladie coelique de l'adulte (48 cas). *Arch. Fr. Mal. App. Dig.*, **64**, 465
20. Jones, P. E. and Gleeson, M. H. (1973). Mucosal ulceration and mesenteric lymphadenopathy in coeliac disease. *Br. Med. J.*, **3**, 212
21. Cluysenaer, O. J. J. and van Tongeren, J. H. M. (1977). *Malabsorption in Coeliac Sprue.* (The Hague: Martinus Nijhoff Medical Division)
22. Bossart, R., Henry, K., Booth, C. C. and Doe, W. F. (1975). Subepithelial collagen in intestinal malabsorption. *Gut*, **16**, 18
23. Cooke, W. T., Fone, D. J., Meynell, M. J. and Gaddie, R. (1963). Adult coeliac disease. *Gut*, **4**, 279
24. Holdstock, D. J. and Oleesky, S. (1973). Successful treatment of collagenous sprue with combination of prednisolone and gluten-free diet. *Postgrad. Med. J.*, **49**, 664
25. Croft, D. N., Loehry, C. A. and Creamer, B. (1968). Small bowel cell-loss and weight-loss in the coeliac syndrome. *Lancet*, **ii**, 68
26. Crosby, W. H. (1961). Concept of the pathogenesis of anaemia applied to disorders of the intestinal mucosa. *Am. J. Dig. Dis.*, **6**, 492
27. Booth, C. C. (1970). Enterocyte in coeliac disease. *Br. Med. J.*, **3**, 725 and **4**, 14

Discussion of chapter 33

Dodge	Did you examine the trace elements status of your patients?
Van Tongeren	No.
Delmont	How was the colon?
Van Tongeren	The colon was normal in both patients, also the gastric wall and gastric mucosa was normal.
Watson	I wonder if your patients lack some kind of trophic hormone? It looks as though nothing is happening to stimulate crypt cell production. I presume that these patients did not have amyloid in their bowel.
Van Tongeren	There was no amyloid and I cannot comment about hormones.
Strober	We frequently see patients with a flat mucosa who are thought to have gluten-sensitive enteropathy and have IgA deficiency.
Van Tongeren	Neither patient was IgA deficient.
Tripp	Was there any change in enterocyte size in association with the hyperplasia and did you look at bone marrow to see if there was corresponding change in bone marrow?
Van Tongeren	Bone marrow was normal in both patients. Some enterocytes were cuboidal and others were cylindrical, so there was some difference in different parts of the small intestine.
Ferguson	This is a serious and not fictitious question. Is there any possibility that either patient was poisoned or exposed to radiotherapy? This looks quite like late results of radiation damage.
Van Tongeren	We have no evidence of poisons. I don't think that radiotherapy could cause such an extensive small bowel lesion.
Challacombe	We see in children a situation associated with protracted or chronic diarrhoea where the mucosa simply cannot regenerate because of the poor nutritional status of the child. Do you think there is a vicious circle of events in patients like this and that we are not properly considering nutritional status? You leave the mucosa with no option but to remain flat.
Van Tongeren	No, I don't believe that because the patient's disease started in an acute situation and secondly, we have fed these patients intravenously for long periods but nevertheless the situation deteriorated and the patients died.
Booth	It is worth, I think, trying total parenteral nutrition in these patients. J. Levi of Northwick Park, has recently had a patient of this sort treated for a prolonged period with total parenteral nutrition and improvement occurred.

34

Malabsorption, villous atrophy, and excessive serum IgA in a patient with unusual intestinal immunocyte infiltration (abstract)

K. BAKLEIN, P. BRANDTZAEG and O. FAUSA

An 11-year-old boy with gastrointestinal complaints of about 4 years' duration, was in 1967 admitted to hospital with severe malabsorption and villous atrophy of the small intestinal mucosa. The clinical symptoms disappeared in association with gluten withdrawal. During the subsequent 10 years, however, the villous atrophy has persisted, and malabsorption tests have been virtually unchanged. Moreover, his serum level of IgA has remained extremely high (58–66 g/l), along with normal IgM and IgG. His IgA is mainly polymeric and shows polyclonal characteristics.

Immunohistochemical investigation has demonstrated that the gastrointestinal mucosa is its major production site. About 96 per cent of the intestinal immunocytes are of the IgA class. An increased number of IgA-producing cells is also present in gastric mucosa, whereas nasal mucosa and bone marrow show no abnormality. The polymeric IgA permeates dermal and mucosal connective tissue in high concentrations and appears in the urine, but there is no marked elevation of secretory IgA levels in duodenal and salivary fluids. Nevertheless, staining of glandular epithelia indicates normal transport of IgA and presence of secretory component (SC), and saliva contains IgA-associated as well as free SC. A defect in its external transport does therefore not seem to be involved in the excessive contribution of dimeric IgA to serum. The possibility is discussed that this case may bear some relation to alpha-chain disease or coeliac disease.

References

Baklien, K., Fausa, O., Brandtzaeg, P., Fröland, S. S. and Gjone, E. (1977). Malabsorption, villous atrophy, and excessive serum IgA in a patient with unusual intestinal immunocyte infiltration. *Scand. J. Gastroenterol.*, **12**, 421

Brandtzaeg, P. and Baklien, K. (1977). Characterization of the IgA immunocyte population and its product in a patient with excessive intestinal formation of IgA. *Clin. Exp. Immunol.*, **30**, 77

Discussion of chapter 34

L'Hirondel	Did you try antibiotics in your patients?
Baklien	We gave tetracycline for four weeks, but we could not find any lowering in the IgA level. We did not do a repeat biopsy for several reasons. We would like to try the effect of more intensive antibiotic therapy.
Booth	Could I ask you, have you done electron microscopy on the plasma cells in the lamina propria? In α-chain disease are the cells quite different to the normal plasma cell?
Baklien	Yes; could I have the last slide please. This is from a patient with α-chain disease and we see the immature appearance of the cells. There is a complete lack of light chain in these cells. In our patients the cells are more mature looking.
Booth	And the difference from myeloma is the nature of the dimer in the serum and the distribution of the cells throughout the body; if it weren't for that you could call it myeloma of the intestine.
Baklien	No, because these cells are polyclonal and that is quite different from myeloma when the cells are monoclonal.
Strober	We have seen a number of patients who are not unlike this. I wouldn't say exactly like this and we have never worked them up as well. The thought has occurred to us that there are other kinds of food protein enteropathy. There is a report for instance of soya bean enteropathy, and there may be other food substances to which patients react in a very specific fashion in the way that a gluten-sensitive patient reacts to gluten. It would be difficult to determine this but one approach would be to put a patient on either parenteral alimentation or an amino acid diet which is available now and see if the patient improves under those circumstances. We have had one case where the patient did improve very dramatically after a period of parenteral alimentation; presumably there was something in the food which we didn't identify which was causing the enteropathy.
Bernier	Is the secretory component present in the duodenal or jejunal juice?
Baklien	There is no difference from what we find in normal patients and the secretory component is bound to IgA and IgM as in normals.
Bernier	In the summary you said you measured it in saliva not in the duodenal or jejunal juice. Do you measure it in the jejunal juice?
Baklien	Yes.

35

Zinc deficiency and coeliac disease

A. H. G. LOVE, M. ELMES, M. K. GOLDEN and D. McMASTER

Nutritional failure is a frequent consequence of intestinal malabsorption. Indeed in the coeliac syndrome this feature may be more impressive than the intestinal symptomatology. Nutrients which have received little attention until recently are the so-called trace elements, e.g. zinc, copper and chromium. Zinc is an essential constituent of many enzyme systems and necessary for protein synthesis. Since it is absorbed primarily through the upper small intestinal mucosa, it is postulated that problems of zinc deficiency may develop and even contribute to certain features of the coeliac syndrome.

Patients with coeliac disease respond both symptomatically and their mucosa structurally to exclusion of gluten from their diet and those who do not are usually inadvertently consuming gluten[1]. Some patients however do not respond to the most rigorous dietary management. The term 'non-responsive coeliac disease' is often applied to this state and it may respond in some cases to treatment with steroids or other immuno-suppressive agents[2]. A typical experience is shown in Figure 35.1. In the present series six patients have been studied who failed to respond to conventional treatment. They have been compared with a similar age group of matched patients who responded to dietary gluten exclusion.

Figure 35.2 shows two estimates of intestinal absorptive function, 5 h D-xylose excretion and ^{14}C fat absorption. It can be seen that the non-responders had significantly poorer absorptive ability. As regards their nutritional state as measured by serum albumin levels, blood urea, serum cholesterol and carotene, there was also a significantly greater degree of nutritional failure in the non-responders (Figures 35.3 and 35.4).

In all six cases of non-responsiveness severe zinc deficiency was noted (Figure 35.5). The values were 37.0±7.5 μg/100 ml as compared with 78.5±10.2 μg/100 ml.

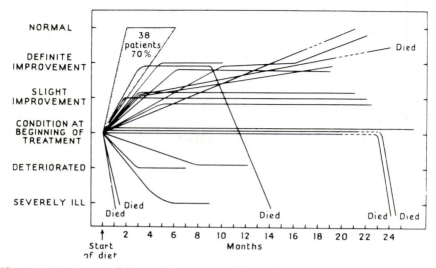

Figure 35.1 Course of illness of non-responding patients to gluten-free diet

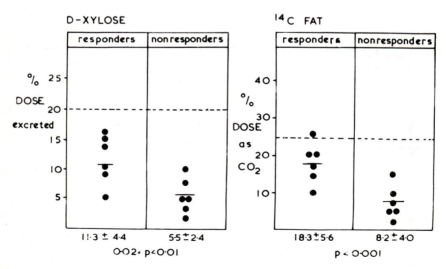

Figure 35.2 Intestinal absorptive characteristics determined by D-xylose excretion and "C" fat absorption

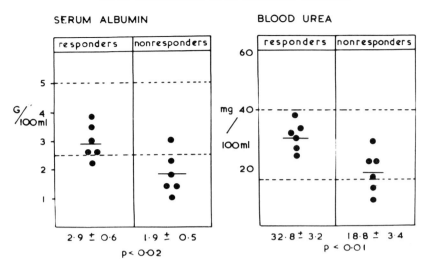

Figure 35.3 Nutritional state as determined by serum albumin and blood urea

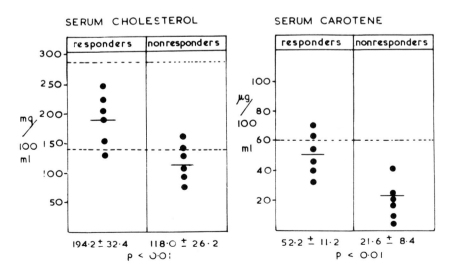

Figure 35.4 Nutritional state as determined by serum cholesterol and serum carotene

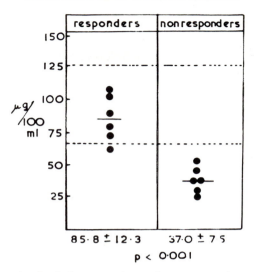

Figure 35.5   Serum zinc levels in responsive and non-responsive cases

In Figure 35.6 is shown the clinical course of one of the non-responsive cases M.A., a female aged 37 years. It can be seen that despite gluten exclusion, prednisone and parenteral feeding, no sustained improvement was produced. In April 1973 when zinc deficiency was discovered, this element was replaced by zinc sulphate (5 mg daily) intravenously. There was an immediate improvement in absorptive ability and nutritional state. Also there was a marked increase in serum alkaline phosphatase levels. This enzyme is zinc dependent. A similar picture was seen in all six patients in this group. Figure 35.7 shows the dramatic improvement in absorptive function produced by zinc replacement therapy as estimated by serial D-xylose excretion measurements. In Figure 35.8 the effects of zinc therapy are seen on serum albumin levels.

Another aspect of intestinal disease which can apparently be modified by zinc nutritional status is appetite. This may be important since weight loss is often better correlated with anorexia than with malabsorption. Figure 35.9 shows the effect of correction of zinc deficiency on food intake in the patients in this series.

Following initial treatment with parenteral zinc, oral zinc supplements were given, zinc sulphate (Zincomed) 220 mg t.d.s. This has produced sustained improvement in well-being, intestinal function and nutritional state in four of the six patients. In the remaining two patients after follow up for 2 and 3 years respectively these patients have died with intestinal lymphoma. It may be therefore that this malignant condition was already contributing to the state of 'non-responsiveness'.   In reviewing recent

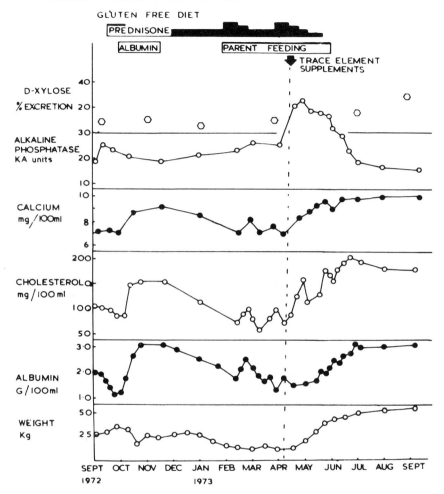

Figure 35.6 Clinical course of one non-responsive patient before and after zinc therapy

cases of coeliac disease seen in this department zinc levels are lower than in a control population, as shown in Table 35.1.

Table 35.1

Patients	Mean ± SD	Range	Significance
Controls	95.0 ± 12.5	76.0–150	
Coeliac disease	78.5 ± 11.3	52.5–105	<0.05
Non-responsive coeliac disease	37.0 ± 7.5	23.0–48.5	<0.001

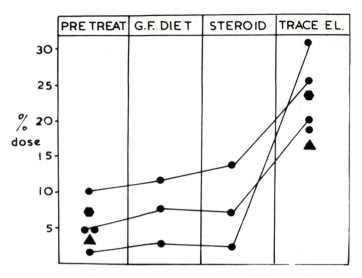

Figure 35.7   Absorptive function determined by D-xylose following zinc therapy

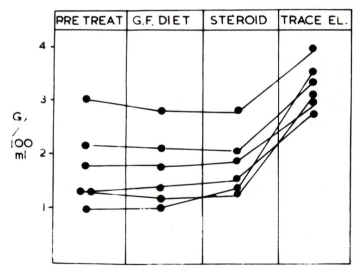

Figure 35.8   Effect on serum albumin levels of zinc therapy

It is concluded therefore that zinc deficiency may play an important role in coeliac disease. Some cases of 'non-responsiveness' may be contributed to by profound zinc deficiency. The mechanism may be through abnormal enterocyte turnover since some of these cases are associated with reduced rather than increased cell turnover[3]. A possible

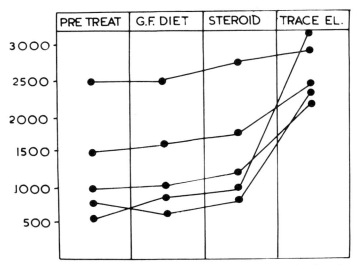

Figure 35.9 Effect of gluten-free diet, steroids and zinc therapy on food intake in kilo-calories/day.

connection with DNA synthesis rate and response has been suggested recently[4] and it is of interest that zinc is necessary for protein synthetic activity. It may be that the slow DNA turnover in these non-responders is a manifestation of zinc deficiency.

It is important to record that two patients who apparently responded to zinc replacement eventually developed lymphoma. It is perhaps worth considering whether zinc replacement in these patients could have increased cell turnover to such an extent as to allow malignancy to occur or whether this condition was present throughout the latter period of their illness. Also one patient on zinc supplementation developed copper deficiency with anaemia, neutropenia and thrombocytopenia[5]. This was probably due to carrier competition at mucosal level. It does however illustrate the importance of considering not just one trace element but the balance between them.

Finally let me say that no member of this symposium need fear the development of zinc deficiency since a highly concentrated dietary source of zinc is available in the Galway Bay oyster.

References

1. Baker, P. G., Barry, R. E. and Read, A. E. (1975). Detection of continuing gluten ingestion in treated coeliac patients. *Br. Med. J.*, **1**, 486
2. Hamilton, J. D., Chambers, R. A. and Wynn-Williams, A. (1976). Role of gluten, prednisone, and azathioprine in non-responsive coeliac disease. *Lancet*, i, 1213

341

3. Croft, D. N., Loehry, C. A. and Creamer, B. Small bowel cell loss and weight loss in the coeliac syndrome. *Lancet,* ii, 68

4. Jones, P. E. and Peters, T. J. (1977). DNA synthesis by jejunal mucosa in responsive and non-responsive coeliac disease. *Br. med. J.,* **1,** 1130

5. Porter, K. G., McMaster, D. Elmes, M. E. and Love, A. H. G. (1977). Anaemia and low serum copper during zinc therapy. *Lancet,* ii, 774

Discussion of chapter 35

Holmes	Did you estimate zinc in the jejunal biopsies?
Love	No. and I think this will be a very interesting study. I think Dr Peters is looking at zinc levels and the methodology of doing this.
Shmerling	Did you assess the patient's ability to taste and smell? Impairment could be one of the reasons why patients with zinc deficiency have such a bad appetite.
Love	Two patients had very marked depression of appetite and taste sensation. One patient when zinc was replaced would consume upwards of 6000 calories per day and would only allow her husband to visit her in hospital if he brought food supplements.
Rey	What was the folate status of your last patient, because it looks as if folate deficiency was present.
Love	Folate was not deficient nor B_{12} and we have taken care of these more common aspects of nutritional failure by supplementation.
Holmes	Have you tried treating these patients with zinc and missing out the gluten-free diet to see if they improved on zinc alone? We heard this morning we should not talk about non-responsive coeliac disease so where do you think this leaves us with respect to the diagnosis, if they do not get better on a gluten-free diet, but do get better on zinc? Is it zinc-induced enteropathy?
Love	No, I feel that a patient should be treated with a gluten-free diet. We should be aware of the possible coexistence of zinc deficiency. It is interesting that zinc is primarily absorbed in the upper small intestine which is most damaged in coeliac disease.
Booth	Can we just get this clear. We have had no evidence presented that there is any change in the morphology of the intestine as a result of giving zinc?
Love	We have been able to re-biopsy three of the six patients and they have shown improvement in the villous stature from flat biopsy to the presence of recognizable villi. We have not measured DNA synthesis and mitotic rate of cells. This might be very interesting because zinc may well be important in protein synthetic activity in the mucosa.
Moynihan	Did you do serial estimations of the hair zinc?
Love	Yes. We have looked at the zinc level in hair at the initial presentation, and when zinc is added the level in the newly grown hair rises.
Moynihan	We studied a young woman with anorexia nervosa, who was zinc-deficient but she was also copper-deficient.
Booth	I would like to ask you something about your acrodermatitis enteropathica patients. How do Professor Love's serum zinc levels compare with the levels in your patients?

Moynihan

Most of the zinc levels in his patients are very much lower than in mine. Zinc is much more important the younger you are and is related to other trace elements. At times of rapid growth, for example, adolescence, additional zinc is required. We don't know anything about the body store of zinc, how much you have got to call on before you show any signs.

Love

I would entirely agree with the comments. I think that serum is only one very easy 'biopsy area' and we really need methods of knowing what the zinc status is and for that matter the status of other trace elements in the patients.

Section VII
The skin and coeliac disease

36

A skin test for coeliac disease

P. M. RAWCLIFFE, B. S. ANAND, R. E. OFFORD, J. PIRIS and S. C. TRUELOVE

INTRODUCTION

Until recently all attempts to find a skin test for coeliac disease yielded negative results. Then Baker and Read[1] tested coeliac subjects with an intradermal injection of Frazer's fraction III of wheat gluten and obtained positive reactions of Arthus-type in 52% of untreated coeliac subjects and in 33% of patients on a gluten-free diet. At about the same time, an independent study was being made in Oxford of the skin reactions to a range of fractions of gluten with which we had been experimenting for some years. It was found that, of 10 coeliac subjects tested, all gave Arthus-type skin reactions to one or more of these fractions whereas 20 healthy control subjects were uniformly negative[2]. Overall, the fraction B2 gave the strongest skin reactions, being positive in all 10 coeliac subjects. This fraction was therefore selected for future study as a possible basis for a useful skin test for detecting likely cases of coeliac disease.

Preliminary observations on skin biopsies suggest that a positive test is characterized by oedema, dilatation of the small blood vessels with some swelling of their walls, and a perivascular infiltration with inflammatory cells which are mainly neutrophil polymorphs. No intravascular thrombosis and no fibrinoid reaction have been observed.

For technical reasons, further evaluation of the test has been slow. Fraction B2 is obtained from fraction B by passing it through a large Sephadex column. The resulting eluate needs to be freeze-dried. As the portion representing fraction B2 amounts to 50 litres, it has been necessary for us to have the freeze-drying carried out away from Oxford and unfortunately this has resulted in delay in obtaining additional supplies of the material.

TECHNIQUE

Four intradermal injections of 0.1 ml are given in random order on the
ventral surface of either forearm, two of control solution and two of
the test solution of fraction B2. People over 70 years are excluded due
to the atrophic state of their skin. The patient is not given any indication
of what reactions are likely to occur. The reactions are read and
measured at 6 h by an observer other than the one who gave the injections.

Table 36.1 Results of skin testing with Oxford fraction B2 in
coeliac disease, Crohn's disease, ulcerative colitis and healthy
volunteers

Condition	No. tested	No. positive	% positive
Coeliac disease	13	13	100.0
Crohn's disease	8	4	50.0
Ulcerative colitis	15	4	26.7
Healthy volunteers	27	3	11.1

Table 36.1 shows the results that have been obtained up to the present
time. It will be seen that all 13 coeliac subjects gave positive results.
However, there are now some positive reactions among the healthy
control subjects and positive reactions are comparatively common
among the patients with Crohn's disease or ulcerative colitis. All the
patients so far tested have not been receiving treatment with corticosteroids or azathioprine.

It is therefore evident that the test is not specific for coeliac disease,
which is disappointing in view of the early results. Nevertheless, the
test may still be valuable provided that it continues to give uniformly
positive results in coeliac subjects. If this proves to be the case, we
consider that it will be useful in at least two situations:

(1) As a screening test to select patients for jejunal biopsy
(2) In family studies of coeliac disease to indicate those relatives of
    coeliac subjects in whom jejunal biopsy is likely to be positive.

Much more extensive studies will be required to show if the test is
uniformly positive in coeliac disease. Dr Anne Ferguson has undertaken
to perform the test on a large number of coeliac subjects and controls,
and Dr Janet Marks is similarly planning to study dermatitis herpetiformis. Fortunately ample supplies of B2 are now available for this
purpose.

From a more fundamental viewpoint, it now looks as though the
skin reaction is a reflection of the leakage of an antigenic moiety of

gluten through the gut wall in sufficient quantities to provoke an immunological response. This would explain why the test has been only occasionally positive in healthy subjects, fairly often positive in patients with inflammatory bowel disease, and uniformly positive to date in coeliac subjects.

References

1. Baker, P. G. and Read, A. E. (1976). Positive skin reactions to gluten in coeliac disease. *Qu. J. Med.*, **45,** 603
2. Anand, B. S., Truelove, S. C. and Offord, R. E. (1977). Skin test for coeliac disease using a subfraction of gluten. *Lancet,* **i,** 118

37

Positive skin reactions to wheat, barley and oats in coeliac disease

P. G. BAKER and A. E. READ

INTRODUCTION

Though positive skin reactions to gluten have been observed previously in coeliac patients[1,2] they have not been accorded a role in the pathogenesis or diagnosis of the disease.

On histological grounds these responses have been regarded as being due to a delayed hypersensitivity to gluten. An Arthus reaction would be equally compatible however, and, since it occurs following complement activation by antigen–antibody complexes, it is supported by the finding of serum gluten antibodies, circulating immune complexes and subnormal C3 or haemolytic complement levels in coeliac patients[3–6] especially those ingesting gluten.

We have, therefore studied skin reactions to gluten and other cereal proteins with particular regard as to whether they are Arthus-mediated.

MATERIALS AND METHODS

Subjects

Fifty-five adults with biopsy-proven coeliac disease, untreated and treated by a gluten-free diet were compared with 52 normal adults as a control group.

Skin testing

Antigen

100 g gluten (BDH) was added to 20 ml water, followed by 2 g pepsin. The mixture was left for 2 h at room temperature, following which 2 g trypsin was added, and the solution again left to stand for 2 h at room temperature. After centrifugation the supernatent was subjected to freeze-drying. The resultant solid was stored at room temperature in a sterile container.

For use in skin testing the peptic–tryptic gluten digest was dissolved in sterile water to give a 1 g per cent concentration, and filtered through a micropore filter immediately prior to use. Sterile water was used as a control solution.

Technique

(i) A drop of antigen solution was placed on ventral aspect of the forearm and pricked into the skin using a sterile hypodermic needle.
(ii) 0.1 ml antigen and control solutions were injected intradermally in three sites on the ventral aspect of the subjects' forearms.
(iii) Reactions were recorded 20 min, five to eight, 24 and 48 hours following the skin challenge intradermally, and 20 min after prick testing. Two diameters at right angles to each other of visible erythematous area were measured using a ruler, followed in some cases by photography.

Further skin testing by this procedure was also carried out using hordein (barley), avenin (oats) and zein (maize).

Skin biopsies

These were obtained in suitable cases from the skin challenge site, five to eight hours after intradermal gluten injection, using a 3 mm skin biopsy tool. Half of the biopsy obtained was placed in formalin and processed for light microscopy, the remainder being stored at −70 °C in a sterile labelled plastic container.

Histological study

Skin biopsies were removed from formalin, embedded in paraffin wax, sectioned, and stained with haematoxylin and eosin. Slides were examined by light microscopy and low power, and photographed.

Immunofluorescence

Reagents

Anti-whole human immunoglobulin was obtained from Burroughs Wellcome, and anti-C3 complement was supplied by Dako Immuno-chemicals. Both were labelled with fluorescein isothiocyanate.

Technique

Skin biopsies stored at −70 °C were placed on a cryostat and cut into slices. These were lifted onto microscope slides, and washed in phosphate-buffered saline. Separate specimens were then treated with the anti-Ig and anti-C3 solutions. After standing at room temperature for 30 min slides were rewashed in phosphate-buffered saline, mounted in fluoromount and examined under blue light using a 'Wild' micro-scope fitted with a camera attachment. For technical reasons it was not possible to photograph all the sections examined.

Circulating cereal antibodies

These were measured using tanned erythrocytes coated with peptic–tryptic digests of gluten, hordein, avenin or zein[7] in all patients studied.

Gluten intake

This was assessed by direct questioning and the use of a prospective dietary questionnaire[7]. Patients ingesting less than 2 g daily of gluten were regarded as having a small intake, whilst those taking more than 2 g were classed in the large intake group. The national average adult daily gluten intake is 7 g. If patients were adhering to their gluten-free diets a nil intake was recorded.

RESULTS FOLLOWING SKIN CHALLENGE

Using gluten

No visible skin reactions were observed in either coeliac patients or controls at the 20 min, 24 h and 48 h time intervals following antigenic challenge. Responses were noted in a proportion of the coeliac patients five to eight hours after intradermal administration of the peptic–tryptic gluten digest. These are shown in Table 37.1, along with the titre of serum gluten antibodies, and gluten intake.

None of the control group had visible skin changes five to eight hours following skin testing, or circulating antibodies to gluten.

Table 37.1 Results at five to eight hours in coeliac patients using P–T gluten digest 1 g per cent intradermally

Case	Sex	Visible skin reaction diameter (cm)	Gluten intake	Serum gluten antibody titre
1	F	2×2	Small	32
2	F	5×4	Large	128
3	F	3×4	Large	256
4	F	3×3	Small	64
5	F	2×2	Large	256
6	F	2×2	Small	64
7	F	2×2	Large	128
8	F	6×4	Small	256
9	F	3×3	Large	128
10	F	3×3	Large	128
11	M	2×2	Large	128
12	M	3×2	Nil	2048
13	M	3×3	Large	1024
14	F	2×1	Large	64
15	F	1×1	Large	64
16	M	3×2	Large	256
16	M	0	Small	0
17	M	4×4	Large	16000
17	M	3×3	Nil	512
18	F	0	Large	32
19	F	0	Large	128
20	F	0	Nil	0
21	F	0	Large	16
22	F	0	Large	512
23	F	0	Small	64
24	F	0	Large	64
25	M	0	Nil	128
26	F	0	Large	1028
27	F	0	Nil	32
28	F	0	Nil	16
29	F	0	Small	16
30	M	0	Small	16
31	F	0	Small	0
32	F	0	Nil	0
33	F	0	Small	0
34	M	0	Large	0
35	M	0	Nil	0
36	F	0	Small	0
37	F	0	Nil	0
38	M	0	Small	0
39	F	0	Small	0
40	M	0	Nil	0
41	F	0	Small	0
42	M	0	Nil	0
43	M	0	Nil	0
44	M	0	Nil	0

Table 37.1 contd.

45	F	0	Large	0	
46	M	0	Nil	0	
47	F	0	Large	0	
48	M	0	Small	0	
49	M	0	Small	0	
50	M	0	Nil	0	
51	F	0	Small	0	
52	M	0	Small	0	
53	F	0	Large	0	
54	M	0	Nil	0	
55	M	0	Large	0	

Skin biopsy histology

Biopsies obtained from normal controls five to eight hours after intradermal antigen challenge were compared with those taken at the same
time interval from coeliac patients displaying positive and negative skin
responses to gluten. Table 37.2 shows the findings in terms of any
cellular infiltrate noted, alongside the visible skin reaction already
recorded in Table 37.1. The histology from a coeliac patient with a
positive test is compared with a normal control in Figure 37.1.

Table 37.2 Relationship between the skin reaction and skin biopsy
findings in control subjects and coeliac patients

Case	Sex	Remarks	Skin reaction diameter (cm)	Skin biopsy histology
AB	M	Control	0	Normal
FD	F	Control	0	Normal
12	M	Coeliac	3×2	Marked polymorph infiltrate
17	M	Coeliac	4×4	Marked polymorph infiltrate
21	F	Coeliac	0	Normal
16	M	Coeliac	3×2	Marked polymorph infiltrate
8	F	Coeliac	6×4	Marked polymorph infiltrate
2	F	Coeliac	5×4	Marked polymorph infiltrate
11	M	Coeliac	2×2	Marked polymorph infiltrate
4	F	Coeliac	3×3	Marked polymorph infiltrate
3	F	Coeliac	3×4	Marked polymorph infiltrate
10	F	Coeliac	3×5	Marked polymorph infiltrate
23	F	Coeliac	0	Normal
51	M	Coeliac	0	Normal
35	M	Coeliac	0	Normal
36	F	Coeliac	0	Normal
26	F	Coeliac	0	Normal
41	M	Coeliac	0	Normal

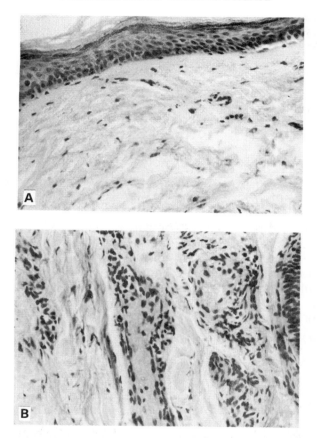

Figure 37.1 (A) Skin biopsy from control subject. Normal histology (× 325). (B) Skin biopsy from coeliac patient having positive skin response to gluten. Marked polymorph and mononuclear cell infiltrate (× 325).

Immunofluorescence

The majority of skin biopsies subjected to histology were also treated with fluoroescein conjugated anti-human immunoglobulin and anti-C3 complement to see whether skin challenge sites contained immunoglobulin or complement deposits. The results are shown in Table 37.4, and an illustration in Figure 37.2.

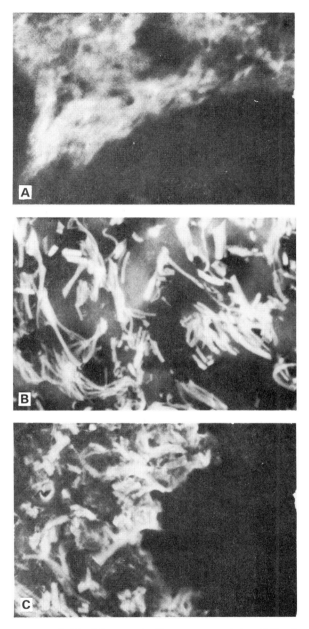

Figure 37.2 (A) Normal skin biopsy. No fluorescent staining following anti-Ig and anti C3 treatment (× 100). (B) Positive Ig staining in skin biopsy of coeliac with positive skin response to gluten (× 100). (C) Positive C3 complement demonstrated in skin biopsy of coeliac having skin reaction to gluten (× 100).

Table 37.3 Relationship between gluten skin reaction size and serum gluten antibody titres

Antibody titre	Mean visible skin reaction area (sq.cm)
< 32	0
32–64	3.1
128+	6.9

Table 37.4 Results of immunofluorescent studies on the skin biopsies of control subjects and coeliac patients

Case	Fluorescence in skin biopsy using	
	anti-immunoglobulin	anti-C3 complement
AB	–ve	–ve
FD	–ve	–ve
12	+ve	+ve
17	+ve	+ve
16	+ve	+ve
8	+ve	+ve
2	+ve	+ve
11	+ve	+ve
4	+ve	+ve
3	+ve	+ve
23	–ve	–ve
51	–ve	–ve
35	–ve	–ve
36	–ve	–ve
26	–ve	–ve
41	–ve	–ve

DISCUSSION

The only skin reactions to cereal antigens, particularly gluten, detected in this study occurred in coeliac patients. These took the form of induration and erythema appearing 2–3 h following intradermal skin challenge, becoming maximal at 5–8 h and fading over the ensuing 12–18 h.

Such a time course is suggestive of an Arthus reaction. This is produced by complement activation following the combination of antigen in the tissues with circulating antibody. Chemicals released locally during the process cause an influx of polymorphs, accompanied by vasodilation and oedema. Histologically therefore, the lesion is typified by the presence of oedema, with, in the early stages, a polymorph and mononuclear cell infiltrate, followed later by an influx of plasma cells and lymphocytes (Figure 37.1). Immunoglobulin and C3 complement deposition can be demonstrated using immunofluorescent techniques (Figure 37.2).

Skin biopsies taken from patients having a visible skin response to gluten were noted at light microscopy to be compatible with an Arthus reaction. Further evidence that these skin reactions were Arthus-mediated was provided by the detection of immunoglobulin and C3 complement in such specimens. Skin biopsies from negative responders did not contain immunoglobulin or C3 complement deposits and no cellular infiltrate could be seen.

Of the 55 patients with coeliac disease, 23 of whom were untreated, 17 (30%) were noted to have positive Arthus-type skin reactions to gluten. Twelve of these were from the group taking a normal diet. Serum gluten antibodies were detected in all 17, which strongly suggests that their combination with intradermal gluten is the mechanism by which complement is activated. The correlation between skin reaction size and antibody titres, coupled with the fact that patients reacting to

Table 37.5 Results at 5–8 h in coeliac patients using P–T cereal protein digests 1 g% intradermally

| Case | Sex | Visible skin reaction size (cm diam.) using | | | Antibody titres | | |
		Hordein	Avenin	Zein	Barley	Oats	Maize
1	F	0	0	0	0	0	0
2	F	0	o	0	10	0	0
3	F	0	0	0	0	0	0
4	F	0	0	0	0	0	0
5	F	0	01	0	0	0	0
66	F	0	0	0	0	0	0
7	F	0	0	0	0	0	0
8	F	0	0	0	0	0	0
9	F	0	0	0	0	0	0
10	F	2×2	0	0	64	16	0
11	M	0	0	0	0	0	0
12	M	0	2×2	0	64	32	32
13	M	0	0	0	64	0	0
14	F	0	0	0	0	0	0
15	F	0	0	0	0	0	0
16							
17	M	4×3	2×1	0	64	32	16
18–55		0	0	0	0	0	0

barley or oats had circulating antibodies to hordein or avenin, supports a concept based on antibody combination with antigen.

Positive responses to barley or oats occurred in only 4% of coeliacs and not at all to maize (Table 37.5). Bearing in mind that untreated coeliacs in the UK consume much more oats than barley, such findings accord with the relative toxicity of these cereals as compared to gluten[8]. Although of little help clinically, this does indicate that positive skin reactions in coeliacs are induced by compounds able to cause the small bowel damage, and provides an avenue for further research.

From a clinical standpoint, we have shown that just over half of a group of patients with untreated coeliac disease developed visible Arthus-type reactions following intradermal challenge with a peptic–tryptic digest of gluten. No false positives were observed.

Refinements of method should improve these encouraging early results, to accord skin testing a valuable place in the diagnosis and management of coeliac disease.

ACKNOWLEDGEMENTS

We would like to thank Mr R. I. Palmer, F.I.M.L.S., Chief Technician, Haematology Department, Bristol Royal Infirmary, for his help and guidance in the work involving immunofluorescence.

References

1. Collins-Williams, C. and Ebbs, J. H. (1954). Role of skin testing in patients with coeliac sprue. *Ann. Allergy,* **189**, 267
2. Asquith, P. (1974). Immunology of coeliac disease. *Clin. Gastroenterol.,* **3**, 213
3. Doe, W. F., Henry, K., Holt, L. and Booth, C. C. (1972). Am immunological study of adult coeliac disease. *Gut,* **13**, 324
4. Alarcon-Segovia, D., Gerskovic, T., Wakin, K. G., Green, P. A. and Scudamore, H. H. (1964). Presence of circulating antibodies to gluten and milk fractions in patients with non-tropical sprue. *Am. J. Med.,* **36**, 485
5. Berger, E., Deschwanden, G. and Mullner, E. (1957). The physiological occurrence of antibodies against foodstuff antigens without demonstrable pathogenic action. *Ann. Pediat.,* **189**, 267
6. Ferguson, A. and Carswell, F. (1972). Precipitins to dietary proteins in serum and upper intestinal secretions of coeliac children. *Br. Med. J.,* **1**, 75
7. Baker, P. G., Barry, R. E. and Read, A. E. (1975). Detection of continuing gluten ingestion in treated coeliac patients. *Br. Med. J.,* **1**, 486
8. Baker P. G. and Read, A. E. (1976). Oats and barley toxicity in coeliac patients. *Postgrad. Med. J.,* **52**, 264

Discussion of chapters 36 and 37

McNicholl   I would like to ask if either of the speakers have had an opportunity of using the skin tests on asymptomatic coeliacs. They
spoke of screening and one would be very interested in its use
in this regard. Have they been able to find any coeliacs as yet
and if so what have the strengths of the reactions been?

Rawcliffe   We have not used it for that purpose yet.

Baker   My story on this is rather anecdotal in that one of the patients
who had a particularly strong skin reaction had completed a dietary
questionnaire showing that she was not ingesting gluten at all.
Now in view of the positive skin reaction we then went back and
questioned her again and apart from having serum gluten antibodies, we also found out that she was ingesting gluten in the
form of wheat-coated potato crisps and gluten-containing mustard
so in that particular case it did prove useful in showing us that
she wasn't adhering to the diet.

Schneider   I would just like to tell Dr Rawcliffe that we have some very preliminary results with a non-digest subfraction of gliadin and have
found similar responses to you with your peptic–tryptic digests.
I was going to ask you whether you had made the same observation
that we had, that the sensitivity is greater at the distal end of the
forearm? We also used the forearm, but we found that the sensitivity tended to be greater at the distal end than at the proximal
end and therefore we always make two injections of our subfraction
so we can compare the two. I also wonder whether he reads his
results at 24 h to exclude delayed type reactions, rather than on
Arthus reactions which we tend to do, and I should also like to ask
him what dilutions he uses because we have made the observation
that the response varies with the dilution and it is by no means
always the stronger concentration which produces the greater
reaction; on the contrary, quite often it is a weaker concentration
which produces a greater reaction.

Baker   Yes, of course I did control work. First of all I should make the
point that I always gave three injections of the control solution as
well as the peptic–tryptic digest and the mean was taken of these.
The other point was that in the early stages I tried to find the optimum concentration and found that with 500 mg% of a peptic–
tryptic digest I got reasonably good results. I was then using 1 g%
dilution but when I went up to 2 g% dilution I found that I did get
some positives, two out of 50 control patients reacting. I didn't
get this when I was using a 1 g% solution which gave rather a higher
pick-up rate than 500 mg% solution.

Rawcliffe	With regard to the site on the arm, I found it more difficult to do an intradermal injection near the wrist because the skin is rather tougher and as I had a feeling that this might introduce a factor that we would want to eliminate, I tended to concentrate a bit further up the arm and so not many of my injections except the early ones were near the wrist. Injections were given mainly on the fleshy part of the forearm, trying to make the test as uniform as possible. We haven't observed all our patients at 24 h. Until recently, we asked them to telephone us at 24 h if they had one, but none have done so. As for the strengths, we do plan to do some dose/response curves because indeed we may not be using an appropriate dose. We are using $500 \mu g$/ml of B2. It is certainly true that sometimes one can get a stronger reaction with a weaker dilution. When we were using Fraction B, we sometimes got a more obvious reaction with 2 mg/ml than we did with 4 mg/ml, and sometimes vice versa.
McCarthy	Could I ask for some details about precautions taken to ensure sterility? The reason I ask is that Dr Stevens and I have done some preliminary studies in which we passed our material through a millipore filter and we had no positive reactions. Now, we are not quite sure what passed through but for what it's worth the results were negative.
Baker	When I first started testing, the precautions were very little and one patient did have a positive reaction at 4 days which responded to penicillin rather than anything else! Since then I have been particularly careful to use a millipore filter to sterilize everything and I haven't had any further trouble.
Rawcliffe	Our material being in very large bulk is in fact prepared at the final stage by the Bencard Allergy Unit and as they apply strict microbiological controls to their preparation, I think we are guaranteed a sterile preparation.
Cooke	Have you noted any keloid formation subsequent to the biopsies? We used Fraction III some eight or nine years ago and from a biopsy on a positive test we produced a keloid formation which took roughly 15 months to settle down. We did not go on with our skin tests because we were not sure what had happened and nobody could help us with the immunology of a keloid. About the Crohn's cases, were they active, were they small bowel, were they large bowel, was there any particular correlation between the site and our positive results?
Rawcliffe	They were all small bowel cases and all except one were well; one was distinctly unwell and had no treatment at the time test was performed; she shortly afterwards went on intravenous steroids. The responses have in the main been fairly weak, in other words 1+ or 2+ on our scale which means up to but not exceeding 10 mm, mostly in the 1+ range. We have not seen keloid formation.
Baker	I used a 3 mm punch biopsy technique and did not have any problems with keloid formation.
Ferguson	Let's get it quite straight, an Arthus reaction is only a test for antibody, probably of the IgG and IgM class and I think it is not fair to say that a skin test like this is easier for the patient than a venepuncture with assay of the antibodies by techniques which were beautifully described yesterday, especially by the group from

Hamburg. I would caution Dr Baker—an injection of 1 mg of antigen intradermally can be a very potent re-immunizing phenomenon and he may well be producing further hypersensitivity in his patients if he re-injects them regularly.

Albert

Dr Baker, you have described in the histological pictures the occurrence of polymorphonuclear cells which indeed are an indication of the reaction of antibodies with antigen as one can judge from transplant rejection data but if you claim that this could be a model for the tissue damage in the gut you see any polymorphonuclear cells in the gut, for instance upon a challenge of the patient.

Truelove

In recent work which has not been published, two patients with treated coeliac disease and one healthy control subject have been challenged by an intraduodenal instillation of fraction B of gluten, which is a toxic fraction, and serial biopsies have been taken repeatedly over the course of 24 h using an indwelling hydraulic biopsy instrument. For the first three to four hours the mucosa is quite unaffected and then at about 4–6 h corresponding to the time that the skin reaction takes place there are dramatic changes in the jejunal biopsy with morphological changes including the presence of many polymorphonuclear cells and also a sudden and precipitous fall in disaccharidase levels. Big changes are seen on electron microscopy and by immunoperoxidase there is a great increase in the number of IgA-containing immunocytes and of IgM-containing immunocytes but no change in the IgG.

Hekkens

I want to know if you have also injected other solutions, such as digests of casein or other proteins and whether you have utilized blanks of the enzymes that you have used for the digestion because it could be that they would also give a reaction. Then you would not know whether the reaction was related to the toxicity of the fractions or of the enzymes.

Baker

Yes, in fact I have used peptic–tryptic digests of soya flour and also rice flour. The point was that I only injected them into the patients who had a positive response. They didn't respond, but it can't really be regarded as a full trial in that only those patients that had a positive skin response were tested.

38

Gluten antibodies in coeliac disease and dermatitis herpetiformis

B. B. SCOTT and M. S. LOSOWSKY

Gluten antibody titres are commonly raised in the serum of patients with coeliac disease, tending to fall on a gluten-free diet. Less attention has been paid to these antibodies in dermatitis herpetiformis. In one study[1] of dermatitis herpetiformis, antibodies were not detected in any patient. This could possibly be due to the frequently milder mucosal abnormality found in dermatitis herpetiformis. This study was designed to assess whether gluten antibody titres in coeliac disease are related to the degree of mucosal abnormality and, by analogy, whether differences in titres between coeliac disease and dermatitis herpetiformis can be ascribed to differences in severity of the mucosal lesion.

Gluten antibodies were measured using a tanned red cell agglutination technique. In the first part of the study, sera from nine untreated coeliac patients with a flat mucosa were compared with sera from four coeliac patients who, although also untreated, had the milder mucosal abnormality of convolutions. The antibody titres were significantly lower in the patients with a convoluted mucosa ($p < 0.05$) thus suggesting that gluten antibody levels in coeliac disease are related to the severity of mucosal abnormality.

In the second part of the study, gluten antibody titres in 22 patients with coeliac disease were compared with titres in 22 patients with dermatitis herpetiformis, individually matched for degree of mucosal abnormality and duration of treatment with a gluten-free diet. In addition, the two groups of patients were well-matched for the presence of the histocompatibility antigen HLA-B8, since we have previously shown that gluten antibody titres are related to the presence of this antigen[2]. Milk antibody titres were also measured as a possible index of the extent of mucosal abnormality. Gluten antibodies were

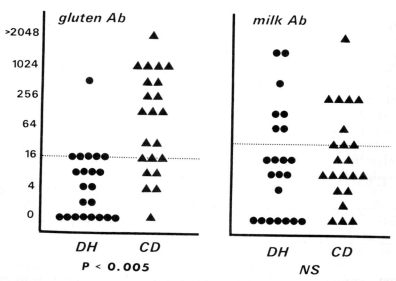

Figure 38.1 Serum gluten and milk antibody titres in the patients with dermatitis herpetiformis (DH) and coeliac disease (CD). Reciprocals of titres are shown

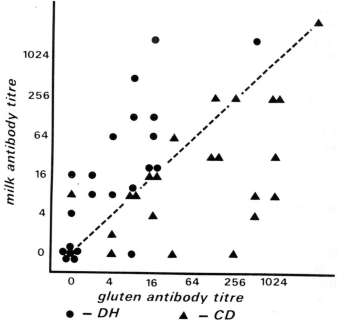

Figure 38.2 Serum gluten antibody titres plotted against the corresponding milk antibody titres in the patients with dermatitis herpetiformis (DH) and coeliac disease (CD). Reciprocals of titres are shown

significantly higher in coeliac disease than in dermatitis herpetiformis ($p<0.005$), but milk antibody titres were similar in the two groups suggesting that they were well-matched for extent of mucosal abnormality (Figure 38.1). Milk and gluten antibodies correlated significantly for each condition, but at any given level of milk antibody (and therefore perhaps at any given severity and extent of mucosal abnormality) the level of gluten antibody was much higher in coeliac disease than in dermatitis herpetiformis (Figure 38.2).

The explanation for lower gluten antibody titres in dermatitis herpetiformis is not known. Theoretically it is due either to decreased production or increased removal of antibody. Decreased production could result from there being a different type of immune response to dietary gluten or possibly to the non-involvement of gluten in some patients with dermatitis herpetiformis. Could some patients be sensitive to a dietary constituent other than gluten? In this context it is interesting that patients have been described with dermatitis herpetiformis apparently precipitated by milk[3,4]. There is also the possibility that the mucosal lesion was less extensive in our patients with dermatitis herpetiformis. Our patients were certainly well-matched for the severity of the proximal mucosal abnormality but there is no simple way of measuring the extent of abnormality. However, the similar milk antibody levels in the two groups suggest that they were well-matched for extent of abnormality if, as has been suggested, milk and other dietary antibodies in serum reflect non-specific absorption through a damaged mucosa. The possibility of increased removal of gluten antibody in dermatitis herpetiformis is supported by the presence of circulating immune complexes and by the deposition of immunoglobulins in the skin. Whatever the explanation for the difference, our results suggest that there is a fundamental difference in the immunological abnormality in dermatitis herpetiformis and coeliac disease.

ACKNOWLEDGEMENT

We thank Dr Janet Marks, Newcastle-upon-Tyne, for supplying sera from some of the patients with dermatitis herpetiformis.

References

1. Graber, W., Laissue, J. and Krebs, A. (1971). Biopsies and serological investigations of the enteropathy in dermatitis herpetiformis. *Dermatoligica*, **142**, 329
2. Scott, B. B., Swinburne, M. L., Rajah, S. M. and Losowsky, M. S. (1974). HL-A8 and the immune response to gluten. *Lancet*, **ii**, 374
3. Pock-Steen, O. Ch. and Niordson, A. M. (1970). Milk sensitivity in dermatitis herpetiformis. *Br. J. Dermatol.*, **83**, 614
4. Engquist, A. and Pock-Steen, O. Ch. (1971). Dermatitis herpetiformis and milk-free diet. *Lancet*, **ii**, 438

39

Fine structural changes in the small intestine in dermatitis herpetiformis

H. F. CHIU and W. C. WATSON

The histopathology of the enteropathy in dermatitis herpetiformis and its response to a gluten-free diet, has been well-documented[1-13]. This is the first report of the ultrastructural changes in this condition.

Multiple jejunal biopsies from five patients with dermatitis herpetiformis were studied with the electron microscope. Biopsy was repeated 72 h after the patients had ingested 20 g of gluten. For controls, jejunal specimens were obtained from two normal subjects before and after gluten challenge as well as from three patients with coeliac disease.

On light microscopy, of the five cases of dermatitis herpetiformis, one showed a normal villous pattern with a mild increase in mononuclear cellular infiltration in the lamina propria (Grade I); one showed minimal villous atrophy (Grade II); two exhibited partial villous atrophy (Grade III); and a completely flat mucosa was present in one (Grade IV). Increased intraepithelial lymphocytes were present in all cases. After gluten challenge, there were no significant alterations in the histological grading. Increased oedema in the villi and pericapillary nodular aggregates of lymphocytes and plasma cells were observed. Estimations of the mucosal enzymes, including maltase, sucrase, lactase and alkaline phosphatase, revealed no significant change after gluten administration.

Ultrastructurally, in dermatitis herpetiformis, the epithelial cells lining the mucosal surface and the tip of the villi were more poorly differentiated than normal (Figure 39.1). Microvilli were irregular, less numerous and often branched. The rough endoplasmic reticulum was distended and vesiculated. The mitochondria were swollen and showed disruption of the cristae. Lysosomes were increased Intraepithelial lymphocytes (theliolymphocytes) were frequently present, mucus cells

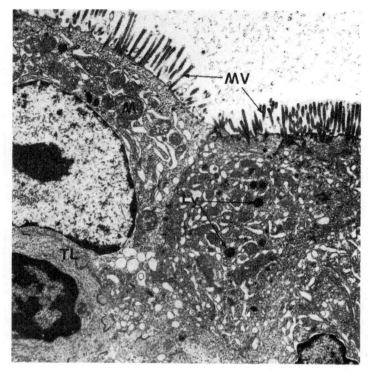

Figure 39.1 Epithelial cells lining the surface of the jejunal mucosa in dermatitis herpetiformis (see description in text). MV: microvilli, M: mitochondria, ER: endoplasmic reticulum, Ly: lysosomes, TL: theliolymphocyte. Magnification × 7500

were decreased. As in coeliac disease, the fine structural features of these surface cells resembled more closely the crypt cells than the mature absorptive cells[4,5]. A prominent change was observed in the basement membrane of the epithelial cells; instead of being linear and delicate, it was replaced by aggregates of granulo-fibrillary materials of irregular thickness (Figure 39.2). This feature was present throughout the mucosal thickness—the villi, surface mucosa and crypts, and could be seen in the specimens which were normal by light microscopy. Electron dense immune-complex deposits in the basement membrane were not found.

Distinctive ultrastructural changes were observed in all five cases 72 h after gluten challenge. In the lamina propria, there was marked oedema associated with increased lymphocytes, histiocytes and plasma cells. There was disappearance of any remnant of the epithelial basement membrane. The basal portions of the epithelial cells came to lie in direct contact with the oedema fluid in the lamina propria (Figure 39.3). The

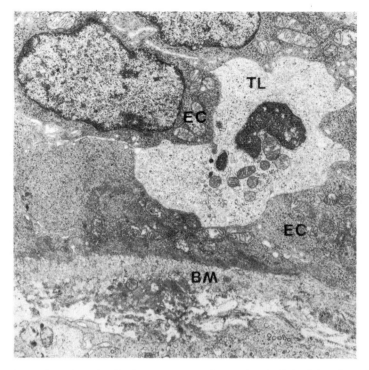

Figure 39.2 Alterations in the basement membrane (BM) of the jejunal epithelium (EC). A theliolymphocyte (TL) is also shown. Magnification × 7300

intercellular spaces between adjacent absorptive cells were distended with oedema fluid. The cytoplasmic organelles showed an advanced degree of injury. Theliolymphocytes were increased and they contained abundant endoplasmic reticulum and mitochondria indicating blastic transformation.

Two conclusions can be drawn from this study:

(1) There are clinical, immunologic, and histological similarities between coeliac disease and the enteropathy of dermatitis herpetiformis. The ultrastructural findings lend support to the concept that both enteropathies are similar and related, at least in part, to gluten sensitivity;

(2) The consistent and severe damage to the basement membrane of the jejunal mucosa in dermatitis herpetiformis is probably a specific feature of this enteropathy. Similar alterations and dissolutions of the basement membrane have been observed in the skin lesions in dermatitis herpetiformis and have been attributed to the attack on the basement membrane by the inflammatory cellular infiltrate[6,7].

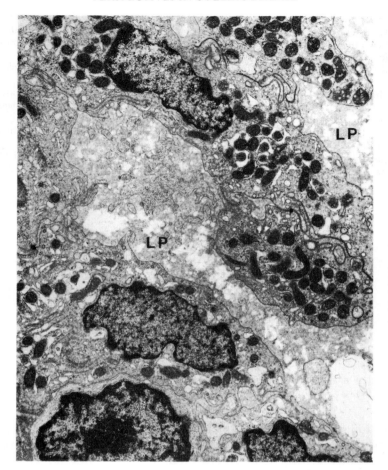

Figure 39.3 Complete dissolution of the epithelial basement membrane 72 h after gluten challenge. Note the oedema fluid in the lamina propria (LP). Magnification × 10 500

ACKNOWLEDGEMENTS

We wish to thank Drs W. Pace and J. Purnes for referring patients with DH.

References

1. Shuster, S., Watson, A. J. and Marks, J. (1968). Coeliac syndrome in dermatitis herpetiformis. *Lancet,* **ii,** 1101
2. Brow, J. R., Parker, F., Weinstein, W. M. and Rubin, C. E. (1971). The small intestinal mucosa in dermatitis herpetiformis. I. Severity and distribution of the

small intestinal lesion and associated malabsorption. *Gastroenterology,* **60,** 355

3. Weinstein, W. M., Brow, J. R., Parker, F. and Rubin, C. M. (1971). The small intestinal mucosa in dermatitis herpetiformis. II. Relationship of the small intestinal lesion to gluten. *Gastroenterology,* **60,** 362

4. Rubin, W., Ross, L. L., Sleisenger, M. H. and Weser, E. (1966). An electron microscopic study of adult coeliac disease. *Lab. Invest.,* **15,** 1720

5. Shiner, M. (1974). Cell distribution in the jejunal mucosa in coeliac disease. In: *Coeliac Disease. Proceedings of the Second International Coeliac Symposium* W. Th. J. M. Hekkens and A. S. Peña (eds.) (Leiden: Stenfert Kroese)

6. Fry, L. and Johnson, F. R. (1969). Electron microscopic study of dermatitis herpetiformis. *Br. J. Dermatol.,* **81,** 44

7. Jakubowicz, K., Dabrowski, J. and Maciejewski, W. (1971). Deposition of fibrin-like material in early lesions of dermatitis herpetiformis. *Ann. Clin. Res.,* **3,** 34

Discussion of Chapters 38 and 39

Holmes	Could I ask Dr Watson whether he controlled his instillation experiments with a completely non-gluten containing protein?
Watson	No, we haven't tried that as yet.
Holmes	So the changes could be possibly due to factors other than gluten intake?
Watson	We have considered ourselves the possibility that some of these are due to artefact, but I don't think these are artefactual changes, they look consistent in the samples.
Marks	Could I ask Dr Scott if one of his suggested explanations for the difference between the patients with DH and with coeliac disease, was that in some patients with DH gluten was not casually involved? I can't now remember the details of the patients whose sera I gave him, but to my knowledge, we haven't yet seen any patients who have not responded to a gluten-free diet.
Scott	As you say, all the patients have responded to gluten withdrawal, so it does really seem unlikely.
Watson	I wonder if Dr Scott is using 'convoluted' as a shorthand description, or is he segregating that group purely on the dissecting microscope appearances?
Scott	They all had the appearance of convolutions on stereomicroscopy. They also had partial villous atrophy on histology, but I was referring to the stereomicroscopic appearance.
Watson	It is my experience that when convoluted specimens are examined histologically, some of them approach towards normality and a smaller number tend towards the appearance of coeliac disease, and this is true also of the cytogenetic status of the crypts as well.
Scott	We find good correlation between the stereomicroscopic appearance and the histology.
Albert	Dr Scott—you have shown a quite nice correlation between the antibodies and the degree of gut lesions, but can you tell us which was first, the hen or the egg?
Scott	I don't know. I imagine the milk antibodies result from the gut lesion, and I'd like to think the gluten antibodies had a different role.
Unidentified speaker	It is very interesting that you found a correlation between the gluten antibodies and the severity of the mucosal lesion, because up till now it has been very difficult to find anything that relates to the severity of the mucosal lesion. Did you go any further into this with measurements such as surface cell heights or lymphocyte infiltration?

Scott	No, we didn't.
Strober	Dr Watson, I wasn't clear whether you were comparing patients with ordinary coeliac disease and patients with dermatitis herpetiformis who had the same degree of light microscopy abnormalities. You say in your conclusion that the membrane lesion might have been more severe in the DH patients. To prove that point you would have to first be given in a blind fashion, specimens from patients of either group of known severity, not knowing which group was which, then pick out which ones were the ordinary coeliac disease and which the dermatitis herpetiformis.
Watson	That is a fair point, but in the literature as it exists at the moment, the description of the basement membrane (which is not given at all in many of the papers) is limited largely to Margot Shiner's description of membrane before and after gluten in a series of patients with coeliac disease that she studied at different times, and it is interesting that her description of the membrane in coeliac disease is virtually identical to what we have seen in our three coeliac patients. The degree of change in DH seems to be quite different.
Cooke	I am not quite sure whether you are talking about coeliac disease complicated by DH or whether you are talking about DH complicated by coeliac disease, and finally where do you draw the line when you get DH occurring in, for example, Crohn's disease; do you think they are all coeliacs or what is the situation? Are these entitled to be called coeliacs? I believe they are, but that is another matter.
Scott	In patients with coeliac disease who have a mucosal abnormality which responds to a gluten-free diet, we call it coeliac disease. If they also satisfy the criteria for DH then they also have DH, and the two co-exist.
Watson	We are really talking about something different, I think. If we are suggesting anything we are suggesting that the patient with DH has an intrinsic abnormality of basement membrane, and that what makes them different, and the ways in which they are different from coeliac disease, is because they have that difference, and gluten can do something to the basement membrane if you like, at lower titres than in CD.
Strober	I want to make my point crystal clear—before you can make that statement, you will have to very carefully compare patients of equal severity, on the basis of light microscopy, and not know which patient you are examining. Before you can say that there is a difference in the lesion at the level of the electron microscope, because there is no difference, that I am aware, of on the basis of light microscopy.
Watson	If you take the patient with coeliac disease, the most severe coeliac has that kind of minimal tri-layer lesion that I have shown on electron microscopy, but the patients with even mild light microscopic changes in DH have that gross thick granule-fibrillary membrane, in the gut in DH; there is quite a striking difference.
Douglas	I think most of us accept the definition that Dr Scott gave, when he said that coeliac disease is a flat mucosa that gets better when you take gluten away. We also have to remember that Fred Weinstein showed extremely nicely, that if you take a patient with

DH, even if his mucosa looks normal, and give him enough gluten, then a high proportion are going to develop a lesion that is identical with that which we accept as coeliac disease, and it gets better again when you take gluten away, so that they have coeliac disease.

40

Investigation of the cellular immunity in infants and children with coeliac disease using the DNCB test

E. ROSSIPAL

INTRODUCTION

We do have proof that antigen–antibody reactions are involved in the pathogenesis of coeliac disease. Evidence for immunological reactions has been provided through complement activation, lowering of complement level by gluten loading and by the existence of gluten antibodies[1-3]. Histological evidence of an immunological reaction in the lamina mucosae of the small intestine in coeliac disease has also been shown[4]. Since reactions of humoral immunity influence cellular immunity, we investigated the status of cellular immunity in infants and children with coeliac disease. For this test we used the DNCB-system (2,4-dinitrochlorobenzene) as proposed by N. J. Catalona in a modified form. We chose DNCB as sensitizing agent for several reasons:

1. Because the percentage of people in normal population who develop sensitivity to DNCB is very high being about 94–98%.

2. Because the extent of cellular allergy in a patient at any one particular time can be ascertained with DNCB. The accidental development of sensitivity to DNCB at some previous time can be ruled out because of the nature of the test substance.

3. Because no humoral antibodies are formed by sensitivity with DNCB; the sensitizing process affects only the cellular immune system.

METHOD AND MATERIAL

The sensitizing procedure was carried out in the following manner. The volar side of the right forearm was wiped off with acetone.

Following this $0.1 \, cm^3$ of DNCB-acetone solution containing $2000 \, ng$ of DNCB was placed on a circular area of $3 \, cm^2$. Then, $0.1 \, cm^3$ of DNCB acetone solution containing $50 \, \mu g$ of DNCB was placed on a second area distal to the first. Afterwards the arm was not allowed to be washed for 24 h. The result of the test was determined after ten days. The result was interpreted as being positive if nodules or erythema with or without infiltration appeared on one or both of the application points. If there was no sensitivity reaction after ten days a booster of $50 \, \mu g$ DNCB was applied to the volar side of the left forearm. The application points on both arms were checked after another two days. A positive result could be either a reaction solely on the left arm, secondarily a reaction solely on the right arm at the application area of $2000 \, \mu g$, or else a reaction on both of these mentioned application areas. In case the results were still negative a final check was made after another two days.

The DNCB solution was kept refrigerated in dark bottles and was renewed every 14 days.

Eighty children with coeliac disease in the age bracket from 7 months to 14 years were tested under different dietary conditions. The diagnosis of coeliac disease was made on the basis of clinical symptoms, a small bowel biopsy, the demonstration of gluten antibodies and by other pertinent biochemical parameters. As a control group, 50 children from the same age bracket but without gastrointestinal disturbances, were used.

RESULTS

Of the 50 children in the control group 46% showed a positive reaction after ten days. Another 48% showed a positive reaction after the booster, while 6% showed a negative result.

The DNCB test was carried out on 42 patients with coeliac disease who were having a gluten-free diet. This group had been on the gluten-free diet for an average period of 20.6 months (2 months–4 years). A total of 66.7% of the patients showed a positive test result 10 days after the application of DNCB. This result shows by the x^2 test a significant difference from the control group. In three of these patients the reaction was a strong one, with the formation of blisters. In another 30.9% there was a positive reaction after a booster, while 2.4% of the patients showed no reaction at all to the DNCB. The DNCB test was carried out in 26 patients with coeliac disease during a period when they were receiving a gluten-containing diet, which averaged 10.2 months' duration, (1 month–3.5 years). Only 30.8% of the children showed a positive reaction 10 days after the DNCB application. The results became positive in another 15.4% after the booster. A total of 53.8% of the children in this test group showed a negative result to the test. This gives by the x^2 test a highly significant difference compared with the control group.

Finally the test was carried out on 12 patients with coeliac disease 1–4 weeks after the introduction of a gluten-free diet. Sixty-seven per cent of the children showed a positive reaction with or without the booster while in 33% the result was negative.

Comparing the results of the different test groups with one another, the patients with coeliac disease who were on a gluten-free diet demonstrated a significantly increased cellular immunity, as indicated by the DNCB test, over the control group of children without gastrointestinal complications. On the other hand, the children with coeliac disease who were on a diet containing gluten showed a significant reduction in cellular allergy by the DNCB test. As the results of the investigation indicate, this reduction in cellular immunity is exhibited for up to four weeks after beginning a diet free from gluten. Eight children with coeliac disease who were previously sensitized to DNCB while on a gluten-free diet, were subjected to a follow-up test over a period lasting up to several months in which they received food containing gluten. It was then shown that the cellular allergy in these children was not essentially altered. Thus a gluten-containing diet seems only to depress the development of a cellular immunity in children with active coeliac disease. An immunity that has already previously been developed seems however not to be influenced. We found that this was true not only for DNCB sensitivity, but also for other previously acquired sensitivities, for example, those to tuberculin, streptodornase and *Candida* antigen.

DISCUSSION

The results indicate compared to a normal control group an increased reactivity of cellular immunity in children with coeliac disease, who had been on a gluten-free diet for at least two months. Introduction of gluten into the diet leads in children with coeliac disease to a significant reduction of cellular immunity as shown by DNCB test. The suppression of the cellular immune system can most likely be explained as the activation of a T-suppressor cell by means of an antigen–antibody reaction[5,6]. The finding that cellular immunity once established, for example to tuberculin, *Candida* antigen or to DNCB is not suppressed, provides evidence that the suppressor effect does not function at the level of the T-effector cell. It might rather be suggested that macrophages activated by T-cells depress blast transformation. The suppression of cellular immunity may be important in the development of complications in untreated coeliac disease such as malignancy and infections.

References

1. Doe, W. F., Henry, K., Holt, L. and Booth, C. C. (1972). An immunological study of adult coeliac disease. *Gut,* **13,** 324
2. Rossipal, E. (1972). Die Bedeutung präzipitierender Antikörper gegen Kleber-proteine in der Pathogenese der Coeliakie. *Pädiatrie und Pädologie,* **7,** 253
3. Doe, W. F., Henry, K. and Booth, C. C. (1974). Complement in coeliac disease. In: W. Th. J. M. Hekkens and A. S. Peña (eds.) *Coeliac Disease,* pp. 189–194 (Leiden: H. E. Stenfert Kroese B.V.)
4. Shiner, M. and Ballard, J. (1972). Antigen–antibody reactions in jejunal mucosa in childhood coeliac disease after gluten challenge. *Lancet,* **i,** 1202
5. Taylor, R. B. and Basten, A. (1976). Suppressor cells in humoral immunity and tolerance. *Br. Med. Bull.,* **32,** 152
6. Asherson, G. L. and Zembala, M. (1976). Suppressor T-cells in cell mediated immunity. *Br. Med. Bull.,* **32,** 158

Discussion of chapter 40

Douglas	I am somewhat concerned about the ethics of these tests, particularly repeated tests in children that have already been sensitized. Did you have informed consent?
Rossipal	We did have informed consent. Repeat testing was with a small dose of 50 micrograms, and as far as I can tell from the literature this does not imply any danger to children.
Mawhinney	Could I ask if you had any opportunity to compare the untreated coeliac children with children whose nutritional status might have been comparable, because I think that any malnourished child might well have a comparable depression of cell-mediated immunity.
Rossipal	The children who had been on a gluten-free diet and showed this increased cellular immunity were not below the 3rd weight percentile, so that they were not malnourished at the time we investigated them.
Mawhinney	What about the children who were on a normal diet when you investigated them?
Rossipal	The children who were on a normal diet were between the 3rd and 10th percentile for weight.
Mawhinney	In untreated patients whom you were not able to sensitize with 2000 μg DNCB and who did not react when you re-challenged them with 50 μg, did you test any of them again with a 50 μg dose after they had been on a gluten-free diet?
Rossipal	No.

Section VIII
Gut hormones in coeliac disease

41

The role of the gastro-entero-pancreatic (GEP) hormones in coeliac disease

K. D. BUCHANAN and F. A. O'CONNOR

INTRODUCTION

It is now recognized that the gastrointestinal tract is a major endocrine organ. It is therefore likely that this endocrine system may have a primary role in some gastrointestinal diseases or may play a secondary role in other disorders. Their primary role is exemplified by tumours arising from the endocrine cells of the gastrointestinal tract e.g. the Zollinger–Ellison syndrome, glucagonomas, insulinomas, etc. However, deficient or excessive secretion of these hormones (apart from the tumour syndromes) could play a primary role in gastrointestinal disorders or may perpetuate the clinical features of a disease by becoming secondarily involved by the disease process. It would be surprising if coeliac disease with often severe mucosal damage would spare the endocrine cells. In this review the present knowledge with respect to endocrine cells of the gastrointestinal tract will be briefly examined. Thereafter the knowledge containing their role in coeliac disease will be reviewed. In addition an attempt will be made to place a variety of hypotheses and point the direction for future research.

THE GASTRO-ENTERO-PANCREATIC (GEP) ENDOCRINE SYSTEM

The term GEP hormones is preferred to the more limiting term of 'gut hormones' or 'gastrointestinal hormones' as the authors consider that the hormones secreted from the pancreas and stomach are frequently the same or similar to the hormones secreted from the intestine. Indeed it may be that the GEP nomenclature may be too limiting in that the distribution of these hormones is now recognized to be very extensive possibly including the brain, the salivary glands and perhaps even the placenta, the kidneys and lungs.

This section is designed merely to highlight certain features of the GEP hormones which may be relevant in the coeliac syndrome . Johnston[11] has recently extensively reviewed the gastrointestinal hormones and their function. GEP hormones consist structurally of three major categories of substances, peptides, amines and prostaglandins. In this review the peptide hormones will mainly be discussed.

Table 41.1   Gastro-entero-pancreatic (GEP) peptide hormones

Established

Insulin
Pancreatic glucagon
Gastrin
Cholecystokinin–pancreozymin (CCK–PZ)
Secretin
Gastric inhibitory peptide (GIP)

Very Nearly Established

Vasoactive intestinal peptide (VIP)
Somatostatin
Pancreatic polypeptide (PP)

Some of the Others

Bombesin, substance P, motilin, gut glucagon-like immuno-reactivity (GLI)

Table 41.1 lists a number of the GEP peptide hormones. This list is far from extensive. It is pertinent to ask when does a GEP hormone become 'established' and what are the requirements necessary to reach these upper echelons. Grossman[8,9] has recently reviewed this problem in addition to discussing what actions of GEP hormones may be regarded as physiological. The criteria to be established would include the complete chemical identity of the peptide, proof of a hormonal role and finally that this hormonal role can be reproduced by infusion of the hormone in doses which are similar to the levels achieved during the physiological event under examination. Needless to say all such studies must be reproducible and should be documented by several laboratories. As many of the techniques involved in establishing these criteria remain in their infancy it is sometimes impossible to be thoroughly satisfied that all criteria have been established. The authors take sole responsibility for the list in Table 41.1 but such a list may not be very greatly different if a consensus of views of all the workers in the field were taken.

Advances in the field in recent years has been largely due to improvements in technology. These include a variety of chemical techniques for purifying and identifying the hormones, techniques of assay of hormones including sophisticated bioassay and radioimmunoassay methods. There have also been extensive studies of the GEP hormones by histological techniques including standard chemical stains, immunological techniques and also ultrastructural studies.

Certain problems in these techniques may be pointed out. Bioassay methods are non-specific and often too insensitive to detect levels of the hormone in the physiological range. The radioimmunoassay methods offer far greater sensitivity and specificity; however immunological measurements may not necessarily mirror the biological event. For this reason a combination if possible of radioimmunoassay and bioassay should be performed. Most GEP hormones exist in multiple molecular species. This may represent a pro-hormone–hormone relationship as is the case for proinsulin and insulin but could also represent degradative biologically inactive products as is the case for C-peptide in insulin production. Alternatively multiple molecular species of hormones may represent entirely separate hormone species with overlapping chemical structure and biological function. The immunological histological techniques are open to the same problems as the radioimmunoassay methods but in addition have their own problems as the fixation and processing of tissue may destroy the hormone or render it structurally dissimilar from the starting material. Quantitation of hormones in endocrine cells is also difficult as the specific immunological methods only stain the cell granules. Therefore if the granules have been recently discharged the appearance may be that of few hormone cells whereas in reality there could be large numbers which are empty. The ultrastructural methods have the obvious difficulties of attempting to decide which hormone belongs to which cell type and only the development of reliable methods of applying specific antisera at the ultrastructural level will help to solve this problem.

Cells which secrete GEP hormones have been termed the APUD (amine precursor uptake and decarboxylation) cells[18] although Dawson points out that even this term may not be satisfactory in that all the cells do not show APUD properties and he suggests that a more non-committal term such as 'endocrine cells' should be preferable[4]. All cells within this family are broadly similar histologically. They tend to be triangular or pear-shaped with their broad base lying at the base of the membrane and their granules predominantly though not exclusively infranuclear. The apex of many reaches the lumen of intestinal glands and is covered by modified microvilli. At the ultrastructural level the cells are differentiated by the size and density of the granules and the presence or absence of a halo between the core and the bounding membrane.

THE ACTIONS OF GEP HORMONES WHICH MAY BE RELEVANT TO COELIAC DISEASE

Table 41.2 lists a variety of actions of GEP hormones which may be relevant in coeliac disease. Exocrine pancreatic function is under hormonal control principally secretin, cholecystokinin–pancreozymin (CCK–PZ) possibly also other hormones including vasoactive intestinal peptide (VIP). CCK–PZ controls gall bladder function. Several hormones may have actions on motility of the gastrointestinal tract including motilin and glucagon-like immunoreactivity (GLI). It is also considered that some hormones may have trophic actions within the gastrointestinal tract and of particular relevance to coeliac disease is the action on mucosal growth.

Table 41.2   Actions of GEP hormones which may be relevant in coeliac disease

Exocrine pancreas (secretin, CCK–PZ)
Gall bladder function (CCK–PZ)
Mucosal growth (gastrin, GLI)
Motility (motilin, GLI)
Enteroinsular axis (GIP)
Direct actions on metabolic functions (insulin, glucagon, secretin, VIP, GIP, etc.)

Not only do GEP hormones have local gastrointestinal functions but it now appears likely that they may have a wider metabolic role. The concept of the entero-insular axis was rekindled by McIntyre and colleagues[25]. Their work showed that there was a greater insulin release after intrajejunal glucose compared to a similar load of glucose given intravenously. The concept therefore arose that there was an enteric factor probably hormonal which stimulated insulin release. In the past few years several hormones have vied for the candidature of the 'incretin'. At the present time it would appear that gastric inhibitory peptide (GIP) provides this role. GEP hormones may therefore affect metabolism through their insulin-releasing properties. In addition some hormones may have direct effects on metabolic functions. VIP for example has hyperglycaemic properties and both secretin and GIP have direct effects on the fat cell.

GEP HORMONES AND COELIAC DISEASE

Table 41.3 gives an extensive list of clinical and chemical abnormalities in coeliac disease. There might appear to be good evidence that the probable and possible disturbances may be due to hormonal abnormalities whereas there is no evidence in the literature that might implicate the 'just possible' disturbances as being hormonally-induced except to indicate that such features as finger clubbing, hyperpigmentation, texture of skin and hair could have an endocrine explanation. So

Table 41.3 Disturbances in coeliac disease which may be
hormonally induced

Probable	Diminished exocrine pancreatic function
	Diminished gall bladder emptying
Possible	Villous atrophy
	Motility
	Diminished insulin secretion
Just possible	Anorexia
	Apathy
	Abdominal distension
	Vomiting
	Dermatitis herpetiformis
	Eczema
	Skin and hair texture
	Hyperpigmentation
	Finger clubbing
	Diminished gastric secretion and emptying
	Increased incidence of DM
	Malignant lymphoma

also could such gastrointestinal effects as gastric secretion and emptying, vomiting, abdominal distension and anorexia. The known association between skin rashes particularly dermatitis herpetiformis and
coeliac disease could have an endocrine basis although immunological
mechanisms appear to be more likely. The increased incidence of
malignant lymphoma in coeliac disease could conceivably be hormonally induced.

Table 41.4 summarizes from a review of the literature what disturbances of GEP hormones have been found in coeliac disease. These
findings are principally produced by three approaches. Firstly by
biological measurements e.g. of the end organ served by the hormone,
the studies being performed during the physiological event which is
thought to stimulate the hormone secretion. Secondly the recently

Table 41.4 Disturbances of GEP hormones in coeliac disease

1. *Biological measurements*
   (a) ↓ GB emptying after fatty meal
   (b) ↓ Exocrine pancreatic function after ID acid usually injection
   of hormone (CCK–PZ or secretin) produced expected result
2. *Blood hormone assays (RIA)*
   (a) ↓ Secretin response to ID acid
   (b) ↓ CCK–PZ response to fat meal
   (c) ↓ GIP response to oral stimulus (unpublished work)
   (d) ↓ Insulin response to oral glucose but not intravenous glucose
3. *Tissue assessment*
   1. Increased enterochromaffin cells
   2. Increased secretin cells

developed radioimmunoassays for GEP hormones have allowed a direct measurement in the blood of hormone levels in the disease and finally there has been an assessment of the histological appearance of the GEP hormone cells in coeliac disease.

It is generally held that exocrine pancreatic function is diminished in coeliac syndrome[10]. Worning and colleagues[21] studied intestinal secretions after ingestion of a standard meal in 25 patients with gluten-induced enteropathy and 16 patients with various intestinal disorders. They found in both groups of patients the secretion of lipase and to a minor degree that of amylase were more markedly reduced than the secretion of the proteolytic enzymes and they thought the effects were explained as a non-specific effect of the malabsorption. Wormsley[20] studied patients with duodenal ulcer, coeliac syndrome and normal subjects by infusing acid into the duodenum and into the jejunum and found impaired secretory responses to both duodenal and jejunal acidification in patients with coeliac syndrome and with duodenal ulcer. Novis and other[16] studied exocrine pancreatic function by means of a secretin–pancreozymin test in 50 patients with coeliac disease. There was no evidence of gross pancreatic insufficiency but pancreatic function was abnormal in 78% of patients. One can conclude therefore that there is disturbed exocrine pancreatic function in coeliac disease although this might not necessarily be only confined to the coeliac syndrome. In addition to hormonal factors being implicated as a cause of the dysfunction, it is also suggested that a combination of other factors may be involved including folic acid deficiency and chronic malnutrition. It is also possible that the end organ response to the hormone may also be diminished. However, from the studies of Wormsley[20] who found that the exocrine pancreas responded normally to infusions of secretin it might be suggested that end organ responsiveness is in fact normal.

With respect to gall bladder function Low-Beer and colleagues[12] showed that of 18 patients with adult coeliac disease 12 had absent or minimal contraction of the gall bladder in response to a fatty meal. In the majority radioactive taurocholate remained in the enterohepatic circulation for longer than normal and metabolized more slowly than normal. They considered that the most likely explanation of these findings was impaired cholecystokinin release by the damaged small bowel mucosa leading to accumulation of bile in an inert gall bladder. Dimagno et al.[6] found that outputs of pancreatic enzymes and gall bladder contents in response to essential amino acids in the duodenum were reduced in sprue. In addition they tested pancreatic lipase and bile acid concentrations after two standard meals and found that the outputs of both of these were diminished. They also found that gall bladder and pancreatic function were normal after intravenous CCK–PZ suggesting that the end organ was normal. The normal end organ responsiveness of the gall bladder however is disputed by the data of Braganza et al.[2] who do suggest that there is impaired response to injected CCK–PZ.

It remained to confirm these hypotheses by direct measurement of hormone levels in plasma. There are three published reports of hormone levels in plasma. Two relate to secretin[1,17] and one relates to cholecystokinin[13]. Using intraduodenal acid as the stimulus, studies from our own laboratory have demonstrated lower levels of plasma secretin as measured by radioimmunoassay in coeliac patients compared with control subjects (Figure 41.1). The absolute fasting levels of

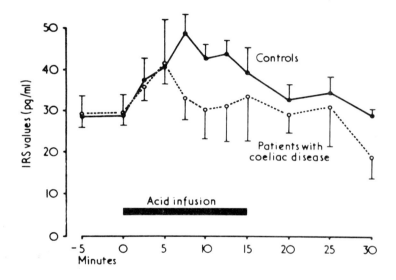

Figure 41.2 Mean (± SE of mean) plasma immunoreactive secretin (IRS) levels after intraduodenal acid in patients with coeliac disease and in controls. (From O'Connor, F. A., McLoughlin, J. C and Buchanan, K. D. (1977) Br Med. J., **1**, 811)

secretin were however not different in the two groups of subjects. There was a suggestion from the data that the more severe the mucosal lesion the more impaired was the plasma secretin response to intraduodenal acid. Similar results have been reported by Bloom[1]. Low-Beer et al.[13] using a newly developed radioimmunoassay for CCK–PZ showed elevated levels of plasma CCK–PZ in coeliac patients as compared to control subjects (Figure 41.2). However, the response to a fatty meal was impaired in the coeliac patients as compared with the control subjects. In the course of their study they also confirmed the previous finding of sluggish gall bladder response to food in patients with coeliac disease.

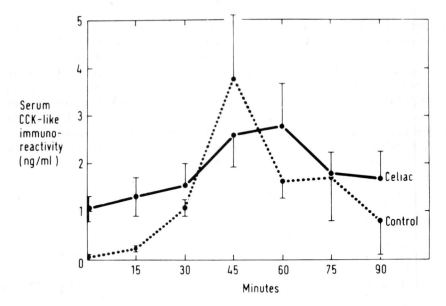

Figure 41.2 Serum cholecystokinin (CCK) levels in coeliac and control groups measured before and at 15 minute intervals after a fatty meal The points and vertical bars show the mean values ± standard error of the mean. (From Low-Beer, T. S., Harvey, R. F. Davies, E. R. and Read, A. E. (1975), *N. Engl. J. Med.*, **292**, 961)

Their data would be consistent with the hypothesis that the gall bladder was lacking in response to endogenous CCK–PZ. Elevated levels of CCK–PZ have also been found in patients with exocrine pancreatic disease although the levels are much more elevated than in coeliac disease (R. F. Harvey, personal communication).

A flat glucose tolerance test is frequently found in patients with coeliac disease. Studies by Maxwell et al.[14] show that after oral glucose there was a flat glucose tolerance in the coeliac patients although the insulin response was perhaps greater than expected from the small rise in blood sugar although it was significantly less than the control subjects. Because the insulin response was greater than expected the authors argue that this might have been due to release of an insulin stimulating factor from the gut. Day et al.[5] have shown that the insulin responses to intravenous tolbutamide in children with coeliac disease were significantly smaller than in the controls. They did not consider that the result could be explained by malnutrition.

Polak and colleagues[19] carried out specific immunological staining techniques to study the endocrine cells in coeliac disease. Only secretin cells were studied by immunological techniques. In 11 out of 16 coeliac patients they found a generalized hyperplasia of the endocrine cells and specifically of the secretin cells. The results may suggest that the secretin cells were abnormally storing hormone and were perhaps unable to release it or else that the hyperplasia was associated with excessive production of secretin. Challacombe and Robertson[3] counted enterochromaffin (EC cells) in the duodenum mucosa of 10 patients with coeliac disease and then controls. They found significantly greater numbers of EC cells in children with coeliac disease. They considered that abnormalities of 5-hydroxytryptamine metabolism in coeliac disease may therefore be the result of hyperplasia of EC cells.

IMPLICATIONS OF GEP HORMONE DISORDERS IN COELIAC DISEASE

What may be the implications of these abnormalities in GEP hormones in coeliac disease? The diminished exocrine pancreatic function would now appear to be due to diminished release of secretin and CCK–PZ from the intestinal mucosa. However, it is not yet completely certain whether the end organ is responsive to CCK–PZ and there appears to be continuing controversy in the literature over this. However, the exocrine pancreatic response to secretin appears to be intact. Now that plasma levels of secretin have been measured in the blood of patients with coeliac disease it would appear that the hyperplasia of secretin cells noted by Polak is due to cells storing their hormone and unable to release the hormone. Impaired exocrine pancreatic and gall bladder function could worsen the malabsorption of coeliac disease, protein and fat absorption being principally affected.

The impaired insulin secretion probably due to a deficient enteroinsular axis in coeliac disease may have important nutritional implications. There is however a suggestion that the impaired insulin secretion may be due to additional factors as insulin response to intravenous stimuli also appears to be diminished in coeliac disease. There is poorly substantiated evidence that coeliac patients have an increased incidence of diabetes mellitus but diminished insulin secretion could seriously impair nutritional status. In addition other hormones which have direct effects on metabolism such as secretin, glucagon and gastric inhibitory peptide may also be implicated in some of the nutritional disturbances in coeliac patients.

Relatively unstudied are the vast array of other GEP hormones. From the scant evidence so far it might appear that there is generally diminished responsiveness of GEP hormones to orally administered stimuli in coeliac disease including GIP (Proceedings of the International Symposium in Gut Hormones, Lausanne, June 1977). The authors are as yet unaware of studies of gastrin, glucagon, pancreatic peptide, vasoactive intestinal peptide, motilin, etc. in coeliac disease. Further studies of these hormones are obviously indicated which may add further to the features of coeliac syndrome which may be hormonally mediated.

One of the most striking diagnostic features of coeliac disease is the intestinal villous atrophy. One could speculate that this may be hormonally induced. Striking giant intestinal villi have been noted in some patients with the glucagonoma syndrome[7] and also in a patient studied by one of the authors (K. D. Buchanan) and F. Stevens in Galway. Gastrin and cholecystokinin also have effects on intestinal growth. One might speculate therefore that the villous atrophy may be the result of hormonal deficiency.

The leading question remains as to whether coeliac disease may be primarily a hormonal disorder. This would appear to be unlikely, the most plausible explanation for the hormonal disturbances being that they are secondary to the mucosal damage. However, once again very much more evidence than is available at present would be required to support that view. It is intriguing to suggest that the gluten-induced enteropathy may not only affect the enterocyte but also the endocrine cell.

References

1. Bloom, S. R., Patel, H. R. and Johnston, D. I. (1976). Failure of secretin release in coeliac disease. *Gut,* **17,** 812
2. Braganza, J. and Howat, H. T. (1972). Gall bladder inertia in coeliac disease. *Lancet,* **i,** 1133
3. Challacombe, D. N. and Robertson, K. (1977). Enterochromaffin cells in the duodenal mucosa of children with coeliac disease. *Gut,* **18,** 373
4. Dawson, I. M. P. (1976). The endocrine cells of the gastro-intestinal tract and the neoplasms which arise from them. *Curr. Top. Pathol.,* **63,** 221
5. Day, G., Evans, K. and Wharton, B. (1973). Abnormalities of insulin and growth hormone secretion in children with coeliac disease. *Arch. Dis Child.,* **48,** 41
6. Dimagno, E. P., Go, V. L. W. and Summershill, W. H. J. (1972). Impaired cholecystokinin–pancreozymin secretion, intra-luminal dilution, and malabsorption of fat in sprue. *Gastroenterology,* **63,** 25
7. Gleeson, M. H., Bloom, S. R., Polak, J. M., Henry, K., Dowling, R. H. and Pearse, A. G. E. (1971). Endocrine tumour in kidney affecting small bowel structure motility and absorptive function. *Gut,* **12,** 773
8. Grossman, M. I. (1977a). How does a candidate hormone become a hormone? Presented at *International Symposium on Gastrointestinal Hormones and Pathology of the Digestive System,* Rome, June 13–15
9. Grossman, M. I. (1977b). Physiological effects of gastrointestinal hormones. *Fed. Proc.,* **36,** 1930
10. Herskovic, T. (1968). The exocrine pancreas in intestinal malabsorption syndromes. *Am. J. Clin. Nutr.,* **21,** 520
11. Johnson, L. R. (1977). Gastrointestinal hormones and their functions. *Annu. Rev. Physiol.,* **39,** 135

12. Low-Beer, T. S., Heaton, K. W., Heaton, S. T. and Read, A. E. (1971). Gall bladder inertia and sluggish enterohepatic circulation of bile salts in coeliac disease. *Lancet*, **i**, 991

13. Low-Beer, T. S., Harvey, R. F., Davies, E. R. and Read, A. E. (1975). Abnormalities of serum cholecystokinin and gall bladder emptying in coeliac disease. *N. Engl. J. Med.*, **292**, 961

14. Maxwell, J. D., McKiddie, M. T., Ferguson, A. and Buchanan, K. D. (1970). Plasma insulin response to oral carbohydrate in patients with glucose and lactose malabsorption. *Gut*, **11**, 962

15. McIntyre, H., Holdworth, C. D. and Turner, D. S. (1964). New interpretation of oral glucose tolerance. *Lancet*, **ii**, 20

16. Novis, B. H., Bank, S and Marks, I. N. (1972). Exocrine pancreatic function in intestinal malabsorption and small bowel disease. *Dig. Dis.*, **17**, 489

17. O'Connor, F. A., McLoughlin, J. C. and Buchanan, K. D. (1977). Impaired immunoreactive secretin release in coeliac disease. *Br. Med. J.*, **1**, 811

18. Pearse, A. G. E. (1968). Common cytochemical and ultrastructural characteristics of cells producing polypeptide hormones (the APUD series) and their relevance to thyroid and ultimobranchial C cells and calcitonin. *Proc. R. Soc. Med. B.* **170**, 71

19. Polak, J. M., Pearse, A. G. E., Van Noorden, S., Bloom, S. R. and Rossiter, M. A. (1973). Secretin cells in coeliac disease. *Gut*, **14**, 870

20. Wormsley, K. G. (1970). Response to duodenal acidification in man. III. Comparison with the effects of secretin and pancreozymin. *Scand. J. Gastroenterol.*, **5**, 353

21. Worning, H., Mullertz, S., Hess Thaysen, E. and Bang, H. E. (1967). pH and concentration of pancreatic enzymes in aspirates from the human duodenum during digestion of a standard meal in patients with intestinal disorders. *Scand. J. Gastroenterol.*, **2**, 81

Discussion of chapter 41

Strober	The question I have is in relation to diabetes—is the diabetes seen in coeliac disease entirely similar to ordinary juvenile diabetes? There is an association between gluten sensitivity and HLA-B8 and there is a similar association in juvenile diabetes. The question is whether the association between these two diseases is on a genetic level, somehow, in some way that we don't understand, related to histocompatibility type and immune responses.
Buchanan	I think the population studies are very difficult to interpret, and from a clinical standpoint from what I got out of reading the papers was that most of the patients were of the juvenile type, and I don't think HLA typing was done. The clinical point is that diabetics of long standing get diabetic diarrhoea and it is important not to label them as having diabetic diarrhoea on an autonomic basis without first considering the possibility of coeliac disease.
Strober	It is worth keeping in mind the possibility that neither diabetes nor coeliac disease are related to each other causally, but are both related to a single underlying genetic abnormality. The second question I had relates to the level of pancreozymin. When I last checked this there was some question about the radioimmunoassay, some people claiming that it was considered a good radioimmunoassay and was valid and others counterclaiming that it was not valid and that clouded the issue as far as coeliac disease was concerned. Do you know anything further about this?
Buchanan	Well, as soon as you use radioimmunoassay you get into deep water. Most radioimmunoassays don't actually measure the specific hormone you think you are measuring. You measure usually a soup of species of hormones and possibly cross-acting titres you don't know anything about, so we are always terribly careful when measuring anything in the blood. We talk about an immunoreactive measurement which means that we are not entirely certain until it is proven that we are actually measuring the thing that is our standard. I think the cholecystokinin pancreozymin assay is a particularly difficult one and I think Dr Bloom and I have great difficulty with it. As far as I can see, there are certain problems with Harvey's assay but a lot of the specificity work appears very good.
Chairman	Could I come in there, Richard Harvey has gone back to using a bioassay and has shown exactly the same thing. There are increased levels of active material as measured by bioassay as with immunoassay.
Albert	I would like to make a further comment on the correlation with

HLA between diabetes and coeliac disease. The data you have shown are interesting in relation to the frequency of coeliac disease among diabetics which was, if I remember correctly, in the order of 1–2% and the frequency of diabetes in coeliac patients which was in the order of 4–5% and that agrees quite well with the differences in association. In coeliac disease the association is about twice as strong with B8 and DW3 as it is for diabetes so the frequencies you have got in your slide would be compatible with a common under-lying genetic mechanism or genetic predisposition. One part of it anyway as we know that the genetic predisposition is composed of different parts. I think that is quite clear, for the diabetes and it is becoming clear for coeliac disease as well.

Cooke   My recollection of our data is that the HLA problem did not really work out. We hoped it would. The paper is in the course of publication at the moment so that you can see the full data in due course.

Dodge   I wonder whether Keith Buchanan would stick his neck out a little and take up his last point. It is possible that the terminal peptide of any of the enterohormones might resemble the peptide sequences in the toxic fractions of gluten and thereby raise the possibility of either blockage or stimulation of a particular hormone.

Buchanan   No comment.

42

Gut hormone profile in coeliac disease: a characteristic pattern of pathology

S. R. BLOOM, J. M. POLAK and H. S. BESTERMAN

ABNORMALITIES IN COELIAC DISEASE

It has been known for some time that pancreatic function in gluten enteropathy is diminished following a test meal. The bicarbonate response to intraluminal acidification and the enzyme response to intraluminal amino acid perfusion[1,2] are similarly greatly reduced. After exogenous administration of cholecystokinin or secretin, however, the response of the pancreas is quite normal. This suggests that the pancreas itself is not diseased but that it lacks the appropriate gastrointestinal signal.

Enterocyte turnover is increased and there is enhanced absorption in the ileum of a variety of substances, e.g. sodium, water, glucose, cortisol, methionine and vitamin B_{12}[3]. There is also an impression that the rate of intestinal transit is reduced in coeliac disease which, together with the adaptive changes in the ileum may tend to reduce the degree of malabsorption. So far, however, no pathophysiological basis of these observations has been found.

GUT HORMONES

The last decade has witnessed a very great increase in our knowledge of gut endocrinology. The number of new hormones discovered is bewilderingly large[4]. It has been established that each hormone has a highly specific cellular localization[5] and well-defined distribution in the alimentary tract[6].

RADIOIMMUNOASSAY AND IMMUNOCYTOCHEMISTRY

Over the last twenty years the ability of high titre antibodies to bind with great affinity and specificity with small peptide hormones has been utilized both to measure them in the circulation and also to localize their producing cells. A number of the early technical problems have been overcome. For example, highly radioactive hormone for use as radio-immunoassay tracer can now be produced without causing the hormone significant structural damage. Antibodies have been raised which combine most avidly with the active site on the hormone and therefore are able to reflect biological activity quite closely. Fortunately the gut hormones are sufficiently distinct in their amino acid sequence to avoid completely any problems of assay cross-reactivity. The localization of endocrine cells by immunocytochemistry has been much advanced by the development of new fixing agents. These are now capable of completely insolubilizing the stored hormone and preserving cellular architecture without causing any loss of the hormone's antigenic site on which the technique depends. These technical advances have now allowed proper investigation of the endocrine pathology of gluten enteropathy.

PATIENTS AND METHOD OF STUDY

Patient groups

Three groups of patients were studied. Six children with partial or sub-total villous atrophy, six children who had been successfully treated with a gluten-free diet and whose mucosal biopsy had returned to normal and 15 control children who had been biopsied because of short stature but whose mucosa was normal formed the first study group[7]. Following duodenal intubation they received a 5 ml/kg 0.5 molar citric acid load infused over 10 min. Blood samples were taken from a small peripheral catheter. The second group of patients were 10 normals, 11 active coeliac patients and 7 patients successfully treated with a gluten-free diet. These patients, who were studied by Dr J. H. Walsh, Birmingham General Hospital, received a 50 g oral glucose load. The third group consisted of 11 adult patients with biopsy-proven active coeliac disease, 13 patients with coeliac disease treated with a gluten-free diet and a good clinical and histological response and 13 age and sex matched normal control subjects. They received a standard test breakfast consisting of two boiled eggs, 60 g bread (toast), 10 g butter, 25 g marmalade and 150 ml of unsweetened orange juice (total 18 g protein, 22 g fat, 66 g carbohydrate, 530 calories).

Methods

Immunocytochemistry

Intestinal mucosal biopsies were obtained in seven patients with active

400

coeliac disease and five controls in a suitable state for immunocyto-chemistry. A conventional Crosby capsule placed at or just beyond the ligament of Treitz was employed and the samples were extremely rapidly harvested and immediately quenched in arcton (Freon) at −156 °C Subsequently the tissue was freeze-dried in a thermoelectric freeze dryer and vapour-fixed[8].

Secretin antiserum was raised in rabbits to pure porcine secretin con-jugated to bovine serum albumin by carbodiimide. After two injections of 50 μg an antiserum was developed, usable at a titre of 1 in 800 000. There was no detectable cross-reaction with other hormones including vasoactive intestinal peptide (VIP), glucagon or gastric inhibitory pep-tide (GIP). Antiserum to cholecystokinin was raised by immunizing rabbits with the synthetic fragment of CCK 9–20[9]. This CCK fragment was coupled to hen egg albumin with glutaraldehyde in a molar ratio of 4.6 to 1. After three injections of 150 μg each an antiserum was raised, usable at a titre of 1 in 8000. As predicted this antiserum showed no cross-reaction with other gut hormones including gastrin. Immuno-cytochemical staining of the tissue sections was carried out by the in-direct (sandwich) method of Coons LeDuc and Connolly[10]. Controls included prior absorption of the antibodies with the corresponding antigen. Quantitative studies were undertaken by means of an Auto-matic Television Image Analyser Computer[11].

Radioimmunoassay

Blood samples for hormone measurement were taken into heparinized tubes with addition of 500 KIU aprotinin/ml. Plasma was rapidly separated and deep frozen within 15 min of the initial venepuncture. Hormone radioimmunoassay was carried out using conventional methodology[12]. The ability of the assays to detect hormone concen-tration changes between individual samples at the 95% confidence level were as follows:–

Secretin	1.5 pmol/l[13]
Gastrin	2 pmol/l[14]
Pancreatic polypeptide (PP)	5 pmol/l[15]
GIP	10 pmol/l[16]
Motilin	5 pmol/l[17]
Enteroglucagon	20 pmol/l[18]

No assay was available which gave reliable values for the numerous circulating forms of cholecystokinin.

RESULTS

Histology

The coeliac biopsies studied showed the conventional changes of subtotal or partial villous atrophy. None of the controls showed even slight abnormalities. The treated coeliac patients appeared indistinguishable from normal.

Immunocytochemistry localized the secretin cells mostly to the intestinal crypts and the CCK cells to both villi and crypts (Figure 42.1).

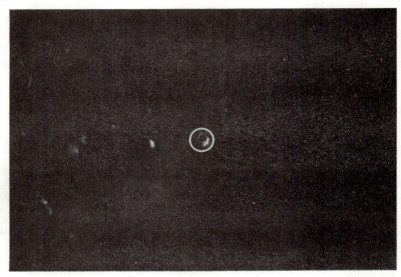

Figure 42.1   CCK cells in small intestine. Control patient × 500

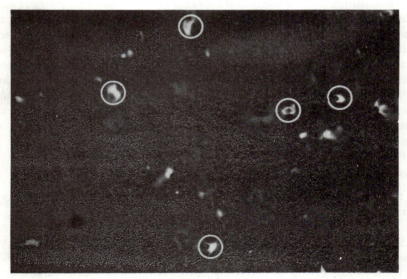

Figure 42.2   CCK cells in childhood coeliac disease × 500

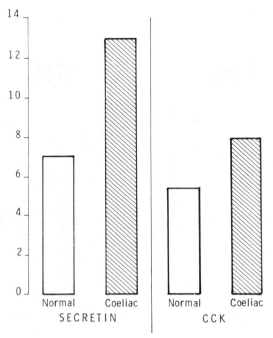

Figure 42.3 Quantitative immunocytochemistry of secretin and CCK cells in coeliac disease: number of cells per mm²

Almost all the coeliac cases showed numerous brightly stained secretin and CCK cells. In contrast, controls showed a much smaller number of cells with a much lower intensity of immunostain (Figure 42.2). Quantitative immunocytochemistry showed a 49% increase in the number of secretin cells (mean 13.0/mm² ± 2.4) (normal mean 7.0/mm²) and a 37% increase in the number of CCK cells (mean 7.9/mm² ± 2.0) (normal mean 5.7 ± 0.8). (Figure 42.3). Differences in the size and hormone content, as estimated by quantitative immunocytochemistry, are shown in Figure 42.4.

Hormone levels

In the healthy control children the intraduodenal acid load resulted in a plasma secretin rise from a basal level of 1.3 ± 0.7 pmol/l to a value of 24.7 ± 3.5 pmol/l at 10 min. The rise was similar in the treated group (0.9 ± 0.6 to 33.8 ± 6.9 pmol/l). On the other hand, children with active disease showed a rise from 1.7 ± 0.9 to only 6.3 ± 1.2 pmol/l. The rise of secretin in this group of active coeliac children was thus greatly reduced ($p < 0.001$)[7]. In the second group of patients, adults studied after an oral glucose tolerance test (OGTT), only enteroglucagon has so far been measured. In the group with active coeliac disease the basal enteroglucagon was 69 ± 15.6 pmol/l and this rose to a mean peak of 206.2 ± 48.1 pmol/l at 60 min. By comparison the controls had a basal level of 31.9 ± 8 pmol/l rising at 60 min to 88.3 ± 28.6 pmol/l. The patients who had been given a gluten-free diet were not significantly different from the control group. In the third group of patients who were studied by means of a test breakfast a wider range of hormone measurement was made. There was a good rise of both gastrin and PP following the meal but the basal and peak values were identical in patients with active disease and healthy controls. In contrast the active coeliac patients showed a marked reduction in the release of GIP. (Figure 42.5) From a basal level of 13.7 ± 0.6 pmol/l they rose to a mean peak of 17.8 ± 1.0 pmol/l at 60 min, whereas the controls had a basal level of 12.5 ± 0.9 pmol/l and at 60 min achieved a value of 24.0 ± 2.9 pmol/l. No significant rise of VIP was found following the meal in any of the subjects and while there was a small rise in motilin, it was not statistically significantly

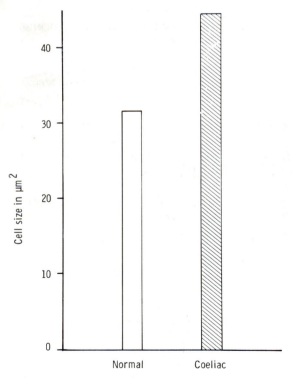

Figure 42.4 Size and hormone content of CCK cells shown by quantitative immunocytochemistry

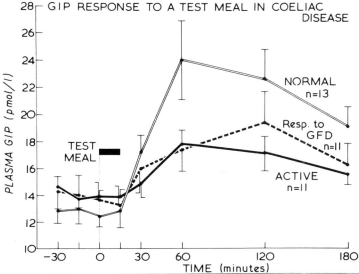

Figure 42.5 Impaired release of GIP in patients with active coeliac disease

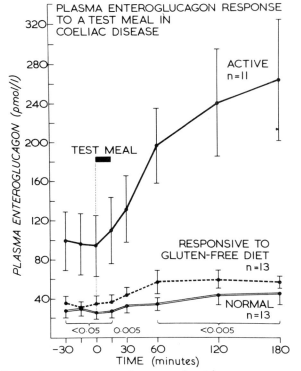

Figure 42.6 Enteroglucagon release after a test breakfast

different between those with active disease and healthy controls. Secretin values after a meal rose in controls and treated patients but only by a mean quantity of approximately 1 pmol/l. This was of insufficient magnitude to achieve statistical significance. As with the patients studied by an oral glucose tolerance test the patients with active coeliac disease having a test breakfast showed both raised basal enteroglucagon values (94 ± 31, controls 28 ± 7 pmol/l) and greatly exaggerated rise after the meal (263 ± 62, controls 45 ± 11 pmol/l at 180 min) (Figure 42.6). These differences were highly statistically significant ($p < 0.005$). Patients with treated coeliac disease had a normal enteroglucagon response to the test breakfast.

DISCUSSION

The finding of increased numbers of secretin[20] and cholecystokinin cells fits well with an apparent failure of release of duodenal hormones. Presumably the normal release mechanisms are in some way interfered with by the acute inflammatory change secondary to gluten sensitivity. A failure of GIP release has been previously demonstrated in a small mixed group of patients with coeliac disease by Creutzfeldt's group[21]. Recently Buchanan and colleagues have been able to confirm our finding of a failure of secretin release following intraduodenal acid[22]. The gut hormones have a well-defined distribution in the alimentary tract. Similarly, gluten enteropathy causes significant damage only in the upper small intestine. Thus one might have predicted the finding of normal release of pancreatic and gastric hormones, diminished release of those from the damaged upper small intestine and increased release of hormones found mostly in the lower small intestine which receives an unusually large quantity of nutriment. The hormone profile reported in these studies fulfils the prediction.

The most striking finding is the gross elevation of enteroglucagon. As this hormone has not yet been purified, its actions have not been fully defined. However, a single patient studied at the Hammersmith Hospital with an enteroglucagon tumour[23] showed two marked abnormalities. Firstly there was a gross retardation of small intestinal transit and secondly a marked hypertrophy of the intestinal mucosa. These changes ·were immediately reversed following tumour removal. It is possible to speculate that the increased turnover of the mucosa and slower transit time seen in coeliac disease is a direct result of the elevated enteroglucagon levels. The mechanism causing the elevated enteroglucagon levels is uncertain however. Enteroglucagon release is caused by triglycerides and carbohydrate and it may therefore seem obvious that the most important factor is the presence of malabsorption allowing unabsorbed fat to appear in the terminal ileum. This does not seem to be the sole factor however, as in a control group of patients with severe malabsorption from chronic pancreatitis the elevation of entero-glucagon was of a much lower order of magnitude (unpublished observations).

Many patients with coeliac disease remain undetected until the development of significant complications. The use of jejunal biopsies as a screening test to improve detection rates in patients with marginal symptomatology has considerable disadvantages. Thus there would be considerable benefit from a diagnostic test based on simple plasma sampling. The delineation of a characteristic hormone profile in coeliac disease now makes this a distinct possibility.

ACKNOWLEDGMENTS

We would like to gratefully acknowledge the assistance of Mr D. Sarson, Mr N. D. Christofides, Mr T. E. Adrian, Miss A. M. West, Mrs S. J. Mitchell and Dr G. R. Greenberg. Gluten-free bread was kindly donated by the Dietetic Department, Hammersmith Hospital. Numerous colleagues have contributed patients and material to these studies which will form the basis of separate publications. Generous support was received from the Wellcome Trust and the Medical Research Council.

References

1. Colombato, L. O., Parodi, H. and Cantor, D. (1977). Biliary function studies in patients with coeliac sprue. *Am. J. Dig. Dis.*, **22**, 96
2. DiMagno, E. P., Go, V. L. W. and Summerskill, W. H. J. (1969). Pancreozymin secretion is impaired in sprue. *Gastroenterology*, **56**, 1149
3. Booth, C. C. (1977). Coeliac disease. *Nutr. Metabol.*, **21**, 65
4. Bloom, S. R.(1977). Gastrointestinal hormones. In: R. K. Crane (ed) *International Review of Physiology, Gastrointestinal Physiology II*, Vol 12, pp. 72–103, (Baltimore: University Park Press)
5. Pearse, A. G. E., Polak, J. M. and Bloom, S. R. (1977). The newer gut hormones. Cellular sources, physiology, pathology and clinical aspects. *Gastroenterology*, **72**, 746
6. Bloom, S. R., Bryant, M. G. and Polak, J. M. (1975). Distribution of gut hormones. *Gut*, **16**, 821
7. Bloom, S. R., Patel, H. R. and Johnston, D. I. (1976). Failure of secretin release in coeliac disease. *Gut*, **17**, 812
8. Pearse, A. G. E. and Polak, J. M. (1975). Bifunctional reagents as vapour and liquid-phase fixatives for immunocytochemistry. *Histochem. J.*, **7**, 179
9. Polak, J. M., Pearse, A. G. E., Szelke, M., Bloom, S. R., Hudson, D., Facer, P., Buchan, A. M. J., Bryant, M. G., Christophides, N. and MacIntyre, I. (1977) Specific immunostaining of CCK cells by use of synthetic fragment antisera. *Experientia*, **33**, 762
10. Coons, A. H., Leduc, E. H. and Connolly, J. M. (1955). Studies on antibody production. 1. A method for the histochemical demonstration of specific antibody and its application to a study of the hyperimmune rabbits. *J. Exp. Med.*, **102**, 49

11. Hobbs, S. E. and Polak, J. M. (1978). Quantitative immunocytochemistry. In: S. R. Bloom (ed.) *Gut Hormones,* Chapter 12, (Edinburgh: Churchill Livingstone Ltd) (In Press)

12. Bloom, S. R. (1974). Hormones of the gastrointestinal tract. In: P. H. Sonksen (ed.) *Radioimmunoassay and Saturation Analysis. British Medical Bulletin,* **30,** 62

13. Häcki, W. H., Greenberg, G. R. and Bloom, S. R. (1978). The role of secretin in man. In: S. R. Bloom (ed.) *Gut Hormones* Chapter 12, (Edinburgh: Churchill Livingstone Ltd) (In Press)

14. Russell, R. C. G., Bloom, S. R., Fielding, L. P. and Bryant, M. G. (1976). Current problems in the measurement of gastrin release. A reproducible measure of physiological gastrin release. *Postgrad. Med. J.,* **52,** 645

15. Adrian, T. E., Bloom, S. R., Besterman, H. S., Barnes, A. J., Cooke, T. J. C., Russell, R. C. G. and Faber, R. G. (1977). Mechanism of pancreatic polypeptide release in man. *Lancet,* **i,** 161

16. Bloom, S. R., Turner, R. C. and Ward, A. S. (1977). GIP release, insulin release and inhibition of gastric acid. *Gastroenterology,* **72,**A-3/813

17. Bloom, S. R., Mitznegg, P. and Bryant, M. G. (1976). Measurement of human plasma motilin. *Scand. J. Gastroenterol.,* **11,** 47

18. Thomson, J. P. S. and Bloom, S. R. (1976). Plasma enteroglucagon and plasma volume change after gastric surgery. *Clin. Sci. Mol. Med.,* **51,** 177

19. Bloom, S. R. Radioimmunoassay of vasoactive intestinal peptide. In: *Methods in Radioimmunoassay,* Jaffe, B. M. and Bierons, S. (eds.) (Academic Press) (In Press)

20. Polak, J. M., Pearse, A. G. E., Van Norden, S., Bloom, S. R. and Rossiter, M. A. (1973). Secretin cells in coeliac disease. *Gut,* **14,** 870

21. Creutzfeldt, W., Ebert, R., Arnold, R., Frerichs, H. and Brown, J. C. (1976). Gastric inhibitory polypeptide (GIP), gastrin and insulin: response to test meal in coeliac disease and after duodeno-pancreatectomy. *Diabetologia,* **12,** 279

22. O'Connor, F. A., McLoughlin, J. C. and Buchanan, K. D. (1977). Impaired immunoreactive secretin release in coeliac disease. *Br. Med. J.,* **2,** 811

23. Bloom, S. R. (1972). An enteroglucagon tumour. *Gut,* **13,** 520

Discussion of chapter 42

Van Tongeren	In coeliac disease more S cells were found in the mucosa and you also mentioned after instillation into the duodenum the increase in secretin in the blood plasma was less. How can you combine these two data?
Bloom	It is what you would expect if you're not getting a release of secretin. The cells are full of it.
Polak	I think from the morphological viewpoint there is an increased number of cells and increased density of fluorescence. A dynamic study should be carried out to combine these findings.
Van Tongeren	You also found an increased content of secretin in the duodenal mucosa.
Polak	Only as judged by qantitative immunochemistry were the cells increased. To check that the cells were unable to secrete you need to carry out dynamic studies. You cannot extrapolate cell data to the dynamic situation.
Bayless	I think Dr Polak is showing that VIP (vasoactive intestinal peptide) is found throughout the intestinal tract, Do you have any stimuli to release it and have you looked at the patterns of VIP say in illnesses such as this?
Bloom	Well, VIP is not released after a meal. We have looked at VIP in our series. There was no change in VIP after a meal either in the active or the treated or the control group, so it didn't look as if it is going to be very helpful. The stimuli that are known to release VIP such as intestinal ischaemia, high doses of intestinal acid and hypertonic solution we have not tried in coeliac disease.
Polak	The morphological data would agree with what Dr Bloom said. VIP is present in endocrine cells throughout the gut, but much the larger bulk of VIP is in the nerves of the gut. Therefore the stimuli for VIP release and abnormality may be completely different to other circulating hormones.
Holmes	This is a comment which involves Dr Buchanan and may involve the Chairman. The idea that the gall bladder is sluggish because there is not a release of cholecystokinin with a test meal may not be strictly true because work done by Howard and colleagues in Manchester using secretin pancreozymin tests shows that a proportion of coeliacs have a sluggishly reacting gall bladder. In this

situation the hormone must be getting to the gall bladder because the pancreas is functioning normally and it may be that the gall bladder has a sluggish motility and shares in some problem of the gastrointestinal tract in coeliac disease.

Buchanan I want to ask Dr Bloom a question. This enteroglucagon material that you talk about—we had the opportunity of studying a lady who infarcted her gut, in fact had lost most of her ileum and she showed very high levels of glucagon-like immunoactivity in her blood and presumably as she didn't have any ileum, it was coming from somewhere else. I should also say that this woman was eventually shown to have coeliac disease and the infarction made the whole clinical picture much more apparent and I think that you are over-simplifying the thinking that this glucagon material is coming from the ileum. It is found in high quantity in the jejunum, colon and also probably in the pancreas so you know I can't really see how you make that statement. Also, the patient that was studied with Dr Stevens had a pancreatic tumour and it was a similar glucagon he was secreting to the one you originally described in 1972. I am asking, are you not over-simplifying? You are making these statements about coming from the ileum and so forth, what evidence have you?

Bloom I suppose the evidence, Keith, is that when you extract the ileum the amount of enteroglucagon present there is higher than anywhere else. There certainly is enteroglucagon in the colon. The amount present in the pancreas is very small but is like the amount of gastrin in the pancreas. This does not stop a gastrin-producing tumour from occurring in the pancreas even though gastrin isn't normally produced from there. It looks as if the pancreas is a tissue which is peculiarly liable to produce endocrine-type tumours. The finding of an endocrine tumour producing glucagon-like materials including enteroglucagon and thus villous hypertrophy isn't perhaps a terribly surprising finding. We have carried out with Professor Dowling in Guy's resection experiments on rats and yes, you are quite right if you resect most of the ileum in controlled experiments the enteroglucagon level in plasma goes shooting up but the enteroglucagon content of the remaining small intestine also shoots up. It is clear that there is a considerable adaptive response of the endocrine cells, especially the enteroglucagon producing cells. If you think of enteroglucagon as a tropic hormone to the gut this is exactly what you would expect. Lose a part of the gut and the rest responds like crazy to try and increase mucosal growth so I completely agree with your finding that after resection of a portion of the gut enteroglucagon goes up. I think this is the same sort of situation as with coeliac disease, you've got an area of the gut that is non-functioning and effectively lost. Enteroglucagon cells respond by hypertrophy and increasing their output thus tending to increase the enterocyte growth rate, but as far as the normal distribution goes the amount of enteroglucagon present in duodenal, gastric and jejunal mucosa is pretty small. I agree that there are a few cells there and they have the potential to hypertrophy after resection of the ileum but the amounts in the ileum and ascending colon are perhaps 90% of the total, so basically that is where it can be said to be localized.

Haffen   Dr Polak, how can you explain the increase in endocrine cells in coeliac mucosa. Is it by mitosis or perhaps by an acceleration of the production from stem cells?

Polak   Well, we cannot explain an increased number of cells by doing immunocytochemistry. We know in immunocytochemistry that we have limits for an endocrine cell. The limit of detection is when the cell becomes visible because it has enough hormone content to be stored. You can't see many more cells because they are still in the quiescent phase of a dynamic cycle. Therefore, by immunocyto-chemistry, as I said before, the fact of finding more cells may imply that they are hyperplastic but equally may imply that they are storing more hormone and may be detected more easily. There-fore, dynamic studies to clarify the problem are required. It has thus been reported that an increase of endocrine cells may or may not be explained by crypt cell hyperplasia.

43

5-Hydroxytryptamine metabolism in patients with coeliac disease

D. N. CHALLACOMBE, P. D. DAWKINS, P. BAKER and K. ROBERTSON

5-HYDROXYTRYPTAMINE METABOLISM IN PATIENTS WITH COELIAC DISEASE

5-Hydroxytryptamine (5-HT) is synthesized from dietary tryptophan by enterochromaffin (EC) cells in the gastrointestinal tract and after oxidative deamination by the enzyme monoamine oxidase, is excreted in the urine as 5-hydroxyindoleacetic acid (5-HIAA). Raised blood levels of 5-HT and increased urinary excretion of 5-HIAA have been reported in adults with coeliac disease, and both blood 5-HT and urinary 5-HIAA fell after the introduction of gluten-free diet[1-7]. L-tryptophan loading tests in adults with coeliac disease further increase the urinary excretion of 5-HIAA and an augmented shunt of the 5-HT to 5-HIAA metabolic pathway was therefore proposed as a possible explanation for these findings[6]. Increased urinary excretion of 5-HIAA was confirmed in children with coeliac disease, and diminished excretion also followed a gluten-free diet[8,9]. Values were expressed as 5-HIAA/creatinine, owing to collecting difficulties in childhood, but urinary creatinine levels were not significantly different in the coeliacs and controls. Estimation of this ratio was proposed as a test to detect children with coeliac disease[8]. Further studies of the small intestine in patients with coeliac disease have therefore been performed to determine the possible origin of the reported abnormalities of 5-HT metabolism.

ENTEROCHROMAFFIN CELLS IN THE DUODENAL MUCOSA

EC cells in sections of tissue obtained by peroral biopsy from the third

and fourth part of the duodenum were stained with alkaline dia-
zonium[10]. Ten children with untreated coeliac disease and ten controls
with a normal duodenal mucosa on light microscopy were studied[11].
EC cell counts were performed by inserting a 1 cm square grid
(Graticules Ltd.) into the × 10 eyepiece of a light microscope and each
section was viewed at a final image magnification of × 250. The grid
(Figure 43.1) contained 81 uniformly distributed points where both
horizontal and vertical lines crossed[12]. In each field the grid points
falling on the epithelium and lamina propria were counted using the
muscularis mucosa as a baseline, as were EC cells within the whole 1 cm
square grid. By systematically moving the microscope stage, each section
was scanned until EC cells within an area covered by 1000 grid points or
'hits' had been counted. Results of EC cell counts in the children with
coeliac disease and in the controls are shown in Table 43.1.

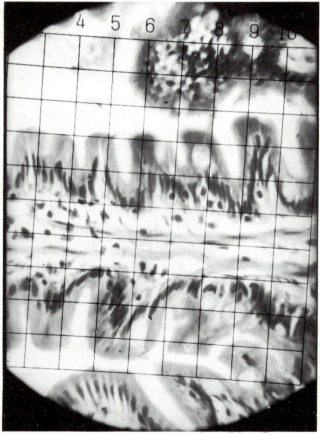

Figure 43.1   The counting grid. Magnification × 175

Table 43.1 Enterochromaffin cells in the duodenal mucosa

Subjects		EC cells/1000 hits
Controls	n=10	Mean count = 41 SD = 18
Coeliacs	n=10	Mean count = 105 SD = 41
Gluten challenge n=4		Pre-challenge:
		Mean count = 37 SD = 14
		Post challenge:
		Mean count 78 SD = 17

Results

Significantly greater numbers of EC cells were present in duodenal biopsies from children with coeliac disease ($p<0.001$). In four children with a clinical history suggestive of coeliac disease but with only minor villous changes in the duodenal mucosa on light microscopy, gluten challenge with 10 g of pure gluten given three times a day for ten days, resulted in more severe histopathological changes and significantly increased the EC cell counts ($p<0.01$).

DUODENAL TISSUE LEVELS OF 5-HYDROXYTRYPTAMINE

Duodenal tissue was obtained by peroral biopsy from four adults and seven children with untreated coeliac disease and tissue levels of 5-HT were compared with levels obtained from four adults and seven children with normal duodenal biopsies[13]. 5-HT was extracted from duodenal tissue[14,15], and was estimated fluorometrically by its reaction with o-phthalaldehyde[16]. The results from patients with coeliac disease and from the controls are shown in Table 43.2.

Results

Duodenal tissue concentrations of 5-HT were significantly greater in patients with coeliac disease than in the controls ($p<0.001$). Values for adults and children were not significantly different in either the controls or in the patients with coeliac disease. Three children with a history suggestive of coeliac disease but with only minor villous changes in the duodenum were challenged with pure gluten for ten days and increased concentrations of 5-HT were found following gluten challenge.

In Figure 43.2 tissue concentrations of 5-HT have been correlated with EC cell counts on the same specimens of duodenal tissue ($r=0.72$). Figure 43.3 shows the correlation between the tissue levels of 5-HT and 5-HIAA (μM)/creatinine (mM) estimated in 8 hour urine collections, ($r=0.85$), from children with coeliac disease and control children.

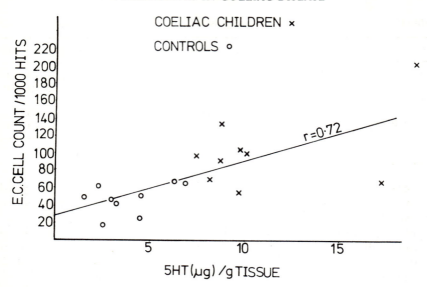

Figure 43.2 EC cell counts (per 1000 hits) related to duodenal tissue concentrations of 5-HT (μg/g of tissue), in coeliacs and controls

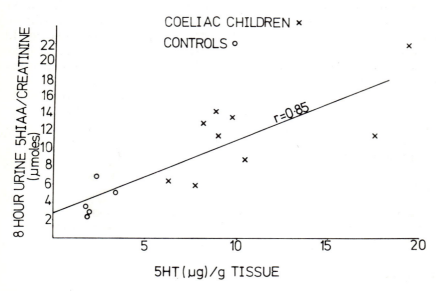

Figure 43.3 5-HIAA (μmoles)/creatinine (mmol) in 8-hour urine collections, related to duodenal tissue concentrations of 5-HT (μg/g tissue wet weight), in coeliacs and controls

Table 43.2 Tissue levels of 5-HT (μg/g tissue wet weight) in the duodenal mucosa

Subjects		Wet weight of tissue (mg)	5-HT(μg/g of tissue)
Controls	n=10	Mean=10.2 SD=5.4	Mean=4.2 SD=2.0
Coeliacs	n=11	Mean=12.7 SD=6.9	Mean=10.8 SD=4.0
Gluten challenge (n=3)			
Pre-challenge		Mean=9.8 SD=1.1	Mean=4.7 SD=2.5
Post-challenge		Mean=12.4 SD=2.2	Mean=7.3 SD=1.8

DISCUSSION

The results suggest that hyperplasia of EC cells is a histopathological feature of the duodenal mucosa in children with untreated coeliac disease. As EC cells were mainly found between epithelial cells in the villous crypts and crypt cell hyperplasia is a feature of the small intestine in coeliac disease, our findings may be secondary to hyperplasia of all crypt cells. Increased tissue levels of 5-HT in patients with coeliac disease may also be secondary to EC cell hyperplasia. Increased urinary excretion of 5-HIAA could result from increased release of 5-HT into the blood and increased breakdown by the enzyme monoamine oxidase. Further studies will however be necessary to determine whether individual EC cells synthesize greater amounts of 5-HT in patients with coeliac disease. Increased duodenal tissue levels of 5-HT may be a response of the small intestine to many dietary factors in susceptible individuals, including dietary gluten, and an association with villous damage in other gastrointestinal disorders has not yet been excluded. Laboratory studies have shown that small doses of 5-HT injected into the rat peritoneum accelerate crypt cell proliferation in the jejunal mucosa and shorten the cell cycle time[17]. Similar abnormalities of cell kinetics have also been reported in the duodenal mucosa of adults with coeliac disease[18,19]. While the response of the small intestinal mucosa to 5-HT in rats may be a species-related phenomenon, a similar response in man could implicate the increased local release of 5-HT in the pathogenesis of the mucosal lesion in coeliac disease.

ACKNOWLEDGEMENTS

We are grateful for the encouragement of our colleagues in this work which was supported by the Research Committee of the South Western Regional Health Authority.

References

1. Haverback, B. J. and Davidson, J. D. (1958). Serotonin and the gastrointestinal tract. *Gastroenterology*, **35,** 570

2. Pimparker, B. D., Senesky, D. and Kalser, M. H. (1961). Blood serotonin in non-tropical sprue. *Gastroenterology*, **40**, 504

3. Scriver, C. R. (1961). Abnormalities of tryptophan metabolism in a patient with malabsorption syndrome. *J. Lab. Clin. Med.*, **58**, 908

4. Sleisenger, M. H. (1961). Clinical and metabolic studies in nontropical sprue. *New Engl. J. Med.*, **265**, 49

5. Warner, R. R. P. and Cohen, N. (1962). Blood serotonin in malabsorption states. *Am. J. Dig. Dis.*, **7**, 553

6. Benson, G. D., Kowlessar, O. D. and Sleisenger, M. H. (1964). Adult coeliac disease with emphasis upon response to the gluten-free diet. *Medicine (Balt.)*, **43**, 1

7. Kowlessar, O. D., Haeffner, L. J. and Benson, G. D. (1964). Abnormal tryptophan metabolism in patients with adult coeliac disease, with evidence for deficiency of Vitamin B6. *J. Clin. Invest.*, **43**, 894

8. Challacombe, D. N., Brown, G. A., Black, S. C. and Storrie, M. H. (1972). Increased excretion of 5-hydroxyindoleacetic acid in urine of children with untreated coeliac disease. *Arch. Dis. Childh.*, **47**, 442

9. Challacombe, D. N., Goodall, M., Gaze, H. and Brown, G. A. (1975). Urinary 5-hydroxyindoleacetic acid in 8-hour urines as an aid in diagnosis of coeliac disease. *Arch. Dis. Childh.*, **50**, 779

10. Pearse, A. G. E. (1960). *Histochemistry, Theoretical and Applied.* Third edition. (London: J. and A. Churchill Ltd.)

11. Challacombe, D. N. and Robertson, K. (1977). Enterochromaffin cells in the duodenal mucosa of children with coeliac disease. *Gut*, **18**, 373

12. Piris, J. and Whitehead, R. (1975). Quantitation of 6-cells in fibre optic biopsy specimens and serum gastrin levels in healthy normal subjects. *J. Clin. Pathol.*, **28**, 636

13. Challacombe, D. N., Dawkins, P. D. and Baker, P. (1977). Increased tissue concentrations of 5-hydroxytryptamine in the duodenal mucosa of patients with coeliac disease. *Gut.* (In press)

14. Snyder, S. H., Axelrod, J. and Zweig, M. (1965). A sensitive and specific fluorescence assay for tissue serotonin. *Biochem. Pharmacol.*, **14**, 831

15. Small, N. A. and Holton J. B. (1970). Determination of platelet serotonin by a fluorometric method. *Clin. Chem. Acta*, **27**, 171

16. Curzon, J. and Green, A. R. (1970). Rapid method for the determination of 5-hydroxytryptamine and 5-hydroxyindoleacetic acid in small regions of rat brain. *Br. J. Pharmacol.*, **39**, 653

17. Tutton, P. J. M. (1974). The influence of serotonin on crypt cell proliferation in the jejunum of rat. *Virch. Archiv. Abt. B: Zellpathol. (Berlin)*, **16**, 79

18. Wright, N., Watson, A., Morley, A., Appleton, D. and Marks, J. (1973). Cell kinetics in flat (avillous) mucosa of the human small intestine. *Gut*, **14**, 701

19. Wright, N., Watson, A., Morley, A., Appleton, D., Marks, J. and Douglas, A. (1973). The cell cycle time in the flat (avillous) mucosa of the human small intestine. *Gut*, **14**, 603

Discussion of chapter 43

Bloom   The results are fascinating. Looking at it wholly from my own viewpoint some EC cells produce motilin. Motilin release, however, does not appear to be abnormal in coeliac disease. There is a rise after a meal and it is approximately the same in the normals so the motilin-producing endocrine cells are presumably not involved.

Booth   I think the thing against 5-HT being involved in cell turnover kinetics is the appearance of the mucosa in the carcinoid syndrome with very high levels of 5-HT. To my knowledge and in biopsies that I have seen the villi are not bigger or abnormal. It would seem therefore that the better explanation would be to say that it is just the same as Julia Polak's observation, there are more cells in hyperplastic tissue and as our French colleague said that this is a reflection of the hyperplasia.

Challacombe   It would be interesting to measure duodenal tissue concentrations of 5-HT in patients with carcinoid tumours. The release of this amine locally rather than the general release which occurs in carcinoid tumours may be more significant in patients with coeliac disease.

Bayless   I wanted to get back to the question I asked Dr Bloom about VIP. I was thinking about the fact that in the small intestine there is a net fluid secretion in untreated coeliacs; I was hoping that he would tell me that the VIP levels were elevated. Serotonin in at least some animal species has been shown to cause net secretion and I wonder perhaps if serotonin would explain the net secretion that we find in our untreated coeliacs. Do you have any comments on that?

Challacombe   These are interesting findings and may be related to our results in coeliac disease.

Polak   I think the information from Dr Challacombe opens up enormous possibilities on gut cellular endocrinology because we know from recent studies that EC cells are a heterogeneous group of cells in the gastrointestinal mucosa. Some of them, as Dr Bloom said, are responsible for the production of motilin, some are also producing substance P and others perhaps unknown substances. Patients with coeliac disease have considerable abnormalities of their EC cells and it would be open for pathologists to disclose what the population of 5-HT producing cells does. In addition to that, perhaps the measurement of substance P in coeliac disease, whether its distribution in tissue or dynamics or release from gut, could be extremely helpful.

Connolly

With such a vast increase in EC cells one might expect to see carcinoid tumours developing in patients with coeliac disease. Recently in our laboratory we have found a patient with carcinoid of the appendix who also had coeliac disease. I wondered, getting back to Dr Holmes' paper this morning, in which he described malignancies being associated with coeliac disease, if some of the other tumours which he didn't specify might indeed have been carcinoid tumours.

Holmes

Yes, we did have one carcinoid.

Dodge

I had the impression from your paper and also in Dr Polak's presentation that there were more EC cells and probably more secretin cells in the crypts of the normal patient than there were in the villi. I wonder whether some of the increased cellularity can't be accounted for by this fact and that you are really introducing an artefact. Perhaps you should be counting only what you see in the crypts of the normals and comparing that with what you see in the crypts of the coeliacs because they haven't got any villi which would dilute your overall cellularity.

Challacombe

The number of EC cells in duodenal biopsies from coeliacs and controls is related by the grid to a standard area of mucosa, using the muscularis mucosa as a baseline. Previous morphometric studies have shown that the absolute amount of tissue in duodenal biopsies from coeliacs and controls does not differ, but that a re-distribution of tissue components occurs in coeliac disease with a lower surface epithelial volume and a greater crypt cell colume. Raised EC cell counts in patients with coeliac disease therefore reflect the crypt cell hyperplasia found in that disorder.

Section IX
Intestinal enzymes in coeliac disease

44

Analytical subcellular fractionation of jejunal biopsy specimens from control subjects and patients with coeliac disease

T. J. PETERS, P. E. JONES, W. J. JENKINS and J. A. NICHOLSON

INTRODUCTION

Morphological studies have described a wide variety of changes in the intestinal mucosa in coeliac disease. Although there is general agreement on the dissecting and light microscopic appearances, ultra-structural studies have revealed abnormalities in nearly all the subcellular organelles of the enterocyte[1-4]. Fragmentation of the brush border membranes, prominent lysosomes, vacuolation of the endoplasmic reticulum and cristolysis of the mitochondria are examples of the lesions described.

The pathogenesis of the coeliac lesion is similarly the subject of controversy. Immunological processes[5], impaired degradation of gliadin[6-8] and an abnormal binding of gliadin[9] or of a glycopeptide[10] to coeliac mucosa have all been implicated as pathogenic mechanisms. How the damage to the enterocyte is initiated and maintained and how this leads to an impairment of its normal absorptive–digestive functions have been little studied.

Since ingestion of gluten induces major changes in the morphology of the small intestine in patients with coeliac disease it is obviously difficult to determine whether any of the biochemical or immunological phenomena demonstrated are secondary to the mucosal damage or whether they reflect an underlying defect in coeliac disease. Careful study of jejunal mucosa from patients who have been treated by strict gluten withdrawal and whose mucosa has a histological appearance indistinguishable from normal should permit the identification of any abnormalities which may be related to the underlying defect in the coeliac mucosa.

Another important aspect for study is that a small proportion of patients with apparent coeliac disease fail to show the expected morphological response to gluten withdrawal. These patients appear to be at particular risk from gastrointestinal malignancies and other complications[11]. At present they can only be identified following careful observation on a strict gluten-free diet. If however biochemical differences could be demonstrated between the gluten-sensitive and the non-responsive groups of patients at the time of initial diagnosis, alternative forms of treatment could be instituted at an earlier stage.

In order to examine some of these problems, a technique has been developed combining analytical subcellular fractionation by sucrose density centrifugation with microanalysis of organelle marker enzyme activities[12–14]. This paper reviews the results of some of these studies which are reported in detail elsewhere[15, 16].

METHODS

Portions of fresh jejunal biopsies are gently homogenized in isotonic sucrose and, after low speed centrifugation, the supernatants are layered onto a sucrose gradient in the Beaufay automatic zonal rotor. After sedimenting the various organelles to their equilibrium densities, some 16 fractions are collected from the rotor. The fractions are assayed for marker enzymes for the principal subcellular organelles and the results expressed as frequency–density histograms. Full methodological details have been published previously[13].

RESULTS

Control studies

Figure 44.1 shows a typical result of such an experiment. Marker enzymes for the following organelles are clearly resolved: 5'-nucleotidase (basal–lateral membrane); alkaline phosphatase (brush border); α-glucosidase (brush border and endoplasmic reticulum); PCMB-resistant β-galactosidase (brush border); N-acetyl-β-glucosaminidase and β-galactosidase (pH 3.5) (lysosomes); catalase (peroxisomes); malate dehydrogenase (mitochondria).

Coeliac disease

Figure 44.2 shows the result of a similar study on a patient with untreated coeliac disease. The most striking abnormalities are present in the brush border. The levels of α-glucosidase (pH 6.0) and alkaline phosphatase are reduced to 37% and 25% of control values respectively. The distribution of the enzymes in the sucrose gradients is also strikingly

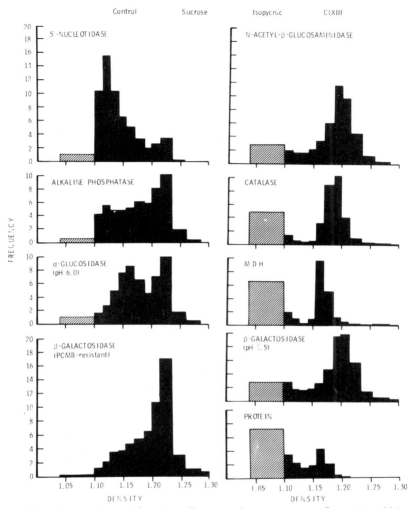

Figure 44.1 Isopycnic centrifugation of post-nuclear supernatant from jejunal biopsy homogenate from a 28-year-old female. The biopsy was histologically normal. Figure shows frequency–density histogram for marker enzymes and for protein. Frequency is defined as the fraction of total recovered activity in the gradient fraction divided by the density span covered. The shaded area represents, over an arbitrary abscissa interval from density 1.05 to 1.10, the activity remaining in the sample layer and presumed to indicate soluble protein. Reproduced from reference 12

abnormal with a loss of the brush border component in the 1.21 density region. Residual activity is found mainly in the gradient fractions corresponding to endoplasmic reticulum and plasma membrane. Apart from an increase in the total level of the lysosomal marker enzyme N-acetyl-β-glucosaminidase and a small reduction in malate dehydro-

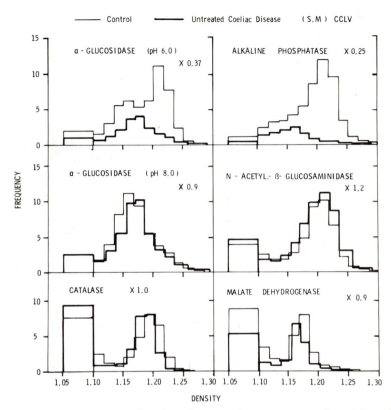

Figure 44.2 Isopycnic centrifugation of post-nuclear supernatant from jejunal biopsy homogenate from a 33-year-old female with untreated coeliac disease. The biopsy showed subtotal villous atrophy. The thin line shows averaged distribution data from control subjects[13] and the thick line shows data for the coeliac patient. Graph shows frequency–density histograms for marker enzymes for principal subcellular organelles. The distributions are adjusted so that the area under the histograms reflects the relative specific activity of each enzyme in the patient's biopsy homogenate compared with control values. Other details as Figure 44.1. Reproduced from reference 28

genase, there are no significant changes in the other organelles.

Figure 44.3 shows the result of a fractionation experiment in the same patient after treatment for 15 months with a strict gluten-free diet; the biopsy was histologically indistinguishable from normal. The two brush border marker enzymes have increased to 70 and 60% of normal levels but there is a persistent quantitative enzymic defect in the microvillus membrane. The other organelles are essentially normal. Further evidence of a persisting brush border abnormality is shown in Figure 44.4. In this figure averaged data from between five and 10 patients are compared to control subjects. Groups of untreated patients treated with a gluten-free diet for up to eight years were studied. Zn^{2+}-

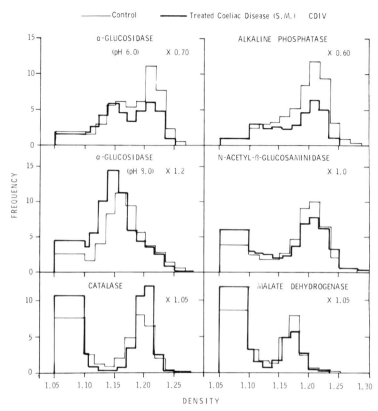

Figure 44.3 Isopycnic centrifugation of post-nuclear supernant from jejunal biopsy homogenate from same patient as shown in Figure 44.2 after 15 months on a strict gluten-free diet. The biopsy was histologically normal. Other details as in Figures 44.1 and 44.2. Reproduced from reference 28

resistant α-glucosidase, a highly specific brush border marker enzyme, is reduced to 12% of control values in untreated coeliac disease with a loss of the brush border component. In the treated group the total activity is 86% of control levels but there remains a persistently reduced level of brush border activity. β-Glucosidase has a dual localization in control subjects with a major soluble component and a smaller brush border component. In untreated coeliac disease the brush border component is completely absent and the soluble activity is reduced to one-quarter of the control level. In the treated patients the soluble component is one-half that of control levels but the brush border component is markedly deficient. N-Acetyl-β-glucosaminidase, the lysosomal marker enzyme, shows elevated levels in untreated coeliac disease with a significant increase in the soluble component but these changes revert to normal in the treated patient. Similarly, lactate

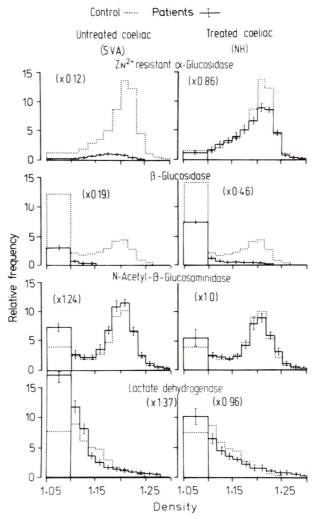

Figure 44.4 Isopycnic centrifugation of post-nuclear supernants from jejunal biopsy homogenates from patients with untreated coeliac disease (——I——) and patients with treated coeliac disease showing normal histology (——I——) compared with control subjects (......). Relative frequency is obtained by multiplying the frequency data by the relative specific activities, shown between parentheses, of the enzymes in the patients' homogenates compared with control subjects. Other details as Figure 44.1. Reproduced in modified form from reference 15

dehydrogenase is markedly increased in the jejunal mucosa from the untreated patients and returns to normal levels with successful treatment.

Figure 44.5 shows the distribution of alkaline phosphatase in the density gradients when biopsies from patients with coeliac disease, either

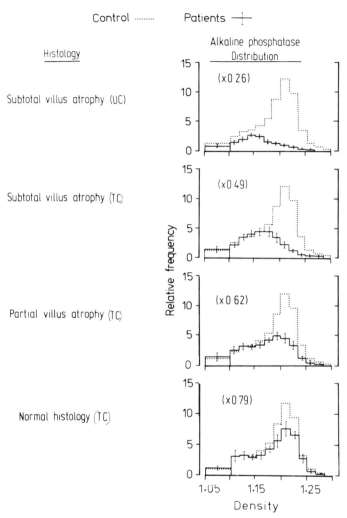

Figure 44.5 Isopycnic centrifugation of post-nuclear supernatants from jejunal biopsy homogenates from patients with coeliac disease (———I———) compared with control subjects (......). Correlations between histological appearance and alkaline phosphatase activities and density gradient distributions are shown. Other details as Figures 44.1 and 44.2. Reproduced in modified form from reference 15

untreated or after receiving a gluten-free diet, are studied. Alkaline phosphatase is reduced to one-quarter of control values with a loss of the brush border peak in the untreated patients. After 4–6 weeks' gluten withdrawal there was no significant improvement in villous architecture with the biopsies showing persistent subtotal villous atrophy. However, the level of alkaline phosphatase had risen to one-half of control values.

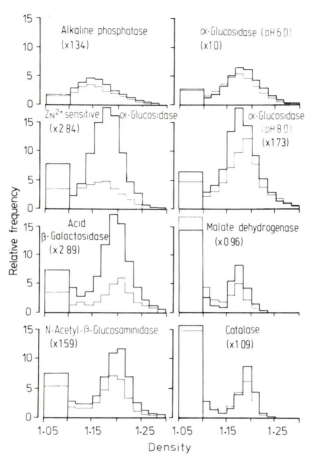

Figure 44.6 Isopycnic centrifugation of post-nuclear supernants from jejunal biopsy homogenates from patients with non-responsive coeliac disease (————) and patients with untreated but responsive coeliac disease (————). Other details as Figures 44.1 and 44.2. Reproduced in modified form from reference 16

The increase in activity in the gradient is in the low density region of the gradient with a modal density of 1.16.

Following a further period of gluten withdrawal, with morphological improvement to partial villous atrophy, there is a further small rise in the level of alkaline phosphatase. Subcellular fractionation studies indicate an increasing density of the alkaline phosphatase-containing membranes with significant activity in the brush border region of the gradient. Following restoration of the villous architecture to normal by prolonged strict gluten withdrawal, a distinct brush border peak is present. However, the total level is only four-fifths of control values, indicating a persistent brush border abnormality.

Non-responsive coeliac disease

Figure 44.6 compares the enzyme levels and the density gradient distributions of the principal organelle marker enzymes in patients with non-responsive coeliac disease with untreated gluten-sensitive patients. Further details are reported elsewhere[16].

Both brush border marker enzymes, alkaline phosphatase and α-glucosidase (pH 6.0) are similarly reduced in activity and have similar density gradient distributions. However the two marker enzymes for the endoplasmic reticulum, Zn^{2+}-sensitive α-glucosidase and α-glucosidase (pH 8.0) show marked differences between the two groups. The non-responsive group has significantly reduced levels, particularly of the more specific marker enzyme Zn^{2+}-sensitive α-glucosidase, compared with the untreated gluten sensitive group. The marker enzymes for mitochondria, malate dehydrogenase and for peroxisomes, catalase, show similar levels and similar gradient distributions in the two groups, although compared to control values they are both significantly reduced. The two lysosomal marker enzymes, acid β-galactosidase and N-acetyl-β-glucosaminidase are significantly elevated in the responsive patients compared with the non-responsive group.

DISCUSSION

Normal jejunal mucosa

The studies reviewed in this paper indicate that subcellular fractionation techniques can be readily applied to portions of peroral jejunal biopsy specimens. By a single-step procedure satisfactory resolution of the principal subcellular organelles of the enterocyte can be readily achieved. The use of certain agents can significantly enhance the resolution of selective organelles. Thus addition of 15 mmol/1 sodium pyrophospate to the homogenizing buffer selectively strips ribosomes from the rough endoplasmic reticulum[7]. Addition of digitonin, 0.2 mg/ml to the homogenization medium has highly specific effects on the various organelles[13]. The basal–lateral and, to a lesser degree, the brush border membranes, show an increase in their median densities and the enzymes associated with the endoplasmic reticulum show a decrease in median density. Lysosomes are disrupted and their constituent enzymes are recovered in the soluble fraction: mitochondria and peroxisomes are unaffected by digitonin at this concentration.

The potential application of these techniques in the investigation of human tissue physiology and pathology are considerable. Studies on the intracellular distributions of gut hormones[18], peptide hydrolases[19,20] and of the turnover of organelle proteins using organ culture techniques[21] are some examples of these applications. Other tissues available for biopsy are also amenable to this approach[14].

Coeliac disease

These subcellular fractionation procedures emphasize the brush border lesion in patients with coeliac disease. Complete loss of the enzyme activity associated with this organelle appears to be typical of untreated mucosa: the residual marker enzyme activity appears to be associated with other cell membranes. Following a short period of gluten withdrawal there is an increase in the brush border marker enzyme before there is a morphological response. The increased activity is not associated with the brush border itself but is found in the endoplasmic reticulum, presumably reflecting *de novo* synthesis of brush border components at this site prior to their transport to the cell surface.

In the treated patient whose biopsy has returned to histological normality there are persisting brush border abnormalities. The marker enzymes for this organelle show reduced levels in the gradient. Particularly striking is the deficit in β-glucosidase but whether this reflects a brush border defect underlying the disease process remains to be determined. It is of course possible that these persistent brush border abnormalities reflect the well-known slow response of certain enzymes, e.g. lactase[22,23] to return to normal levels following gluten withdrawal. However, study of biochemical processes in biopsies from coeliac patients in this category should reveal abnormalities important in the pathogenesis of the coeliac lesion.

Changes in the other organelles, including increased cytosol and lysosomal marker enzymes and decreased levels of mitochondrial and peroxisomal enzymes, found in untreated coeliac disease, all return to normal levels in the treated patients.

Non-responsive coeliac disease

The present studies in conjunction with previous reports showing reduced protein[21] and DNA[24] synthesis clearly distinguish this group of patients from those with gluten-sensitive coeliac disease. The reduced level of endoplasmic reticulum marker enzymes in the non-responsive group is in agreement with the reduced rate of protein synthesis compared with the responsive group reported in these patients.

The significance of the lysosomal changes is not clear. The non-responsive group has received a strict gluten-free diet and it is possible that in the coeliac lesion the abnormal binding of gluten or glycopeptides to cell membranes[9,10] is followed by internalization of this protein with sequestration within lysosomes. The differences in lysosomes between the two groups could therefore reflect the effect of dietary gluten rather than an underlying abnormality.

The fundamental intestinal defect in the non-responsive group is uncertain. Immunological processes may inhibit the normal crypt cell proliferation which is typical of the coeliac lesion, so that a state of hypoplastic rather than hyperplastic enteropoiesis is achieved[25]. The biochemical abnormalities may therefore reflect the differences in cell turnover. Alternatively the enterocytes formed in non-responsive coeliac disease may lack certain synthetic abilities and the endoplasmic reticulum abnormalities may reflect an underlying abnormality. It is therefore of interest that corticosteroids have a remarkably beneficial effect in this group of patients[16]. This class of drug has, amongst other effects, an action in enhancing protein synthesis by the small intestine[26,27] and the endoplasmic reticulum abnormalities in non-responsive coeliac disease are rapidly corrected by prednisolone[16].

The studies reviewed in this paper illustrate how analytical sub-cellular fractionation procedures in combination with organelle marker enzyme microassays can increase our understanding of coeliac disease. Used in combination with other procedures, e.g. gluten challenge, jejunal organ culture, further insight into this intriguing syndrome should be achieved.

ACKNOWLEDGEMENTS

The expert technical and secretarial assistance of Ms Jean de Luca, Ms Janet Heath, Ms Gill Wells and Mr Peter White is gratefully acknowledged. This work is supported by the Medical Research Council and The Wellcome Trust.

References

1. Trier, J. S. and Rubin, C. E. (1965). Electron microscopy of the small intestine: a review. *Gastroenterology*, **49**, 574
2. Rubin, W., Ross, L. L., Sleisenger, M. H. and Weser, E. (1966). An electron microscopic study of adult celiac disease. *Lab. Invest.*, **15**, 1720
3. Shiner, M. (1967). Ultrastructure of jejunal surface epithelium in untreated idiopathic steatorrhoea. *Br. Med. Bull.*, **23**, 223
4. Shiner, M. (1974) Electron microscopy of jejunal mucosa. *Clin. Gastroenterol.*, **3**, 33
5. Booth, C. C., Peters, T. J. and Doe, W. F. (1977). Immunopathology of coeliac disease. Ciba Foundation Symposium, **46**, *Immunology of the Gut*, pp. 329–346
6. Fraser, A. C. (1956). Discussion on some problems of steatorrhoea and reduced stature. *Proc. Roy. Soc. Med.*, **48**, 1009
7. Phelan, J. J., Stevens, F. M., McNicholl, B., Fottrell, P. F. and McCarthy, C. F. (1977). Coeliac disease: the abolition of gliadin toxicity by enzymes from *Aspergillus*

niger. Clin. Sci. Mol. Med., **53,** 35

8. Townley, R. R. W., Bhathal, P. S., Cornell, H. J. and Mitchell, J. D. (1973). Toxicity of wheat gliadin fractions in coeliac disease. *Lancet,* **i,** 1363

9. Rubin, W., Fauci, A. S., Sleisenger, M. H. and Jeffries, G. H. (1965). Immuno-fluorescent studies in adult celiac disease. *J. Clin. Invest.,* **44,** 475

10. Douglas, A. P. (1976). The binding of a glycopeptide component of wheat to intestinal mucosa of normal and coeliac human subjects. *Clin. Chim. Acta,* **73,** 357

11. Barry, R. E. and Read, A. E. (1973). Coeliac disease and malignancy. *Q. J. Med.,* **42,** 665

12. Peters, T. J. (1976). Analytical subcellular fractionation of jejunal biopsies from human subjects. *Biochem. Soc. Trans.,* **4,** 1142

13. Peters, T. J. (1976). Analytical subcellular fractionation of jejunal biopsy specimens: methodology and characterisation of the organelles in normal tissue. *Clin Sci. Mol. Med.,* **51,** 557

14. Peters, T. J. (1977). Application of analytical subcellular fractionation techniques and tissue enzymic analysis to the study of human pathology. *Clin. Sci. Mol. Med.,* **53,** 505

15. Peters, T. J., Jones, P. E. and Wells, G. (1978). Analytical subcellular fractionation of jejunal biopsy specimens: enzyme activities, organelle pathology and response to gluten withdrawal in patients with coeliac disease. *Clin. Sci. Mol. Med.* (In press)

16. Peters, T. J., Jones, P. E., Jenkins, W. J. and Wells, G. (1978). Analytical subcellular fractionation of jejunal biopsy specimens: enzymic activities, organelle pathology and response to corticosteroids in patients with non-responsive coeliac disease. *Clin. Sci. Mol. Med.* (In press)

17. Tilleray, J. and Peters, T. J. (1976). Analytical subfractionation of microsomes from the liver of control and Gunn strain rats. *Biochem. Soc. Trans.,* **4,** 248

18. Bryant, M. G., Bloom, S. R., Jones, P. E. and Peters, T. J. (1978). The study of hormone storage granules by analytical subcellular ultracentrifugation. In S. R. Bloom (ed.) *Gut Hormones,* (In press) (Edinburgh: Churchill-Livingstone)

19. Nicholson, J. A. and Peters, T. J. (1977). Subcellular distribution of di- and tri-peptidase in human jejunum. *Clin. Sci. Mol. Med.,* **52,** 16P

20. Nicholson, J. A. and Peters, T. J. (1977). Subcellular distribution of di-, tri-, tetra-, and penta-peptidase in human jejunum. *Gut,* **18,** A960

21. Jones, P. E., L'Hirondel, C. and Peters, T. J. (1976). Studies on protein, enzyme and DNA synthesis in normal and coeliac jejunal mucosa in organ culture. *Gut,* **17,** 812

22. Pena, A. S., Truelove, S. C. and Whitehead, R. (1972). Disaccharidase activity and jejunal morphology in coeliac disease. *Q. J. Med.,* **XLI,** 457

23. Peters, T. J., Batt, R. M., Heath, J. R. and Tilleray, J. (1976). The microassay of intestinal disaccharidases. *Biochem. Med.,* **15,** 145

24. Jones, P. E. and Peters, T. J. (1977). DNA synthesis by jejunal mucosa in responsive and non-responsive coeliac disease. *Br. Med. J.,* **1,** 1130

25. Booth, C. C. (1970). The enterocyte in coeliac disease. *Br. Med. J.,* **3,** 725

26. Batt, R. M. and Peters, T. J. (1976). Effects of prednisolone on the small intestinal mucosa of the rat. *In vivo* galactose absorption, enzymology, lysosomal membrane fragility, morphology and cell kinetics in jejunum and ileum. *Clin. Sci. Mol. Med.,* **50,** 511

27. Scott, J., Batt, R. M. and Peters, T. J. (1977). Mechanism of action of prednisolone on the absorptive–digestive functions of the rat small intestine. *Gut,* **18,** A967

28. Peters, T. J. and Seymour, C. A. (1978). Human tissue analysis by analytical sub-cellular fractionation techniques in combination with enzymic microassays. *Enzyme* (In press)

Discussion of chapter 44

Tripp   Do you have any evidence, such as electron microscopy, that the alterations in alkaline phosphatase peak might be due to some alterations in structure of brush border membranes?

Nicholson   That is a possible explanation but we have not examined it.

Schmitz   Have you attempted to do enzyme studies on isolated enterocytes? This in my opinion would be more meaningful because since the intestinal epithelium is so greatly reduced it is not surprising that the only changes you observed were in brush border enzymes such as alkaline phosphatase. I feel that some of your findings might as easily be got from crude homogenates.

Nicholson   It would be marvellous if we could study isolated enterocytes. You appreciate however if we isolate enterocytes from mucosal biopsies we would have very little material for our studies. By means of subcellular fractionation of the whole homogenate we are able to pinpoint the subcellular organelle where the enzyme activity changes before and after treatment of coeliac patients. This is not possible by studying enzyme levels in crude homogenates.

45

Peptidases of the human intestinal brush border membrane

E. E. STERCHI and J. F. WOODLEY

INTRODUCTION

In the 1950s, Frazer[1] proposed that coeliac disease may be caused by a lack of a peptidase enzyme, i.e. be an enzyme deficiency disease. Despite intensive investigation since then, this 'missing peptidase' hypothesis has not been validated. Cornell and Townley[2] reported a possible peptidase deficiency in biopsies of children with coeliac disease, but this observation has not been confirmed. On the contrary in 1970, Douglas and Booth showed that the pattern of digestion of gluten peptides by normal mucosa and coeliac mucosa was the same, and they therefore concluded that there was no missing peptidase. Fottrell et al.[3] also showed that the pattern of peptidases on starch gel electrophoresis was the same in normal intestine and that from coeliacs in remission. Both these studies however were carried out using biopsies and thus enzymes from all the cell organelles would be present. It is well-known that the lysosomes contain a wide spectrum of protein hydrolysing activities, and that the cytosol of intestinal cells contains many peptidases. Thus, using whole cell homogenates, the lack of a particular peptidase from one part of the cell may be masked by similar activities in another organelle.

As there is little evidence that intact protein or large peptides enter cells, and as most of the terminal stages of digestion take place in the gut lumen and at the brush border membrane surface, it would seem logical to suggest that any 'missing peptidase' might be located in the brush border membrane. Such is the case with other malabsorption diseases associated with missing enzymes, e.g. sucrase/isomaltase deficiency[4].

We therefore decided to investigate the peptidase enzymes present in highly purified preparations of human brush border membranes, and to examine the specificity of the enzymes, in the hope that such information may define the role, if any, in coeliac disease.

MATERIALS AND METHODS

Sections of small intestine were obtained at surgery, washed immediately in physiological saline and frozen with solid carbon dioxide. The tissue samples were stored at -20 °C until required. The brush border membranes were purified by differential and density gradient centrifugation. The details of the method are shown in Figure 45.1; α-glucosidase, the brush border marker enzyme, and N-acetyl glucosaminidase, a lysosomal marker enzyme, were assayed by measuring fluorimetrically the release of methylumbelliferone from the appropriate derivatives used as substrates. Lactate dehydrogenase was measured by following fluorimetrically the conversion of NADH to NAD.

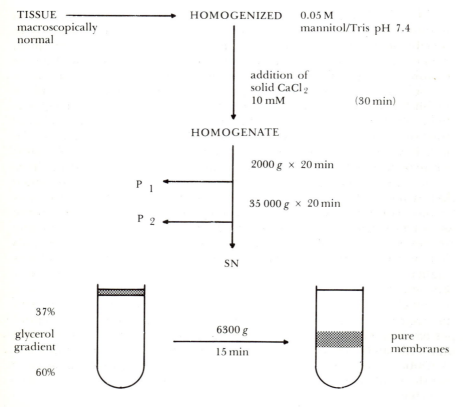

Figure 45.1   Purification of human brush border membranes

Peptidase activities were assayed by measuring the release of amino acids from small peptides, utilizing the L-amino acid oxidase method of Donlon and Fottrell[5]. Where β-naphthylamide derivatives were used as substrates, i.e. for amino peptidase A (α-L-glutamyl-β-naphthylamide), amino peptidase M (L-leucyl-β-naphthylamide), diaminopeptidase IV (glycyl-L-prolyl-β-naphthylamide) and γ-glutamyltranspeptidase (γ-glutamyl-β-naphthylamide), the release of β-naphthylamine was measured fluorimetrically. Protein was estimated by the method of Lowry *et al.*[6]

The enzymes were released from the membranes by use of Triton X100, papain and sodium dodecyl sulphate (SDS) and electrophoresed in polyacrylamide by the methods of Davis and Ornstein[7], and Neville[8]. After electrophoresis, the gels were sliced and the slices assayed for the various peptidase activities.

RESULTS

The distribution of the marker enzymes in the membrane preparation is shown in Table 45.1. The membrane fraction shows an increase in specific activity of 24 for α-glucosidase, and is essentially free from contamination with lysosomal or cytosol enzymes. It was important to establish that the membranes were pure in this respect in that both cytosol and lysosomes contain peptidase enzyme activities. The yields of brush border activity in the membrane were low but enrichment was high. The homogenate, the purified membrane fraction, and the cytosol fraction were assayed for a number of peptidase activities. The results are shown in Table 45.2, expressed as specific activities (μmoles substrate hydrolysed mg protein^{-1} min^{-1}), A number of points emerge from these results. Firstly, the purified brush border membranes contained hydrolytic activity against all the peptides listed, though there was clearly considerable variation in specific activities including some activities which were negligible in some preparations. This may be due to many factors, notably the nutritional state of the individual. Secondly, it is apparent that in general, specific activity against tripeptides is higher in the brush border than the activity against similar dipeptides. For example in the case of both phenylalanyl-glycylglycine, and tyrosylglycylglycine, the specific activity is twice that obtained with phenylalanylglycine and tyrosylglycine. In the case of the tetrapeptide tested (Phe-Gly-Gly-Phe) the specific activity is even greater, being approximately ten times that obtained with phenylalanylglycine. A similar effect has been observed in hydrolytic activity of guinea pig brush borders against glycine containing peptides[9].

Table 45.3 shows the enrichment of various peptidases in the membrane fraction. Clearly the degree of enrichment of any enzyme in

Table 45.1 Marker enzyme activities in fractions

Fraction	Protein %	α-Glucosidase (brush border marker)			N-acetyl-β-D-glucosaminidase (lysosome marker)			Lactate dehydrogenase (cytosol marker)		
		Specific activity ×̄	Increase in specific activity	Recovery %	Specific activity	Increase in specific activity	Recovery %	Specific activity	Increase in specific activity	Recovery %
	[9]*	[5]	[5]	[5]	[4]	[4]	[4]	[5]	[5]	[5]
Homogenate (H)	100	41.8 (29.1–60.2)	1	100	9.2 (4.83–14.5)	1	100	15.3 (13.3–19.2)	1	100
Low speed pellet (P_1)	39.5** (14–61)†	48.1 (34–69.5)	1.1 (0.9–1.26)	47.5 (28.1–50.5)	1.66 (1.1–3.4)	0.22 (0.12–0.31)	8.5 (4.1–12.6)	2.4 (0.12–3.17)	0.17 (0.01–0.5)	11.1 (1.2–34.9)
High speed supernatant (S_2)	60.8 (46.1–78)	4.5 (0.95–9.12)	0.14 (0.08–0.176)	6.3 (1.9–11.9)	13.4 (6.2–19.5)	1.46 (1.3–1.7)	86.2 (79.2–95)	19.2 (12.2–22.9)	1.26 (0.76–1.76)	87.1 (39.6–148)
Brush border membrane	0.372 (0.19–0.64)	9.56 (504–1734)	23.6 (9.6–28.8)	8.62 (5.3–14.6)	1.21 (0–2.57)	0.21 (0.149–0.3)	0.064 (0–0.12)	2.95 (0–5.9)	0.224 (0.15–0.31)	0.46 (0–1.24)
	100.7††			57.4			95.2			98.7

* = Number of fractions
** = Mean
† = Range
†† = Total recovery
×̄ = Specific activity (μmoles substrate hydrolysed/mg protein/hour)

Table 45.2 Peptide hydrolase activities in fractions

Substrate	Homogenate × specific activity	Soluble (S_2) specific activity	Brush border specific activity
L-Leucyl-L-leucine [6]*	0.6**(0.17–1.05)†	0.4 (0–0.86)	1.9 (0–5.0)
L-Leucyl-glycine [4]	0.34 (0–1.03)	0.54 (0–1.03)	1.05 (0–2.41)
L-Phenylalanyl-glycine [5]	0.089 (0.02–0.144)	0.061 (0–0.1555)	0.83 (0.485–1.23)
L-Tyrosyl-glycine [4]	0.049 (0–0.11)	0.007 (0–0.016)	0.52 (0–0.91)
L-Tyrosyl-L-tyrosine [4]	0.055 (0–0.123)	0.018 (0–0.052)	0.39 (0–0.7)
L-Leucyl-L-leucyl-L-leucine [6]	0.66 (0.139–1.36)	0.077 (0–0.236)	6.28 (1.56–13.3)
L-Leucyl-glycyl-glycine [4]	0.18 (0–0.593)	0.076 (0–0.236)	1.41 (0–2.73)
L-Phenylalanyl-glycyl-glycine [6]	0.167 (0.037–0.297)	0.093 (0–0.18)	2.49 (0.79–5.36)
L-Tyrosyl-glycyl-glycine [4]	0.094 (0–0.179)	0.006 (0–0.023)	1.03 (0–2.44)
L-Tyrosyl-L-tyrosyl-L-tyrosine [4]	0.083 (0–0.182)	0.015 (0–0.061)	0.91 (0–1.72)
L-Phenylalanyl-glycyl-glycyl-L-phenylalanine [4]	0.52 (0.023–1.76)	0.014 (0–0.057)	8.15 (0.42–28.1)
L-Leucyl-β-naphthylamide [3]	0.174 (0.12–0.216)	0.027 (0.01–0.056)	4.1 (1.7–7.12)
α-Glutamyl-β-naphthylamide [5]	0.025 (0.017–0.048)	0.0045 (0–0.0073)	0.38 (0.192–0.75)
γ-Glutamyl-β-naphthylamide [5]	0.069 (0.0151–0.175)	0.037 (0.001–0.13)	0.76 (0.287–1.55)
Glycyl-L-prolyl-β-naphthylamide [5]	0.147 (0.0141–0.28)	0.138 (0.01–0.27)	1.73 (0.617–3.39)

× = μ moles substrate hydrolysed mg protein^{-1} min^{-1}
* = No. of fractions
** = Mean
† = Range

441

Table 45.3 Purification and recovery of peptide hydrolases in brush border fractions

Substrate	Brush border membrane		Soluble (S_2)
	Increase in specific activity × (H = 1)	Recovery % (H = 100%)	Recovery % (H = 100%)
L-Leucyl-L-leucine [6]*	8.35** (1.27–29.2)†	1.34 (0,00–6.1)	39.8 (0.00–117)
L-Leucyl-glycine [3]	5.35 (2.34–11)	1.6 (0.63–2.3)	96.4 (19.8–193)
L-Phenylalanyl-glycine [5]	14.6 (4.45–29.6)	2.51 (0.72–4.51)	35.1 (0.00–73.7)
L-Tyrosyl-glycine [3]	14.3 (5.9–35)	1.23 (0.73–1.99)	10.8 (0.00–25.8)
L-Tyrosyl-L-tyrosine [3]	13.6 (3.8–31.4)	2.88 (0.62–6.5)	59.2 (0.00–170)
L-Leucyl-L-leucyl-L-leucine [6]	18.9 (1.15–27.6)	2.95 (0.31–5.76)	7.15 (0.00–19.5)
L-Leucyl-glycyl-glycine [3]	10.0 (4.6–20.8)	2.1 (0.69–4.3)	42.9 (5.15–105)
L-Phenylalanyl-glycyl-glycine [6]	17.6 (5.6–35.5)	3.55 (2.1–6.1)	36 (0.00–90)
L-Tyrosyl-glycyl-glycine [3]	17.7 (4.1–42)	1.39 (1.09–1.95)	7.8 (0.00–22.8)
L-Tyrosyl-L-tyrosyl-L-tyrosine [3]	16.6 (5.4–34.9)	3.54 (0.89–7.2)	5.17 (0–15.5)
L-Phenylalanyl-glycyl-glycyl-L-phenylalanine [4]	16.9 (9.4–24.2)	4.83 (2.1–11)	2.8 (0.00–11.2)
L-Leucyl-β-naphthylamide [3]	23.3 (9.5–33)	4.8 (2.3–9.5)	8.6 (3.6–16.3)
α-Glutamyl-β-naphthylamide [5]	14.2 (11.3–18.6)	2.6 (0.19–5.13)	13.9 (2....73–22)
α-Glutamyl-β-naphthylamide [5]	13.4 (6.7–18.1)	2.64 (0.52–5.2)	30.3 (1.1–77.4)
Glycyl-prolyl-β-naphthylamide [5]	18.8 (2.5–43.8)	3.22 (0.21–5.98)	40.1 (3.6–71.7)
α-Glucosidase [5]	23.6 (9.6–28.8)	8.62 (5.3–14.6)	6.3 (1.9–11.9)

× = μmoles substrate hydrolysed mg protein^{-1} min^{-1}
* = No. of fractions
** = Mean
† = Range

the membrane fraction, expressed as an increase in specific activity compared with the homogenate, reflects the distribution of location of the enzyme between brush border membrane and cytosol. Most of the enzymes are located in both fractions. Where the specific activity in the membrane fraction approaches that of α-glucosidase, the brush border marker enzyme, we conclude that the particular activity is predominantly located in the brush border membrane although precise quantitation is difficult from this data. Aminopeptidase M, measured using L-leucyl-β-naphthylamide shows a very similar distribution and enrichment as α-glucosidase and might therefore be assumed to be located exclusively in the brush border membrane. In general the tripeptidase activities show a greater enrichment in the brush border than the dipeptidase activities, suggesting that the activities are due to different enzymes, and that the tripeptidase activity is associated more with the brush border membrane and the dipeptidases with the cytosol or other cellular organelles. This confirms observations made by other workers[10], where it is suggested that only between 0–10% of the cellular dipeptidase activity is of brush border membrane origin. Quite clearly the human brush border membranes contain a number of peptidases active against di- and tripeptides and synthetic β-naphthylamide substrates and so we decided to solubilize and separate the activities by different methods of solubilization on polyacrylamide gel electrophoresis to resolve precisely the number of different peptidases present in the membrane fraction.

The brush border enzymes were solubilized with papain, and the resulting supernatant electrophoresed on polyacrylamide gels. The gels were sliced and assayed for peptidases with both peptide and naphthyl-amide substrates. The results are shown in Figure 45.2. The activities were resolved into four peaks. Peak 1, 2, 3, corresponded to the enzymes diaminopeptidase IV, (DAP IV), γ-glutamyl transpeptidase and aminopeptidase A. Peak 4 showed activity against a number of di- and tripeptide substrates and leucyl-β-naphthylamide. It was not clear whether this peak contained a number of seperate peptidase activities with differing specificity but similar electrophoretic mobilities or a 'master' peptidase with wide specificity. In an attempt to resolve this question, the brush border membranes were solubilized with Triton X-100 and the resulting supernatant electrophoresed, and the gels sliced as before. Figure 45.3 shows the results of such an electrophoresis. Following Triton solubilization five peaks were obtained. Peaks 1, 2, 3 again showed resolution of DAP IV, γ-glutamyl transpeptidase, and aminopeptidase A. As with papain solubilization, peak 4 contained both di- and tripeptidase activity with different substrates. However, an additional peak, peak 5, showed additional activity against leucyl-β-naphthylamide and alanyl-β-naphthylamide. Such activity is associated with aminopeptidase M. This suggested that the peak 4 observed after

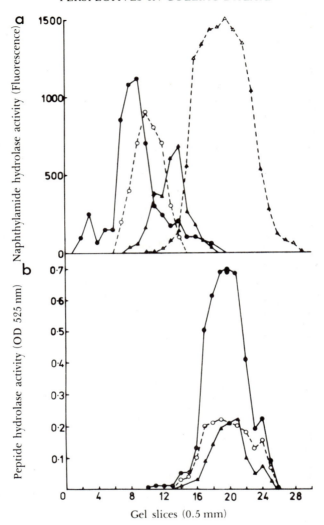

Figure 45.2 Peptidase activities in polyacrylamide gels after papain-solubilization.
a) △----△ Leucyl-β-naphthylamide; ▲——▲ α-Glutamyl-β-naphthylamide,
O----O γ-Glutamyl-β-naphthylamide, ●——● Glycyl-prolyl-β-naphthylamide
b) ●——● Leucyl-leucyl-leucine, O----O Tyrosyl-glycyl-glycine, ▲——▲ Tyrosyl-glycine

papain solubilization may have contained more than one enzyme. Finally the membranes were solubilized with 0.25% sodium dodecyl sulphate (SDS) and electrophoresed. Although many enzymes are labile after treatment with SDS, including activities against β-naphthylamide

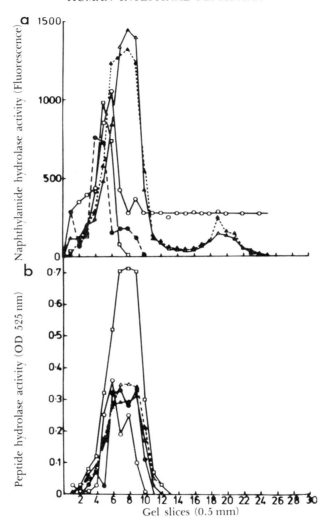

Figure 45.3 Peptidase activities in polyacrylamide gels after Triton X100 solubilization. a) △———△ Leucyl-β-naphthylamide, ▲----▲ Alanyl-β-naphthylamide, ○———○ γ-Glutamyl-β-naphthylamide, □———□ Glycyl-prolyl-β-naphthylamide, ●----● α-Glutamyl-β-naphthylamide.
b) □———□ Leucyl-leucyl-leucine, △----△ Phenylalanyl-glycyl-glycyl-phenylalanine, ○———○ Phenylalanyl-glycine, ▲———▲ Tyrosyl-glycyl-glycine, ●———● Phenylalanyl-tyrosine

substrates, some peptidase activities could be recovered in slices, but not quantitatively. Figure 45.4 shows the pattern of activity in SDS gels of some leucyl di- and tripeptides. Peak 1 showed activity against the

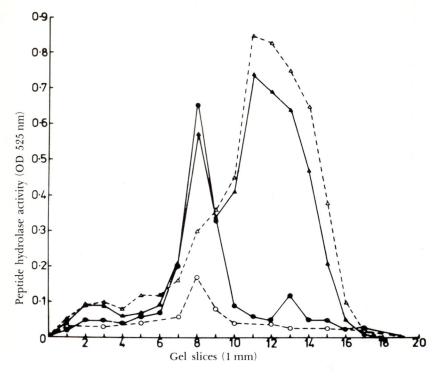

Figure 45.4 Peptidase activities in SDS-polyacrylamide gels after SDS solubilization. ●——● Leucyl-leucyl-leucine, ▲——▲ Leucyl-leucine, ○——○ Leucyl-glycyl-glycine, △——△ Leucyl-glycine

two tripeptides leucyl-leucyl-leucine and leucyl-glycyl-glycine and also the dipeptide, leucyl-leucine. Peak 2, however, showed only activity against the dipeptides leucyl-glycine and leucyl-leucine. This was also confirmed by incubating the peak slices with the substrates and separating the products on thin layer chromatography. It was also evident from this procedure that the enzyme(s) in peak 1 would hydrolyse leucyl-glycyl-glycine, but not leucyl-glycine, clearly indicating a specificity for the tripeptide. This evidence suggests that there are at least two peptidases hydrolysing the peptide substrates used, as well as the three (peaks 1, 2, 3) seen with both Triton and papain solubilized brush border membranes.

DISCUSSION

Evidence presented in this paper suggests that the human intestinal brush border contains at least five discrete peptidase enzymes, some of which have wide specificity against peptidase substrates. Exactly how many peptidases are present is still to be resolved, but it can be concluded that the brush border membrane is capable of hydrolysing a wide range of peptide substrates. Brush border membrane peptidases have been studied in a number of species by different workers. Comparisons are frequently difficult because of the multiplicity of substrates used. Maroux et al.[11] have purified an aminopeptidase from pig and shown that this one enzyme is responsible for essentially all the peptidase activity of the brush border membrane in that species. Recently, Shoaf et al.[12] have purified four separate peptidases from rat brush border membranes. These enzymes have considerable overlapping specificities, but the authors did not assay the enzymes with the substrates for DAP IV, aminopeptidase M or γ-glutamyl transpeptidase, and so there may be up to six or seven discrete peptidases in the rat brush borders. Donlan and Fottrell[13] showed that a crude brush border fraction from guinea pig contained up to four peptide hydrolases. In all these species as in the human, many of the peptide hydrolases have a dual subcellular location, i.e. being present in both the cytosol of the enterocytes and in the brush border membrane. Our results with human tissue suggest that the activities against dipeptides are predominantly located in the cytosol, whereas activities against large tri- and tetra-peptides are principally located in the brush border membrane. It is assumed that the function of these membrane-bound peptidases is to hydrolyse peptides during the terminal stages of digestion, either to amino acids which are then transported into the cells by specific carrier systems or to dipeptides which can also be transported into the cells, to be finally hydrolysed by the cytosol dipeptidases.

The fact that the human brush border membrane contains such a number of peptide hydrolases with broad specificity may be relevant to the 'missing peptidase' hypothesis for coeliac disease. We believe that it would be highly unlikely that the lack of any one of the multiple peptidases could produce the degree of damage seen in coeliac mucosa. It is likely that the hydrolytic function of any one enzyme could be compensated for by others present, particularly given the apparent wide specificity of the enzymes. One possible exception is the enzyme γ-glutamyltranspeptidase, which is specific in its activity, although its function is not clear. In 1970[14], Cohen et al. reported, with a small sample of cases, that the enzyme was partially reduced (50%) in coeliacs in remission. Again, whole biopsies were used, and not a membrane fraction, and it was not clear whether it was a secondary or primary effect.

More substantial evidence against the 'missing peptidase' hypothesis has come from the recent work of Phelan et al.[15], who have demonstrated that the toxicity of gliadin resides in a side-chain component, probably carbohydrate, and that this toxicity can be enzymically removed. This removal does not involve peptidase attack, and the protein chain of the gliadin remains intact. The basis of Frazer's 'missing peptidase' hypothesis[1] was that the toxicity of gliadin could be destroyed by an extract of hog intestine. However, the fact that it was a water extract of intestinal mucosa meant that in addition to the peptidases it was assumed to contain it would have many other types of enzymes present, notably carbohydrases from lysosomes, which could have removed the carbohydrate side-chains, and thus as indicated by Phelan *et al.*[15], the toxicity.

While the evidence of Phelan *et al.*[15] and the demonstration in this paper of multiple peptidase activity in the human intestinal brush border are contrary to the 'missing peptidase' hypothesis, final refutation of the theory is not possible until we have compared the brush border membrane peptidases in the normal with those in the membranes prepared from the mucosa of coeliac patients in remission. Such work is now in progress in our laboratory.

SUMMARY

The brush border membrane of human intestine contains at least five peptide hydrolases, several of which have broad specificity. This, and evidence of non-peptidase removal of gliadin toxicity, suggest that the 'missing peptidase' hypothesis for the aetiology of coeliac disease is untenable. Final confirmation however depends on a comparison between peptidases in brush border membranes from normal mucosa and those from coeliac patients in remission.

ACKNOWLEDGEMENT

The financial support of the Wellcome Trust is gratefully acknowledged.

References

1. Frazer, A. C. (1956). Discussion on some problems of steatorrhea and adult coeliac disease. *Proc. Roy. Soc. Med.,* **49**, 1009
2. Cornell, H. J. and Townley, R. R. W. (1973). Investigation of possible intestinal pepidase deficiency in coeliac disease. *Clin. Chim. Acta,* **49**, 181
3. Fottrell, P. F., Dolly, J. O., Dillon, A., Mitchell, B. and McNicholl, B. (1970). Multiple forms of peptidases in intestinal mucosa from children with coeliac disease In: C. C. Booth and R. H. Dowling (eds.) *Coeliac Disease.* (London and Edinburgh: Churchill Livingstone)
4. Preiser, H., Menard, D., Crane, R. K. and Cerda, J. J. (1974). Deletion of enzyme protein from brush border membrane in sucrase–isomaltase deficiency. *Biochem. Biophys. Acta,* **363**, 279
5. Donlon, J. and Fottrell, P. F. (1971). Quantitative determination of intestinal peptide hydrolase activity using L-amino acid oxidases. *Clin. Chim. Acta.* **33**, 345
6. Lowry, O. H., Rosebrough, N. J., Lewis Farr, A. and Randall, R. J. (1951). Protein measurement with the folin phenol reagent. *J. Biol. Chem.,* **193**, 265

7. Davis, B. J. and Ornstein, L. (1961). Disc electrophoresis. (Distillation Products Industries, Rochester, USA)
8. Neville, D. M. and Glossmann, H. (1971). Molecular weight determination of protein-dodecyl-sulfate complexes by gel electrophoresis in a discontinuous buffer system. *J. Biol. Chem.*, **246** (20), 6328
9. Peters, T. J. (1973). The hydrolysis of glycine oligopeptides by guinea-pig intestinal mucosa and by isolated brush borders. *Clin. Sci. Mol. Med.*, **45**, 803
10. Peters, T. J. (1970). Intestinal peptidases. *Gut*, **11**, 720
11. Maroux, S., Louvard, D. and Barratti, J. (1973). The amino peptidase from hog intestinal brush border. *Biochem: Biophys. Acta*, **321**, 282
12. Shoaf, C. R., Berks, R. M. and Heizer, W. D. (1976). Isolation and characterisation of four peptide hydrolases from the brush border of rat intestinal mucosa. *Biochim. Biophys. Acta*, **445**, 694
13. Donlon, J. and Fottrell, P. F. (1972). Studies on substrate specificity and subcellular localisation of multiple forms of peptide hydrolases in guinea pig intestinal mucosa. *Comp. Biochem. Physiol.*, **41B**, 181
14. Cohen, M. I., McNamara, H., Blumenfield, D. and Arias, I. M. (1970). The relationship between glutamyl transpeptidase and the syndrome of coeliac sprue. In: C. C. Booth and R. H. Dowling (eds.) *Coeliac Disease* (London and Edinburgh: Churchill Livingstone)
15. Phelan, J. J., Stevens, F. M., McNicholl, B., Fottrell, P. F. and McCarthy, C. F. (1977). Coeliac disease: the abolition of gliadin toxicity by enzymes from *Aspergillus niger. Clin. Sci. Mol. Med.*, **53**, 35

Discussion of chapter 45

Hauri

When you use the term tripeptidase activity, are you sure you have determined only tripeptidase activity because in your system one of the products, a dipeptide, would be a substrate for a dipeptidase?

Woodley

The term tripeptidase as I used it refers to the greater specificity of the enzyme for tripeptides rather than dipeptides. The enzyme I described does not apparently hydrolyse dipeptides, only tripeptides. When I referred to hydrolysis I implied the N-terminal releases of amino acids and not complete hydrolysis.

Nicholson

Subcellular fraction techniques have shown in humans, at least, that nearly 100% of dipeptidase activity resides in the cytosol fraction and this is of particular importance for researchers involved in purifying brush border membranes. The slightest contamination by cytosol will affect the results and one might be purifying a cytosolic enzyme in the belief that it is a brush border enzyme. Professor Fottrell's group have shown that this occurs with dipeptidases and they have outlined that great caution must be exercised in the interpretation of work of this kind. Another point is that during solubilization of the enzymes with papain, are you concerned that enzymic artefacts may arise due to fragmentation by this enzyme?

Woodley

I accept your comment about cautiously interpreting possible cytosol contamination of brush border membranes. The figure of nearly 100% of dipeptidase activity in the cytosol of the entero-cyte depends of course on the substrate used and this is one of the problems when studying peptidases. Although we have shown that the activity of a cytosol enzyme such as lactate dehydrogenase is very low, in our brush border membrane preparation, we are aware of the possibility that other cytosol enzymes may combine with brush border. The use of papain to solubilize enzymes does pose difficulties. It has been widely used to solubilize enzymes from the brush border and has in general been reasonably successful. The action of papain is well-defined by Maroux's group in Marseilles. We accept that artefacts may arise with papain but we are using it in combination with other techniques.

46

Cell surface glycosyltransferases of the enterocyte in coeliac disease

M. M. WEISER and A. P. DOUGLAS

INTRODUCTION

Two major theories have been proposed for the aetiology and patho-genesis of coeliac disease: a primary immune defect and a peptidase deficiency. We have recently proposed an alternative mechanism in which the defect in coeliac disease expresses itself as an altered cell surface membrane glycoprotein and the reaction with gluten is viewed as a lectin-type of toxic reaction[1]. To evaluate this hypothesis, studies were initiated to isolate lectin-like factors from gluten[2] and to evaluate glycosyltransferases and endogenous acceptors on the cell surface of intestinal epithelial cells[3,4]. Previous studies with rat intestinal isolated epithelial cells indicated that it was the undifferentiated crypt cell which was high in cell surface membrane glycosyltransferase:endogenous acceptor activities while the villus cell demonstrated only high sialyl-transferase:endogenous acceptor activity. The present report utilizes techniques similar to those used in the animal studies to evaluate the glycosyltransferase activities of isolated cells from human small bowel biopsies. These preliminary studies suggest an intrinsic difference in cell surface galactosyltransferase: endogenous and exogenous acceptor activities in patients with coeliac disease.

[1] This study was supported in part by USPHS grant CA-16703, M. M. Weiser and the Wellcome Trust, London (A.P.D.)
[2] Requests for reprints should be addressed to M. M. Weiser, G.I. Lab, Massachusetts General Hospital, Boston, Massachusetts 02167, USA
[3] Present address: Division of Gastroenterology, University of Southern California School of Medicine, Los Angeles, California 90033, USA

METHODS

Patients

The 20 patients in this study had been or were being evaluated for coeliac disease by the Gastroenterology Group, Department of Medicine, Royal Victoria Infirmary, Newcastle-upon-Tyne, England.

Small bowel biopsies were done for diagnostic purposes or for evaluation of therapy. All patients gave informed consent and all procedures conformed to current regulations regarding human investigation. The major diagnostic and investigative use of the biopsy material was explained to each patient as well as all benefits and risks of the procedure.

Six patients had mild gastrointestinal complaints, no evidence of malabsorption by chemical or radiological criteria, and had normal histology of their small bowel biopsies. Fourteen patients had radiological and chemical evidence of malabsorption and either their present biopsies or past biopsies were consistent with coeliac disease. Two of these patients had been untreated at the time of small bowel biopsy and represent newly-diagnosed cases. They subsequently responded clinically to a gluten-free diet. The other 12 patients represented biopsy-compatible, gluten-free diet responsive patients with coeliac disease. Table 46.1 indicates the time each patient had been on a gluten-free diet, the histology at the time of this study and the patient's HLA type. Small bowel biopsy was performed after fluoroscopically determining that the biopsy capsule was at or beyond the ligament of Treitz. The Crosby small bowel biopsy instrument was used. The tissue was removed from the capsule with 3 to 5 minutes after biopsy. A portion was taken for histology and the rest used for isolated cell preparations.

Isolated cell preparations

A system very similar to that outlined by Weiser[3] was used. The small bowel tissue obtained by biopsy was placed in a petri dish (Falcon 9 cm dia.) in which solution A[3] had been placed and warmed to 37 °C. The tissue was incubated for 15 min at 37 °C in an oven. Solution A was then removed and the tissue covered with 0.05 M sodium phosphate buffer in 0.154 M NaCl, pH 7.0 plus 1 mM dithiothreitol and incubated for 10 min at 37 °C. Cells were then removed by gentle agitation using a Pasteur pipette to create solution movement around the tissue. The isolated cells were then aspirated with the Pasteur pipette and placed

Table 46.1 Clinical characteristics and intestinal epithelial cell surface galactosyltransferase activities of coeliac patients and patients with functional disorders

Patient	Length of time on gluten free diet (months)	Histology	HLA type	Cell surface galactosyltransferase activity	
				Endogenous	Exogenous
				(cpm/mg prot/h)	
A. Coeliac Disease					
DE	14	N[1]	1–8/29–12	6060	14900
Wh	6	PVA[1]	ND[1]	3680	4750
Gl	38	N	2–8/2–7	4690	14900
Ki	5	N	2–13/9–18	1620	32680
Sm	40	N	1–8/2–15	7410	10580
Ha	4	TVA[1]	1–8/2–8	9900	35500
Sc	33	N	1–28/8–W15	5760	20600
Le	13	N	1–8/2–W40	7630	22420
Da	7	N	ND	5440	11150
Po	15	PVA	1–8/1–8	7700	25600
Ba	8	TVA	1–8/1–8	2880	22200
Ho	58	N	3–7/9–8	3890	5570
Wa	0	TVA	2–12/1–8	6670	39600
We	0	TVA	1–8/11–12	8000	16500
				5809 ± 609[2]	19776 ± 2871[2]
B. Functional GI Disorder					
Ma	—	N	ND	3300	5840
Br	—	N	ND	2521	11500
Wr	—	N	ND	4140	4270
El	—	N	ND	3910	20950
Li	—	N	ND	756	1790
Ca	—	N	ND	5500	6280
				3355 ± 658[2]	8438 ± 822[2]
			Normal vs. coeliac patients	$p < 0.05$	$p < 0.05$

[1]TVA = Total villous atrophy
PVA = Partial villous atrophy
N = Normal
ND = Not done
[2]Mean ± SEM

in a graduated conical centrifuge tube (12 ml capacity; 15 mm dia × 12 cm) which was sitting in ice. This gentle agitation was repeated twice and the solutions combined in the conical centrifuge tube. The cells were collected by centrifugation (200 g, 5 min) and washed twice with 0.1 M cacodylate buffer, pH 7.2, and 0.154 M NaCl and finally resuspended in this wash buffer. Protein concentration varied from 0.1 to 1.0 mg/ml. The volume used to suspend cells depended on the estimated yield versus the number of desired assays.

Glycosyltransferase assays

These assays were performed similar to those previously described[4,5]. To a 0.04 ml suspension of intact cells in 0.1 M cacodylate-HCl buffer, pH 7.2, containing 0.154 M NaCl was added 0.01 ml of 0.1 M $MnCl_2$ and 0.01 ml of the various radioactive nucleotide sugars. In order to maximize enyme concentration, two nucleotide sugars were usually added in one assay tube. When this was done, one sugar was labelled with ^3H and the other with ^{14}C. The combinations and final concentrations were: CMP-[4-^{14}C]sialic acid, 2.1 mM, 2.7×10^6 cpm per μmole with UDP-N-acetyl-[1-^3H]galactosamine, 0.8 μM, 2.9×10^{10} cpm per μmole; GDP-[U-^{14}C]mannose, 8.9 μM, 1.24×10^9 cpm per μmole with UDP-[1-^3H]galactose, 2.1μM, 10^{10} cpm per μmole; GDP-[U-^{14}C]fucose, 5.8μM, 8.3×10^8 cpm per μmole with UDP-N-acetyl-[6-^3H]glucosamine, 1.52μM, 1.5×10^{10} cpm per μmole. When enzyme activity with exogenous acceptor was evaluated only one nucleotide sugar was added. The exogenous acceptors were sialyl-free fetuin and sialyl-free, galactosyl-free fetuin prepared as previously described[6]. These acceptor stock solutions usually contained 50 μmoles of acceptor sites per ml and 0.01 ml was added to the assay. Buffer (0.1 M cacodylate-HC1, pH 7.2, 0.154 M NaCl) was added to bring the final volume to 0.1 ml. The assay was incubated for 60 min at 37 °C and the reaction terminated by the addition of 2 ml of 5% cold trichloroacetic acid and the product collected by filtration through glass fibre filters, 2.4 cm in diameter (Reeve Angel grade 934AH) and washed with 10 ml of cold 5% trichloroacetic acid followed by 10 ml of absolute ethanol (at −5 to −20 °C). Collection of filter and preparation for counting was as previously described[4]. A zero time, 0°C control was subtracted from each as non-specific background and this usually represented less than 5% of incorporated radioactivity.

MATERIALS AND GENERAL METHODS

Radioactive materials were purchased from New England Nuclear and Amersham-Searle. Fetuin was purchased from GIBCO. Protein was determined by the method of Lowry et al.[7]

RESULTS

Intestinal epithelial cell surface glycosyltransferase activities

Approximately 90% or more of the isolated cells excluded Trypan blue. The cell surface of these cells was tested for glycosyltransferase: endogenous acceptor activities (sialyl-, galactosyl-, fucosyl-, N-acetylgalactosaminyl-, mannosyl-, and N-acetylglucosaminyl-transferase activities). In addition, two glycosyltransferase:exogenous acceptor activities were also measured (sialyltransferase: sialyl-free fetuin and galactosyltransferase[1]: sialyl-, galactosyl-free fetuin activities). Only galactosyltransferase : endogenous and exogenous acceptor activities were significantly elevated in patients with coeliac disease (Table 46.1, Figure 46.1). These increased galactosyltransferase activities showed no significant correlations with extent of villous atrophy, HLA type or time on a gluten-free diet (Table 46.1).

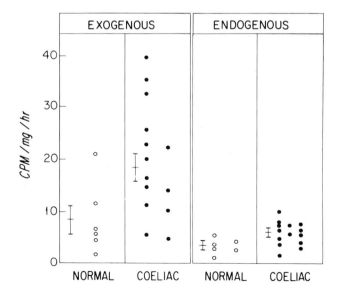

Figure 46.1 Intestinal cell surface galactosyltransferase activity. Exogenous refers to activity with sialyl-, galactosyl-free fetuin. Bars indicate the mean ± SEM

Kinetics of the cell surface glycosyltransferase

There are no available commercial sources for many non-radioactive sugars. Therefore, when a large series of glycosyltransferases are tested and compared, most are assayed at nucleotide sugar concentrations below saturation levels. In this initial study it was elected to test for glycosyltransferase activities with those concentrations of nucleotide sugars available as the radioactive compound in order to survey as many glycosyltransferase activities of the human intestinal cell surface as possible. Exogenous acceptors for sialyl- and galactosyltransferases were used at saturating concentrations. Galactosyltransferase:exogenous acceptor activity was shown to be linear with time for both coeliac and normal cells. Galactosyltransferase:endogenous acceptor activity tended to level off for the normal cell (Figure 46.2) suggesting a limited number of available acceptor sites. However, isolated intestinal cells from coeliac patients showed almost a linear increase with time for galactosyltransferase:endogenous acceptor activity. Thus, the increased galactosyltransferase:endogenous acceptor activity for coeliac cells may be an indication of an increased number of endogenous acceptor sites on the coeliac cell as well as an increase in enzyme activity.

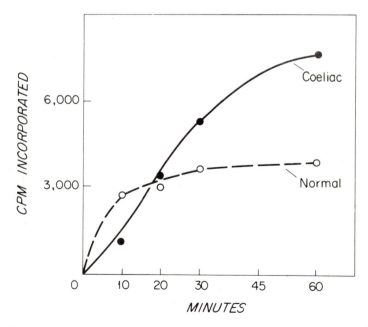

Figure 46.2 Galactosyltransferase: endogenous acceptor activity of isolated human intestinal cells; activity versus time of incubation. (●) Coeliac intestinal cells, (○) normal intestinal cells

DISCUSSION

The studies presented here represent an initial survey to detect differences between the normal and the coeliac intestinal epithelial cell surface. Earlier studies of rat intestinal mucosa[4] suggested that the normal undifferentiated crypt cells had tenfold higher levels of cell surface glycosyltransferase:endogenous activities than did the differentiated villous cell. Evidence was presented that this represented an increase in both enzyme activity (as assayed with exogenous acceptor) and in endogenous acceptors. Thus, the immature, mitotically active crypt cell surface had characteristics more of a Golgi membrane, and it was suggested that the source of new surface membrane in a dividing cell would be the Golgi membrane. In active coeliac disease, the epithelium has a higher rate of turnover, higher mitotic index, and a tendency to be less mature with distorted microvilli and decreased activity of microvillus enzymes. For these reasons, the untreated coeliac epithelial cell has been viewed as a less mature cell and therefore should have cell membrane characteristics more like that of the crypt cell. If the results of studies with rat mucosa[4] are applicable to human mucosa then the untreated or unresponsive coeliac epithelial cell surface should have increased cell surface glycosyltransferase activity as well as increased number of endogenous acceptors. Such changes would fit a recently proposed alternative mechanism for gluten toxicity in coeliac disease[1]. That is, if gluten acts as a lectin in a toxic reaction with the intestinal epithelial cell one must postulate a difference in the glycoprotein of the epithelial cell surface of coeliac patients and that this difference might be exaggerated in any undifferentiated cell, normal or coeliac, where more 'incomplete' glycoproteins have been demonstrated[4]. What was expected was that all of the glycosyltransferase: endogenous acceptor activities would be elevated on the less differentiated, untreated coeliac epithelial cell. However, only galactosyltransferase activity (with either endogenous or exogenous acceptors) was significantly elevated (Table 46.1, Figure 46.1). Furthermore, the amount of endogenous acceptors on the coeliac cell was abundant enough not to be significantly rate-limiting as was observed for the normal cell (Figure 46.2).

Since we have no data on differences between human villous and crypt cell surface, the increased galactosyltransferase activities observed for the coeliac epithelial cells may still be an indication of differences between normal immature and differentiated cells in human intestinal mucosa. Against that was the finding of no correlation between the increased cell surface galactosyltransferase activities and the pathology of the biopsy (Table 46.1). Coeliac patients with normal biopsies also showed high cell surface galactosyltransferase activities.

Although the data presented here suggest a primary abnormality in cell surface galactosyltransferase: endogenous and exogenous acceptor activities, a number of problems in methodology preclude any strong conclusions. First, only non-saturating concentrations of nucleotide sugars were used in order to enable us to assay a number of glyco-syltransferases. Second, activity with exogenous acceptors was evaluated for only sialyl- and galactosyltransferases. This was due partly to avail-ability of acceptors and partly to the amount of cells. Third, the degree of 'leakiness' of the cells for the nucleotide sugars was not specifically evaluated although the cells excluded vital dye. Fourth, the effect of cell surface hydrolytic enzymes on acceptor or nucleotide sugar integrity was not evaluated. Lastly, the number of patients tested, while affording enough to validate statistical comparisons was not a large series, nor were patients repeatedly tested.

In conclusion, preliminary data suggest that patients with coeliac disease, treated and untreated, with normal and abnormal small bowel histology, have increased epithelial cell surface galactosyltransferase: exogenous and endogenous acceptor activity. Furthermore the increase in endogenous acceptor activity suggests more 'incomplete' glyco-proteins on the cell surface and these incomplete glycoproteins could serve to specifically bind a lectin-like compound which we have pro-posed for gluten[1] in initiating the toxicity to the epithelial cell in coeliac disease.

ACKNOWLEDGEMENT

We are grateful to Dr David Roberts who provided the HLA data. We especially thank Dr Kurt J. Isselbacher for his helpful criticisms and review.

References

1. Weiser, M. M. and Douglas, A. P. (1976). An alternate mechanism for gluten toxicity in coeliac disease. *Lancet*, **i,** 567
2. Douglas, A. P. (1976). The binding of a glycopeptide component of wheat to intestinal mucosa of normal and coeliac human subjects. *Clin. Chim. Acta,* **73,** 357
3. Weiser, M. M. (1973a). Intestinal epithelial cell surface membrane glycoprotein synthesis. I. An indicator of cellular differentiation. *J. Biol. Chem.,* **248,** 2536
4. Weiser, M. M. (1973b). Intestinal epithelial cell surface membrane glycoprotein synthesesis. II. Glycosyltransferases and endogenous acceptors of the undiffer-entiated cell surface membrane. *J. Biol. Chem.,* **248,** 2542
5. Podolsky, D. K., Weiser, M. M., Westwood, J. C. and Gammon, M. (1977). Cancer-associated serum galactosyltransferase activity. Demonstration in an animal model system. *J. Biol. Chem.,* **252,** 1807
6. Podolsky, D. K. and Weiser, M. M. (1975). Role of cell membrane galactosyl-transferase in concanavalin A agglutination of erythrocytes. *Biochem. J.* **146,** 213
7. Lowry, O. H., Rosebrough, N. J., Farr, A. L. and Randall, R. J. (1951). Protein measurement with the Folin phenol reagent. *J. Biol. Chem.,* **193,** 265

Discussion of chapter 46

Albert   Are you implying that the defect in coeliacs is the opposite to the missing enzyme hypothesis, for example, that there is an excess of some factor or factors on the cell surface?

Weiser   Our studies to date indicate that there are more incomplete glycoproteins on the mucosal cell surface of patients with treated and untreated coeliac disease. Although our results are preliminary they do show differences in cell surface galactosyltransferase: endogenous and exogenous acceptor activities in coeliac patients compared with controls.

Nicholson   This is an imaginative hypothesis but I am concerned about some of the data. One of the problems in the system you described is the possibility of leakage of your substrate into the cell where I understand glycosyltransferase activity is high. Any such leakage might affect the interpretation of your data.

Weiser   The question of leakage of substrates in to the cells or of enzyme out of cells is a valid point about which we are aware. However, such leakage is difficult to totally control. The cells in this study did not release enzyme activity after 60 minutes' incubation and they generally remained resistant to uptake of vital dyes. We realize that this is not a specific test for 'leakiness' to other factors.

Trier   Are you measuring the specific activity of these enzymes in isolated crypt cells or is it a common pool including crypt and villous cells?

Weiser   This is a common cell pool and we did not try to separate crypt from villous cells.

47

Mucosal adenylate cyclase and sodium–potassium stimulated adenosine triphosphatase in jejunal biopsies of adults and children with coeliac disease

J. H. TRIPP, J. A. MANNING, D. P. R. MULLER,
J. A. WALKER-SMITH, D. P. O'DONOGHUE, P. J. KUMAR and
J. T. HARRIES

INTRODUCTION

Many, though not all, patients with coeliac disease (CD) have loose stools or diarrhoea at the time of diagnosis or during relapse associated with ingestion of gluten. Perfusion studies in adults with CD[1-8] have demonstrated transport defects of certain organic solutes which are absorbed by an Na^+-coupled process, such as glucose, alanine and glycine. A deficit of solute-induced increases of Na^+ and water absorption has also been reported[8], as well as actual secretion of electrolytes and water in some patients[1,4,6-8].

Sodium–potassium stimulated adenosine triphosphatase, (Na^+-K^+)-ATPase, is of fundamental importance in the transport of Na^+ and water across the intestinal mucosa[9], and is the rate-limiting enzyme for solute stimulated absorption of Na^+ and water[10]. The enzyme is situated at the lateral and basal membranes of the enterocyte, as is the enzyme adenylate cyclase. Adenylate cyclase catalyses the formation of the second messenger 3',5' cyclic adenosine monophosphate (cAMP) from ATP, increased levels of cAMP in the enterocyte being associated with active secretion of electrolytes and secretion of water[11]. Increased activity of this enzyme accounts for the massive jejunal secretion that occurs in cholera and probably also in pancreatic cholera (the Verner–Morrison syndrome)[11].

The activities of these two enzymes have been determined in portions of small intestinal biopsies obtained from children and adults with coeliac disease, in order to assess their importance in the pathophysiology of jejunal secretion in CD. Aliquots of mucosa were stored for enzyme assay from biopsies obtained during the routine clinical management of the patients concerned. Biopsies were obtained in children using a two-port modified Crosby Kugler capsule[12] and in adults using a Crosby capsule from the duodeno-jejunal flexure.

Table 47.1 Details of subjects studied

Group	Number	Biopsy findings	Diarrhoea
Controls	28	Normal	None
Coeliacs:			
Remission	15	Normal	None
Active	31	PVA: 13 SVA: 18	17

PVA indicates partial villous atrophy
SVA indicates subtotal villous atrophy

SUBJECTS AND METHODS

Subjects

Table 47.1 shows the number of subjects studied, and these are grouped according to the presence or absence of diarrhoea and the morphological appearances of the biopsy on light microscopy. There were six adults in each of the groups, the remainder being children aged 11 months to 14 years. The control group comprised patients who were being investigated for suspected malabsorption but who were subsequently proven to be normal. All the patients in remission were on gluten-free diets and were completely asymptomatic. Nine of the patients with active CD were new patients and were later proven to have permanent gluten intolerance (i.e. CD). Sixteen biopsies were obtained following gluten challenge, and in six children after they had initiated their own challenge by breaking the diet.

Enzyme assays

Mucosa was snap frozen at the time of biopsy, stored at $-70\,°C$ and homogenized at the time of assay in a glass Dounce homogenizer taking care not to include any muscularis mucosa present. The methods used to assay (Na^+–K^+)-ATPase and adenylate cyclase will be reported in detail elsewhere, and are briefly summarized. (Na^+–K^+)-ATPase was assayed by measuring the total ATPase activity in a medium containing Na_2ATP as substrate with optimal concentrations of Mg^{2+}, Na^+ and K^+, and subtracting from this the activity of the Mg^{2+} ATPase measured in the absence of K^+ and the presence of 1 mM ouabain. The assay was performed in a total volume of $625\,\mu l$ at pH 6.6 at 37 °C for 30 min, and the released inorganic phosphate measured by the method of Fiske and Subba Row[13].

Adenylate cyclase activity was measured by the formation of cAMP from ATP under basal conditions and in the presence of an optimal stimulating concentration of sodium fluoride. Activation (%) of cyclase was calculated as the per cent of fluoride stimulated activity present in the basal assay, i.e.

$$\frac{\text{Basal activity}}{\text{Fluoride stimulated activity}} \times 100$$

cAMP was measured by a saturation analysis technique (after Gilman[14]) using a protein kinase prepared from rabbit muscle.

Statistical analysis

The data from the different groups of patients have been compared by Student's t test. The sequential data obtained from serial biopsies have been compared by paired t tests using a one-tailed test since the results in this paired data were forecast from the group data.

RESULTS

(Na^+–K^+)-ATPase activity was no different in controls compared with patients with CD in remission, but was reduced by approximately 50% in patients with active disease ($p<0.001$; Table 47.2). The mean values for patients with and without diarrhoea were similar, but those with subtotal villous atrophy had a greater reduction in mean activity (57%) compared with patients with partial villous atrophy (45%); this difference was statistically significant ($p<0.025$).

Basal adenylate cyclase activity was increased (>2 SD of control mean) in 11 (35%) of the 31 patients with active disease, and 10 of these patients

Table 47.2 Mucosal (Na^+-K^+)-ATPase and adenylate cyclase in patients with coeliac disease

Activity	Controls (28)[1]	Remission (15)	Active (total) (31)	Active with diarrhoea (17)
(Na^+-K^+)-ATPase[2]	2.80±0.18	2.67±0.13	1.33±0.07‡‡‡	1.32±0.10‡‡‡
Basal adenylate cyclase[3]	13.05±0.54	13.37±0.78	16.78±0.92‡	17.7±1.86*‡
Fluoride-stimulated adenylate cyclase[3]	136.0±7.3	129.8±8.6	145.9±7.4	160.1±10.8
% Activation adenylate cyclase[4]	9.74±0.40	11.13±0.67	12.0±0.64**	11.06±0.77

[1] Numbers of subjects; [2] μmol Pi/mg protein^{-1}h^{-1}; [3] pmol cAMP/mg protein^{-1}min^{-1}; [4] Basal/Fluoride stimulated × 100

Statistical differences from controls: * $p<0.05$ ** <0.01 *** <0.001
Statistical differences from remissions: + $p<0.05$ ++ <0.01 +++ <0.001
All values expressed as mean ± 1 SE

had diarrhoea. The mean activity was increased in the group with active disease as compared with either controls or patients in remission ($p<0.05$, Table 47.2); the patients in remission had similar activities to the control group. Although fluoride-stimulated activity was increased in the patients with active disease, the increase was only significant in those with diarrhoea ($p<0.05$). The per cent activation of cyclase was increased in all patients, but only reached statistical significance ($p< 0.05$) in those with active disease.

In serial biopsies of 10 patients, two following the introduction of a gluten-free diet and eight before and after varying periods (six days to three months) on a gluten-containing diet, there were significant reductions in (Na^+-k^+)-ATPase activity and increases in basal adenylate cyclase activity in all patients (Figure 47.1). There were significant but not consistent increases in fluoride-stimulated activity, and in the per cent activation of cyclase. In all patients the morphological appearances of the mucosa altered in association with the change of gluten intake.

Both the adults and children behaved in a similar fashion with respect to alterations in the activities of the two enzymes.

DISCUSSION

The results of the present study indicate that the activities of (Na^+-K^+)-ATPase and adenylate cyclase are altered in a paradoxical fashion in patients with active coeliac disease. (Na^+-K^+)-ATPase was equally reduced in patients with and without diarrhoea, and were lowest in those patients with subtotal villous atrophy. In contrast, high basal adenylate cyclase activities (>2 SD of control values) were found

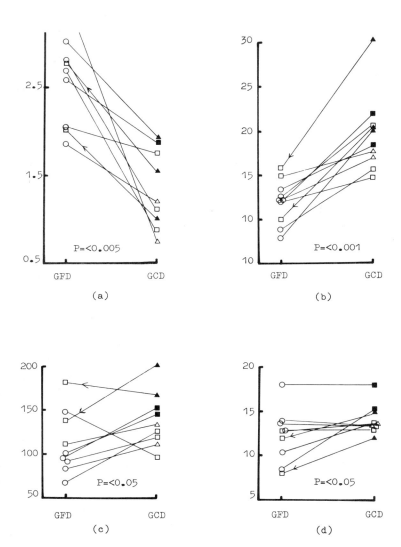

Figure 47.1 Serial mucosal (Na^+–K^+)-ATPase and adenylate cyclase activities in patients with coeliac disease while on gluten-free or gluten-containing diets. (a) (Na^+–K^+)-ATPase: μmol Pi/mg protein^{-1} h^{-1}, (b) Basal adenylate cyclase: pmol cAMP/mg protein^{-1} min^{-1}, (c) Fluoride-stimulated cyclase: pmol cAMP/mg protein^{-1} min^{-1}, (d) % Activation of cyclase: Basal activity/Flouride-stumulated activity × 100

O = normal morphology; □—■ = partial villous atrophy; △—▲ = subtotal villous atrophy. Solid symbols indicate that the patient had diarrhoea at the time of biopsy

predominantly in the group with diarrhoea, and increased activities were equally distributed between patients with subtotal villous atrophy (7 of 18) compared with those with partial villous atrophy (4 of 13). Fluoride-stimulated activity was slightly but significantly increased in the group with diarrhoea, and to a lesser non-significant degree in the patients with active disease as a whole. The per cent activation of cyclase was significantly increased in those with active disease. Both enzyme activities were no different to control values in patients in remission. Serial biopsies in individual patients consuming gluten-free or gluten-containing diets confirmed the effect of dietary gluten in reducing (Na^+-K^+)-ATPase and increasing adenylate cyclase (basal, fluoride and % activation) activities. The absolute values in individual patients frequently fell within the normal range, but in every instance (Na^+-K^+)-ATPase activity decreased and basal adenylate cyclase increased while the patient was on a gluten-containing diet.

These studies were carried out using a homogenate of the whole of the mucosa (avoiding inclusion of muscularis mucosae) so that interpretation of the results in relation to enterocyte enzyme activities presents some problems. There are several alternative possibilities that might explain the changes observed. These include quantitative alterations in the ratio of enterocytes to tissue protein, and alterations in the activities of the enzymes in individual enterocytes (e.g. due to cell membrane damage, biochemical alterations of activity and immaturity of enterocytes). If it is assumed that there is a decreased number of enterocytes per unit of tissue protein in active disease then this, together with the increased number of mononuclear cells in the lamina propria, would tend to reduce the specific activity of enterocyte enzymes as measured. The reduction in (Na^+-K^+)-ATPase could be explained on this basis, secondary to damage to the enterocyte cell membranes or secondary to biochemical changes in the cell, as was envisaged by Bayless et al.[16] to explain reduced lactase activity in the absence of ultrastructural changes in the brush border of the surface enterocytes in CD. None of these possibilities, however, is likely to account for the increased specific activities of cyclase observed in the present study.

A unifying hypothesis to account for all the observed changes, and reduced lactase activity, would be that these changes were the result of the known immaturity of surface enterocytes in active CD[17,25]. Previous studies have established that crypt cells have lower specific activities of (Na^+-K^+)-ATPase[18,19], and Hamilton and co-workers have suggested that a relative immaturity of the surface enterocytes in rotavirous diarrhoea of infant pigs may on this basis account for the diarrhoea[20]. Other studies have shown that crypt cells have increased basal and fluoride-stimulated adenylate cyclase activity[21,22], and from the results of Schwartz et al.[21] it can be calculated that cyclase shows a greater degree of activation in the crypt cells.

These alterations in the enzyme activities of the enterocyte may provide a unifying explanation of the phenomena observed in perfusion experiments that have been reported in adults[1-8]. These studies have reported malabsorption of glucose, glycine and alanine which are all absorbed in association with Na^+, together with a lack of the normally seen solute stimulated absorption of water and Na^+. The active extrusion of Na^+ from the enterocyte into the lateral space which is achieved by (Na^+-K^+)-ATPase is probably the rate-limiting step in solute stimulated Na^+ absorption[10], so that a reduction in (Na^+-K^+)-ATPase activity could account for these observations. Actual secretion of water and Na^+ cannot be accounted for on the basis of reduced (Na^+-K^+)-ATPase activity unless there is a process of active secretion occurring at the same time as absorption. There is some evidence that in cholera, secretion takes place primarily from the crypts[23] and if this is so, as seems likely, the crypt cells secrete large volumes of fluid in response to a smaller change in cAMP concentration than is seen in the villous cells[21,24]. Field[23] has suggested that any individual enterocyte may be able to either secrete or absorb but it is perhaps more attractive to believe that the primitive crypt enterocyte may be the secreting cell, and the mature villous enterocyte the absorptive cell. This allows for the possibility that the whole mucosa may both secrete and absorb at any given time, a situation which was suggested in 1963 by Schedl and Clifton[1] whose perfusion data in patients with CD demonstrated a discordance between glucose and Na^+ absorption. This discrepancy was, they suggested, explained by the presence of simultaneous secretion and absorption in the mucosa, the defect in Na^+ absorption unmasking the secretory process. If the crypt cells are indeed normally secreting, the increased adenylate cyclase and reduced (Na^+-K^+)-ATPase activities of these cells would be appropriate. A decrease in the maturity of the enterocyte would result in this cell being more of a secretory cell than normal with lower (Na^+-K^+)-ATPase and higher adenylate cyclase activities such as we have observed. This cell would secrete water and electrolytes and would not demonstrate glucose-stimulated absorption, the situation described in the perfusion studies in CD.

In contrast to the perfusion studies where no improvement in the abnormalities was found after dietary treatment, we observed a return to normal of enzyme levels in patients in complete remission. This discrepancy might be at least partially due to incomplete remission in the adult studies, since Schmid et al.[4] did not report the biopsy appearances at the time of remission and the biopsy specimens obtained from the patients of Russell et al.[5] were not classified as normal.

ACKNOWLEDGEMENTS

J.H.T. gratefully acknowledges the National Fund for Research into Crippling Diseases for financial support. J.T.H. thanks the Wellcome Trust for a Travel Grant to visit the Department of Physiology, Vanderbilt University, Nashville, Tennessee, to learn the assay techniques for adenylate cyclase and cyclic AMP, and is indebted to Dr Roger Johnson for his patient help during that time. We also acknowledge the support of the Medical Research Council. The authors thank their colleagues who performed many of the jejunal biopsies including Drs David Candy, Anne Kilby, Vic Larcher and David Ogilvie.

References

1. Schedl, H. P. and Clifton, J. A. (1963). Solute and water absorption by the human small intestine. *Nature (Lond.)*, **199**, 1264
2. Holdsworth, C. D. and Dawson, A. M. (1965). Glucose and fructose absorption in idiopathic steatorrhoea. *Gut*, **6**, 387
3. Fordtran, J. S., Rector, F. C., Locklear, T. W. and Ewton, M. F. (1967). Water and solute movement in the small intestine of patients with sprue. *J. Clin. Invest.*, **46**, 287
4. Schmid, W. C., Phillips, S. F. and Summerskill, W. H. J. (1969). Jejunal secretion of electrolytes and water in non-tropical sprue. *J. Lab. Clin. Med.*, **73**, 772
5. Russell, R. I., Allan, J. G., Gerskowitch, V. P. and Robertson, J. W. K. (1972). A study by perfusion techniques of the absorption abnormalities in the jejunum in adult coeliac disease. *Clin. Sci.*, **42**, 735
6. Kumar, P. J., Silk, D. B. A., Rousseau, B., Pagaltsos, A. S., Clark, M. L., Dawson, A. M. and Marks, R. (1974). Assessment of jejunal function in patients with dermatitis herpetiformis and adult coeliac disease using a perfusion technique. *Scand. J. Gastroenterol.*, **9**, 793
7. Silk, D. B. A., Kumar, P. J., Perrett, D., Clark, M. L. and Dawson, A. M. (1974). Amino acid and peptide absorption in patients with coeliac disease and dermatitis herpetiformis. *Gut*, **15**, 1
8. Bernier, J. J., Soule, C., Galian, A., Rambaud, J. C., Modigliani, R. and Matuchansky, C. (1975). Intestinal absorption of water, electrolytes and glucose in adult coeliac disease. A study by the intestinal perfusion technique. *Arch. Françaises des Maladies de l'Appareil Digestif*, **64**, 495
9. Dahl, J. L. and Hokin, L. E. (1974). The sodium potassium adenosine triphosphatase. *Annu. Rev. Biochem.*, **43**, 327
10. Simmons, N. L. and Naftalin, R. J. (1976). Factors affecting the compartmentalisation of sodium ion within rabbit ileum in vitro. *Biochim. Biophys. Acta*, **448**, 411
11. Kimberg, D. V. (1974). Cyclic nucleotides and their role in gastrointestinal secretion. *Gastroenterology*, **67**, 1023
12. Kilby, A. (1976). Paediatric small intestinal biopsy capsule with two ports. *Gut*, **17**, 158
13. Fiske, C. H. and Subba Row, Y. (1925). The colorimetric determination of phosphorus. *J. Biol. Chem.*, **66**, 375
14. Gilman, A. G. (1970). A protein binding assay for adenosine 3'5'-cyclic monophosphate. *Proc. Natl. Acad. Sci. USA*, **67**, 305

15. Lowry, O. H., Rosenbrough, N. J., Farr, A. L. and Randall, R. J. (1951). Protein measurement with phenol reagent. *J. Biol. Chem.*, **193**, 265
16. Bayless, T. M., Rubin, S. E., Topping, T. M., Yardley, J. H. and Hendrix, T. R. (1970). *Coeliac Disease*. Booth, C. C. and Dowling, R. H. (eds.) pp. 76–90 (London: Churchill Livingstone)
17. Shiner, M. (1974). *Coeliac Disease*. Hekkens, W. Th. J. M. and Peña, A. S. (eds.) pp. 121–137. (Leiden: H. E. Stenfert Kroese B.V.)
18. Charney,, A. N., Gots, R. E. and Gianella, R. A. (1974). (Na^+-K^+)-stimulated adenosine triphosphatase in isolated intestinal villous tip and crypt cells. *Biochim. Biophys. Acta*, **367**, 265
19. Gall, D. G., Chapman, D., Kelly, M. and Hamilton, J. R. (1977). Na^+ transport in jejunal crypt cells *Gastroenterology*, **72**, 452
20. Kerzner, B., Kelly, M. H., Gall, D. G., Butler, C. V. M. and Hamilton, J. R. (1977). Transmissable gastroenteritis: sodium transport and the intestinal epithelium during the course of viral enteritis. *Gastroenterology*, **72**, 457
21. Schwartz, C. J., Kimberg, D. V. and Ware, P. (1975). Adenylate cyclase in intestinal crypt and villous cells: stimulation by cholera enterotoxin and prostaglandin E. *Gastroenterology*, **68**, 94
22. Quill, H. and Weiser, M. M. (1975). Adenylate and guanylate cyclase activities and cellular differentiation in rat small intestine. *Gastroenterology*, **69**, 470
23. Field, M. (1974). Intestinal secretion. *Gastroenterology*, **66**, 1063
24. De Jonge, H. R. (1975). The response of the small intestinal crypt and villous epithelium to cholera toxin in rat and guinea pig. Evidence against a specific role of the crypt cells in cholaragen induced secretion. *Biochim. Biophys. Acta*, **381**, 128
25. Rey, J., Schmitz, J., Rey, F. and Jos, J. (1971). Cellular differentiation and enzymic deficits. *Lancet*, **ii**, 218 (Correspondence)

Discussion of chapter 47

Trier   I think one other possible explanation for the increase in adenylate cyclase and perhaps also to some degree the reduction in Na^+–K^+-ATPase is that, certainly in the case of adenylate cyclase you have many more inflammatory cells in the coeliac mucosa. Such inflammatory cells have been shown to contain substantial amounts of adenylate cyclase activity. I also wonder if you are referring to basal cyclase activity or stimulated activity?

Tripp   The activity being measured was basal adenylate cyclase activity. I agree that inflammatory cells do have adenylate cyclase activity but the specific activity is in fact lower than that found in enterocytes. Increases in the number of inflammatory cells would therefore reduce the specific activity of adenylate cyclase as measured in the present assay.

Section X
Clinical section

Excretion of ... amino acid ... in ... coeliac disease ...

48

Excretion of pyrrolidonylpeptides and amino acid conjugates in a patient with coeliac disease and cystic fibrosis

E. A. K. WAUTERS and J. H. van de KAMER

In coeliac patients the peptidase activity of the atrophied small intestinal villi is decreased. As a consequence peptides—originated from nutritional proteins by the action of gastric and pancreatic enzymes—are further broken down insufficiently. Indications are present that these peptides are absorbed and excreted with the urine. An increase of bacterial metabolites from non-absorbed amino acids has also been demonstrated in the urine.

Both phenomena were investigated in a child suffering from coeliac disease as well as from cystic fibrosis of the pancreas, the expectation being that clearer results could be obtained, the proteolysis being twice disturbed. We mainly focused our attention as regards the peptides on the pca-peptides since these will arise easily from gliadin containing such a high content of glutamine, which is cyclized at 37 °C to pca.

At the time of the experiments the patient was 17 years of age. Cystic fibrosis of the pancreas was diagnosed at the age of 4. Moreover, when the girl was 8 years old the diagnosis of coeliac disease was made on the basis of the ESPGAN criteria of Interlaken. At first the patient kept to the rules of her diet correctly, but afterwards it became clear that she had defaulted. Hence at the onset of the experiments it was not surprising to find that the intestinal mucosa was severely damaged, the disaccharidase activities being far below normal.

The outline of the experiments is shown in Figure 48.1.

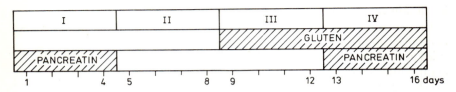

Figure 48.1 Outline of the experiments

During the whole of the four four-day periods of experiments, the diet remained unchanged, in respect of the protein intake. In the gluten period wheat products were administered up to a daily gluten intake of approximately 750 mg/kg body weight. Pancreatin was added to the diet in the first and the last period, but not in the second and third. A small intestinal biopsy was performed on the first and the sixteenth day of the experiment

E.G. (CD and CF)	– GLUTEN	+ GLUTEN
MICROSCOPY	SUBTOTAL VILLUS ATROPHY	TOTAL VILLUS ATROPHY
LACTASE (4.7 ± 2.0)	0.2	0.1
SACCHARASE (8.8 ± 3.6)	2.7	0.8
ISOMALTASE (6.1 ± 2.6)	3.6	2.4
MALTASE (29 ± 10)	8.5	4.9

Figure 48.2 Jejunal mucosa before and after loading with gluten; histology and disaccharidase activity

(Figure 48.2) It appears that the already damaged mucosa deteriorated further following the addition of gluten to the diet.

Since the substances in the urine on which we particularly wanted to focus our attention—pca-peptides and amino acid conjugates—are of an acid character, they could be collected in the water eluate of a Dowex 50 W × 2 column in the acid form. This water eluate was analysed by Sephadex G-10.

The result of two such analyses of the urine of the sixth day from the period with gluten and of the fourth day of the period without gluten is shown in (figure 48.3).

474

By analysis of reference substances the presence of pca-peptides and of the amino acid conjugates phenylacetylglutamine and hippuric acid could be demonstrated. This finding was confirmed by analysis of the three peaks after hydrolysis: the first peak — presumably pca-peptides — proved to be composed of acid, neutral and basic amino acids, the second one — presumably phenylacetylglutamine—after hydrolysis showed only glutanic acid whereas hydrolysis of the third peak — presumably hippuric acid—yielded only glycine. Apart from the above-mentioned amino acids, the presence of phenylacetic acid and benzoic acid

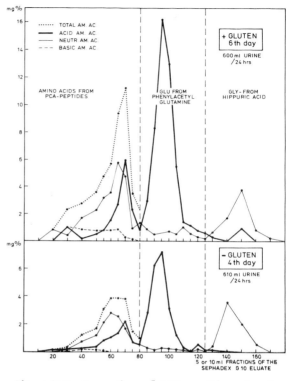

Figure 48.3 Separation of PCA-peptides, phenylacetylglutamine and hippuric acid in the H_2O-eluate of A dowex 50 W × 2 (H^+) column by sephadex G-10

in the second and third peak could be demonstrated after trimethyl silylation followed by gas chromatographic analysis. By separate analysis of the Dowex 50 W × 2 water eluate it also appeared that parahydroxyphenylacetic acid and parahydroxybenzoic acid were present.

The excretion of these acids increases when the diet contains gluten (Figure 48.4). In order to study the influence of gluten on the excretion of pca-peptides, these peptides were calculated as the sum of the composing amino acids by substracting from the total amino acid content of the Dowex 50 W × 2 water eluate the amino acids present in phenylacetylglutamine and hippuric acid. Figure 48.5 makes it clear that an increasing amount of pca-peptides is excreted in the urine after administering gluten.

mg/24 hrs - SLIDING MEAN

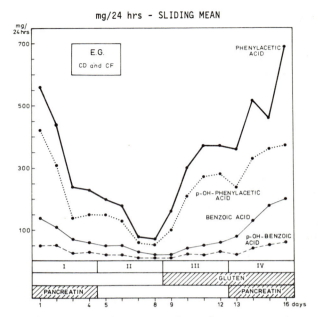

Figure 48.4 Urinary excretion of some organic acids·

mg/24 hrs - SLIDING MEAN

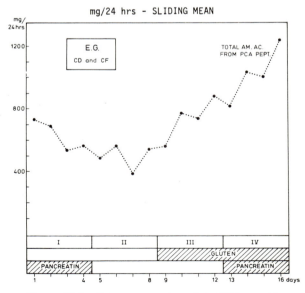

Figure 48.5 Urinary excretion of the PCA-peptides, expressed as total amino acids

SUMMARY

In this patient the amount of pca-peptides as well as of amino acid conjugates excreted in the urine increases when gluten is added to the diet. No influence of pancreatin could be demonstrated. Together with other investigators we are inclined to assume that the increase of the excretion of the amino acid conjugates is caused by bacterial metabolism in the large intestine of non-absorbed amino acids, as a consequence of the disturbed proteolysis in the small intestine. After resorption and conjugation with glutamine and glycine respectively, excretion in the urine takes place.

As for the pca-peptides the following may be worth mentioning. It may be deduced from the G-10 analysis that apart from di- and tripeptides tetra- and pentapeptides are also excreted. Presumably this phenomenon points to an absorption of these peptides. Consequently one would be inclined to think of immunological or toxicological reactions induced by the pca-peptides.

Discussion of chapter 48

Eggermont	In treating a coeliac patient, how many days does it take before these peptides disappear from the urine?
Wauters	We haven't analysed these peptides in coeliac patients, but are working on this now. We have seen in coeliac patients that it takes a long time for the normal excretion of what we call the acetyl amino acids, but we believe now that the glutamine, which remains higher after the start of the gluten-free diet, originates from the excretion of phenylacetylglutamine, which we saw was low in this patient during the period on a gluten-free diet, presumably because she had gluten before the start of the experiment.
Cluysenaer	You were talking about a possible absorption effect in these patients with coeliac disease but it might be that these peptides are 'non-absorbed peptides', having been secreted by the intestine, because as you know, there is protein-losing enteropathy in coeliac disease.
Wauters	The protein-losing enteropathy in this child at the time of our experiment was not measured by means of chromium chloride excretion. I think a longer period is needed to show this protein loss.

49

The 0.1 mol D-xylose absorption test – a gliadin toxicity assay

FIONA M. STEVENS, D. W. WATT, MARY A. BOURKE and
C. F. McCARTHY

INTRODUCTION

In the search for the toxic moiety of gluten, numerous fractions have
to be assessed. Intestinal biopsy studies, before and after fraction
feeding, require considerable toleration and cooperation on the part of
the patient. Although the biopsy signs of toxicity (histological and
biochemical) are usually obvious if present, the absence of toxic change
may indicate either a state of decreased sensitivity to toxic material in
a particular individual or the non-toxicity of the material under test.

The initial promise of *in vitro* toxicity assay, utilizing the organ culture
system has not been fulfilled as no parameter of toxicity has received
universal acceptance.

For the preliminary screening of gluten fractions a simple inexpensive
reliable *in vitro* technique measuring absorptive capacity has been
sought, which is acceptable to the patients.

The 0.1 mol (15 g) D-xylose absorption test has been shown to
differentiate the coeliac from non-coeliac patient[1], and its reproducibility
and performance as a gliadin toxicity assay has been assessed.

PATIENTS AND METHODS

The D-xylose absorption tests were carried out as detailed elsewhere[1].
Repeat tests in the same individual on the same diet were performed in
five untreated coeliac patients, three treated coeliac patients and eight
controls.

Adult coeliac patients in remission were studied before and after
feeding gliadin fractions. The initial xylose absorption study X_1 was
performed no more than 36 h before commencing fraction feeding. A

Table 49.1 Patient and study data

Patient	Age	Sex	Gliadin preparation	Duration of GFD (months)	Duration of feeding (days)	Gliadin eaten (g)
A	21	F	treated gliadin	14	4	45
	21		untreated gliadin	14	3	50
B	19	M	treated gliadin	34	6	47
C	22	M	treated gliadin	20	6	47
	21		untreated gliadin	10	5	48
D	51	F	untreated gliadin	4	4	40

subsequent xylose absorption study X_2 was performed within 24 h of completing fraction feeding. Patient data, length of time on the gluten-free diet prior to study, time interval after commencing feeding and the amount of each particular fraction consumed before X_2 is shown in Table 49.1. Intestinal biopsies were available before and after feeding enzyme-treated gliadin to patients A, B and C and before and after feeding untreated gliadin in patient D. (Biochemical and morphological data on these biopsies is presented in a previous communication — paper 5).

RESULTS

The variability of D-xylose absorption in the same individual on the same diet is shown in Figure 49.1. The abscissa represents the value obtained in the first test and the dots represent the difference between the first and second readings in an individual patient at the times indicated. From these figures a standard error of estimate SEE has been derived, (vertical bar alongside scatterogram). The reproducibility of the test is greatest at 75 and 90 min. Great variability is seen at 30 and 60 min, possibly related to the rate of gastric emptying, and the variability is high at 120 min as the xylose has passed beyond the area of maximal absorption.

In Figure 49.2 are the changes in xylose absorption in patient A

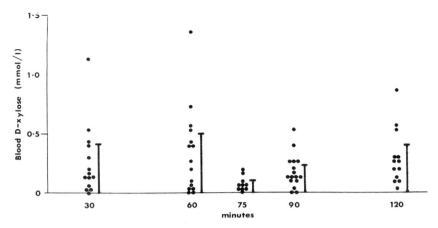

Figure 49.1 Variability of the 0.1 mol D-xylose absorption tests on the same individuals. The abscissa represents the initial xylose value. The variation, from the original, of the subsequent value in each individual is represented by a single dot. The vertical lines alongside the scatterogram shows the standard error estimate (SEE) at each time indicated.

following feeding enzyme-treated gliadin and untreated gliadin. Although there is a lower blood D-xylose level at 30 and 60 min after the feeding of enzyme-treated gliadin, the changes are within the 2 SEE of the test (approx. = 95% confidence limits). However, when untreated gliadin was fed, depression beyond the acceptable limits was seen at 60 and 90 min. No results were available at 75 min.

In Figure 49.3, the changes in xylose after feeding eznyme-treated gliadin in patient B are shown. Follwing feeding treated gliadin no changes outside the range of experimental error were seen.

In Figure 49.4, the changes in xylose blood levels after feeding enzyme-treated gliadin and untreated gliadin in patient C are shown. Although a lower blood xylose level was found at 30 and 60 min after feeding enzyme-treated gliadin, the changes are within the limits of the test. When untreated gliadin was fed, depression greater than acceptable within the limits of the test was found at 90 and 120 min.

In Figure 49.5 are shown the blood xylose changes found in patient D after feeding untreated gliadin. A depression of xylose absorption beyond the confidence limits of the test was found throughout the test.

The enzyme-treated gliadin fed to patients A, B and C produced no deterioration in morphological measurements, although it caused depression in activity of lactase and sucrase in two of the three patients. Untreated gliadin fed to patient D caused histological and biochemical damage. No mucosal histological or enzyme data is available, after

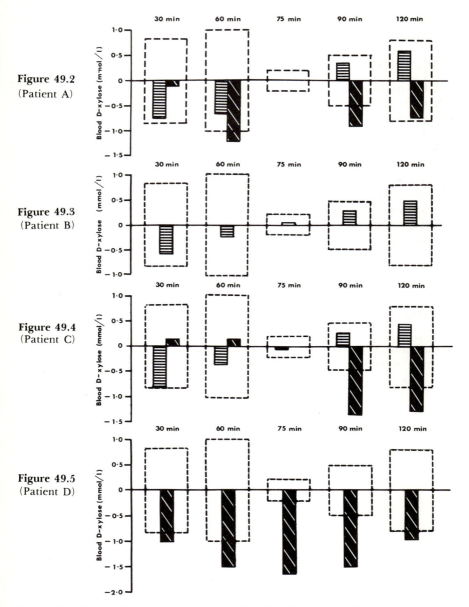

Figure 49.2
(Patient A)

Figure 49.3
(Patient B)

Figure 49.4
(Patient C)

Figure 49.5
(Patient D)

Figures 49.2–49.5 Changes in xylose blood levels after feeding gliadin preparations. Figures 49.2, 3, 4 and 5 represent patients A, B, C and D respectively. ▤ after treated gliadin; ◨ after untreated gliadin; ▬ ▬ ▬ ± 2 SEE (derived from Figure 49.1). The abscissa represents the xylose value in X_1. A positive deflection indicates an increased concentration; a negative deflection indicates a decreased concentration in the subsequent xylose value in X_2.

feeding untreated gliadin to patients A and C, but it is assumed that this material would be causing structural and functional damage.

DISCUSSION

The 0.1 mol D-xylose absorption test has proved acceptable to patients. When the test is repeated in the same individual the variability in blood xylose levels at 75 and 90 min is small.

Using the D-xylose absorption test as an index of toxicity, the results reflect the morphological picture after feeding enzyme-treated gliadin or untreated gliadin.

A depression of xylose blood levels was noted at 30 min and 60 min in all patients fed enzyme-treated gliadin, although this depression always fell within the confidence limits of the test, it may indicate either a slowing of gastric emptying or minimal damage to the mucosa as indicated by the fall in activity of lactase and sucrase.

References

1. Stevens, F. M., Watt, D. W., Bourke, M. A., McNicholl, B., Fotterell, P. F. and McCarthy, C. F. (1977). The 15 g D-xylose absorption test: its application to the study of coeliac disease. *J. Clin. Pathol.*, **30,** 76

Discussion of chapter 49

Peña	At the last meeting of the B.S.G. in April, the Birmingham group suggested that if you correct the xylose level for surface area you can increase the value of the test. Have you considered doing that? The second question is how long have you been giving your treated gliadin, have you given, for example, more than one day and have you done your test then?
Stevens	We have not corrected the blood xylose levels for surface area. With our test already we obtain good separation between coeliac and non-coeliac patients. We do not consider the test useful as a screening method for coeliac disease but rather as an assay of change in absorptive capacity during feeding studies. We feed our treated and untreated gliadin over a period of five days. I doubt if any significant change in body surface area would occur over this short period.
Rey	I am a little surprised by this result with the xylose test. After a week or a month or several months of normal diet many patients show no histological lesion. In your study you find each time a fall in xylose absortion after a very few days of a gluten-containing diet.
Stevens	Are your patients mainly children who have been on a strict gluten-free diet for many months prior to challenge?
Rey	Yes, they are children between two or three years old and 15 or 18.
Stevens	Some of the patients in our study, who are slightly older than yours may have been on a strict-gluten-free diet for only a short period prior to study, although a strict gluten-free diet had been recommended several years previously. I have reason to believe that the majority of young adult coeliac patients cheat fairly frequently. When they receive notification to come to hospital they return to as strict gluten-free diet for the two weeks before study.
Sinaasapel	We challenged one of the patients I showed yesterday with gliadin for one day; he had a xylose one hour test before the challenge which was 50 mg %, and the day after the challenge was 20 mg %. In our hands the test is reproducible.
Nusslé	Like J. Rey I am also surprised by your results. I have studied with the one-hour xylose test 50 children with a flat mucosa and untreated coeliac disease. In 10 cases that is 20% of cases there were normal values of xylose after 60 minutes. The reflection of the state of the mucosa seems to be problematical.
Stevens	Can I ask you, did you look at fasting level or do you just do a one-hour level?
Nusslé	One hour.

Stevens	A fasting reference sample is an essential part of the test. Other pentoses found in the diet produce a positive colour with p-bromoaniline used to assay blood xylose. In addition xylose is a normal constitutent of the diet, being found in fruit and cereals.
Nusslé	The children were fasting before the xylose test.
Stevens	Even though patients are fasting, they continue to absorb from the intestinal contents for many hours after a meal. In this study a fasting xylose of 0.73 mmol/l (10.9 mg%) was recorded in a patient.

50

The patient's view of a gluten-free diet

R. E. BARRY, C. HENRY and A. E. READ

INTRODUCTION

Gluten is present in a large number of foodstuffs where it might not be expected. Consequently, the dietary instructions given to a patient starting a gluten-free diet have become extremely complex. One wonders how many gastroenterologists would answer correctly the question posed by Figure 50.1. Because of the complexity of the gluten-free diet, new patients are faced with a large number of problems in the course of their treatment which must influence their ability or desire to comply with the treatment. We have studied the eating patterns learned by patients taking a gluten-free diet and the problems they have experienced in the hope that the insight so gained, may enable us to anticipate, and thus avoid, the more frequent pitfalls.

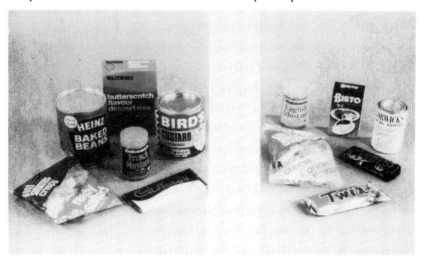

Figure 50.1   Which side is gluten-free?

PATIENTS STUDIED

Sixty-two patients were included in the study. They attended our Coeliac Clinic consecutively and were interviewed by an experienced dietician after first completing a formal questionnaire on their dietary habits and disease-related problems. Patients not taking a gluten-free diet or admitting to more than the occasional lapse were excluded from the study.

The patients' interest and concern for their condition is indicated to sme extent by the high proportion (85%) who were active members of the local branch of the Coeliac Society.

EATING HABITS

Patients fell into two distinct categories in the way in which their gluten-free diet was taken:

(a) Diet by Omission: 10% of patients merely omitted all gluten containing foods from a normal diet. It might be expected that these consisted of single patients living alone, but this was not so. This group seemed to consist of a representative cross-section of the whole patient population. All but two patients taking a diet by omission did so because of a dislike for the taste of gluten-free foods, particularly bread, but a further four patients felt that the inconvenience of preparing gluten-free bread was a factor in their decision.

(b) Diet by Substitution: 90% of patients excluded gluten containing foods but substituted a similar food which was free from gluten. Bread was the major substitute. A total of 58% used a commercially available bread mix; 26% baked their own gluten-free bread from gluten-free flour, whilst 16% used a commercially prepared tinned bread, but all except two of these used this preparation for toasting only.

It became apparent to us, in the course of this study, that in a few patients of a particular personality trait, the institution of a gluten-free diet appeared to trigger the development of somewhat obsessional atitudes to food which in some cases bordered on the eccentric, or even bizarre (Figure 50.2).

PROBLEMS OF THE GLUTEN-FREE DIET

The problems volunteered by patients in order of frequency were as follows:—

1) Holidays

A total of 58% of patients who coped adequately with their gluten-free diet in a home environment found that they experienced considerable difficulties when away from home. Holidays were a major source of concern. Forty-two per cent did not consider holidays to pose a problem and the remainder coped with their gluten-free diet by:—

MILLET AND MUSHROOM CASSEROLE

    cu   millet (raw)   4 tbs oil
onions, chopped   about 2 pints hot water
    lb. mushrooms,chopped   or stock
                                   1 tsp. salt or kelp

 aute mushrooms in oil 5 minutes   Set aside Saute
chopped onions until browned and set aside Toss millet
in same oil and stir well till all grains are coated
Remove. Mix with mushrooms and onions and pour hot
water over the mixture. Turn into an oiled casserole
Cover and bake in moderate oven, 350°F , Regulo 4 about
60 minutes, adding little more liquid if needed
Sprinkle with chopped chives or parsley before serving

PUMPKIN PUDDING AND POPCORN

Cut up one small pumpkin in wedges, after removing
seeds and membranes Steam on rack over a little
boiling water in a covered pan, till tender - about
15 minutes Remove skin and mash smoothly with a
little lemon juice and honey to taste. Turn into
an oiled pie dish, dot with freshly popped corn and
brown lightly in oven. Serve with top of the milk.

CARROT AND CHIVE CUTLETS

    cups basic rice(cooked)   2 tbs powdered milk
  tbs. chopped chives   1 egg, beaten
  large carrot, grated finely
  tbs. finely chopped peanuts 2 tbs oil
  tsp. salt or kelp   Maizemeal to coat

 ash rice with fork till quite smooth Mix in chives,
carrot, peanuts, powdered milk and salt Shape into
 utlets, set aside on plate to dry Dip in egg and
coat with maizemeal Heat oil in pan and fry cutlets
until lightly browned on both sides

PEA SHELL POTAGE

2 lb. fresh young pea shells   Pinch of salt and
1 onion (small) or   Barbados sugar
        3 shallots   ½ pint of milk
1 sprig of mint

Wash the shells, and drop them into enough salted
sugared boiling water to cover. Peel and chop
onion and add. Boil till softish. Allow to cool
in bowl then add mint. Liquidize and strain through
sieve

CREAMED BRAINS WITH CHEESE

1 lb. brains prepared and diced   ½-1 tsp salt (depends on
1 cup milk   cheese)
1 tbs. powdered milk   4 tbs. cheese, grated
                                  2 tbs. finely chopped parsley

Mix powdered milk smoothly with fresh, and bring to
boiling point. Drop in diced brains and simmer till brains
are tender, about 15-20 minutes. Stir in salt, turn out
 n to dish, sprinkle with grated cheese and parsley
and serve with saute potatoes and yellow or green vegetable.

HERB MEATCAKES

  lb. better quality minced beef. 1 beaten egg
  tbs. chopped chives
  tsp. dried thyme   2 tbs. rice or soya flour.

 ix all together in bowl very well and shape
 nto thin, flat cakes. Coat with rice flour
 r soya flour. Grill, bake or saute in oil
 ill nicely brown on both sides.

Figure 50.2

   a) taking a self-catering holiday
   b) giving hoteliers prior notice of their requirements
   c) staying only with a relative

2) Constipation

The frequency of bowel movements declines considerably on a gluten-free diet since many patients suffer from diarrhoea in the untreated state. However, in an unpublished review of 86 cases of coeliac disease in our care, we found that 33% of patients irrespective of the age of onset presented *not* with an acute malabsorption syndrome, but with the insidious onset of such symptoms as anaemia, gradual weight loss, aphthous ulceration, oedema and skin troubles. Some of these patients regarded themselves as constipated before being treated with a gluten-free diet but after six months' treatment 28% of patients complained of constipation which in some cases was so severe that the patient felt obliged to stray from their diet!

3) Obesity

The risk or fear of obesity emerged as a significant problem particularly among female patients. Table 50.1 shows the mean weight gain in male and female patients, six and 12 months after starting a gluten-free diet. There is no difference between the males and females in the first six months of treatment. Subsequently, the rate of weight gain between the

Table I Effect of gluten-free diet on weight

	Males	Females
Mean ($\pm$ SD) weight gain after 6 months' diet	5.78 $\pm$ 4.2 kg	6.43 $\pm$ 5.5 kg
Mean ($\pm$ SD) weight gain after 12 months' diet	1.89 $\pm$ 3.8 kg	−0.13 $\pm$ 3.4 kg

two sexes diverges. Males continue to gain weight though at a smaller rate after their initial rapid rise, but females tend to decrease in weight. We believe that this is due to an active effort by female patients to reduce or reverse their weight gain for fear of obesity.

4) Expense

This emerged as an unexpected problem in 21% of patients. The reasons given for the additional expense incurred by a gluten-free diet were:−

a) The increased fuel costs for those baking gluten-free bread and pastries frequently;

b) the prepared and processed foods which were known to be gluten-free tend to be the more costly brand names;

c) protein foods, particularly meat, taken in lieu of bread are considerably more expensive.

5) Other less frequent problems

These included yearning for normal foods, problems when dining out and when entertaining at home, and ignorant General Practitioners who, in some cases, would refuse prescriptions for gluten-free products.

It was clear from the survey that many of the problems experienced by patients on a gluten-free diet are avoidable or remediable when examined critically. Consider again the problem of constipation, the magnitude of which we had previously failed to appreciate.

Wheat fibre is the major natural source of fibre in the normal gluten-containing diet. The gluten-free diet must of necessity be free from wheat fibre with the result that this diet may frequently be grossly fibre depleted even when, as is our custom, oats are not routinely excluded. We have studied the intestinal transit time in 10 patients who complained of constipation while on such a diet. Intestinal transit time was measured by the method of Cummings and Wiggins (1976). Patients were then treated with an alternative source of non-wheat cereal fibre and the transit time measured again after four weeks' treatment. The fibre source used was defatted rice bran (Figure 50.3) kindly supplied by Riviana Foods Inc. The symptomatic relief obtained on this treatment was dramatic (Figure 50.4). The results are shown in Table 50.2. For the group as a whole, the mean transit time fell from 62 h to 45 h ($p < 0.01$). Normal transit time by this method is approx-

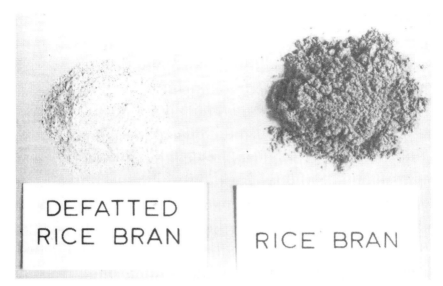

Figure 50.3 Defatted rice bran (left) used to treat constipation in this study. The composition is presented in the Addendum. Normal rice bran (right) has a very short shelf life because of its tendency for its fat content to go rancid. Defatted rice bran retains the bulking properties of rice bran and has a very long shelf life and finer texture.

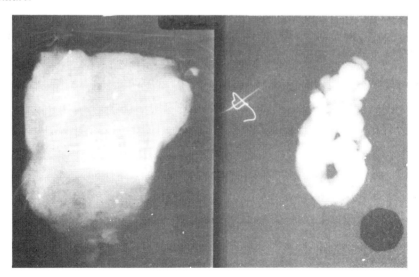

Figure 50.4 X-ray of stool from patient on a gluten-free diet before (right) and after four weeks of treatment (left) with defatted rice bran 25 g daily. The size on the right is indicated by the shadow of a 50p coin. The radio opaque markers from which transit time may be calculated can be seen.

Table 50.2   Effect of rice bran on intestinal transit time in patients on a gluten-free diet

Patient number	Gluten-free diet alone	Gluten-free diet plus rice bran
1	37.3 h	29.0 h
2	59.1	68.2
3	37.0	30.0
4	83.5	63.2
5	55.8	33.0
6	73.7	41.0
7	63.5	34.2
8	87.0	67.8
9	62.0	49.7
10	67.2	34.9
Mean ± SD	62. ± 16.8	45.1 ± 15.9
	$p < 0.01$	

imately 36 h. We can, therefore, strongly recommend defatted rice bran as a cheap and very effective way of treating the constipation of coeliac disease.

CONCLUSION

A wider appreciation by physicians of the problems experienced by patients on a gluten-free diet may help to alleviate these problems and improve patient compliance.

Addendum

Composition of defatted rice bran (Lynn, 1969)		
	Defatted rice bran %	Commercial rice bran mix %
Protein	17.0–21.0	11.0–13.0
Moisture	8.0–12.0	9.0–12.0
Fat	0.5– 2.5	13.0–15.0
Crude fibre	6.0– 8.0	7.0–11.0
Ash	9.5–12.5	11.0–13.5
Ash Composition		
Silica	4.0– 5.5	20.0–27.0
Calcium	12.5–15.0	13.0–16.0
Magnesium	1.5– 2.5	1.8– 4.0
Potassium	12.0–15.0	10.0–14.0

References

Cummings, J. H. and Wiggins, H. S. (1976). Transit through the gut measured by analysis of single stool. *Gut*, **17**, 219

Lynn, L. (1969). In: *Protein Enriched Cereal Foods for World Needs*. Milner, M. (ed.) St. Paul. MN: American Assoc. of Cereal Chemists

Discussion of chapter 50

Unidentified speaker	We don't seem to see as much constipation in Australia and America. A large problem for coeliacs is the failure of many commercial products to indicate whether they contain gluten or not.
Barry	Thank you for your comment; perhaps I should point out that my experience of coeliac disease is not in fact limited to England. I would agree that the incidence of constipation in England is probably higher than in many other areas but the magnitude of the problem was something which we just didn't appreciate until we actually looked for it; may I just suggest that if you look actively for constipation you may find it. There is of course a fad in England at the moment for people to eat anything as long as it comes out of a donkey's nose bag, but this sort of approach is very difficult for a coeliac.
Leighton	I want to point out that a great many of the troubles that you mention can be cured by all coeliacs joining a Coeliac Society; in our Society we have holiday sheets, we have a list of holidays in the UK and we have holiday hints for those going abroad; for those going to foreign restaurants, we have sheets with appropriate phrases.

51

Chronic inflammatory neuromuscular disorders associated with treated coeliac disease

J. J. BERNIER, A. BUGE, J. C. RAMBAUD, G. RANCUREL, J. J. HAUW, C. L'HIRONDEL and D. DENVIL

Neurological disorders occurring during the course of adult coeliac disease (ACD) are usually thought to be the consequence of a deficiency state secondary to malabsorption. However chronic neurological disorders may sometimes develop in ACD without any recognized deficiency[1]. We are reporting three cases of this peculiar disease which occured in three women on a gluten-free diet. Symptoms at the time of presentation and pathological findings in two of these patients have been reported previously[2]. They were suffering from a mainly

Table 51.1 Main neurological findings

Patients	1 4 limbs	2 inf. limbs	3 sup.limbs
Hypoaesthesia			
temperature	+	+	+
proprioceptive	+	+	+
vibration	+	+	+
Paraesthesia	+	+	+
Tendon reflexes	0	0	0
Ataxia	+	+	+
Lighting pain	+	+	+
Proximal muscle decreased power	+	+	0
Muscle pain	+	+	+
Babinski	0	+	0

sensory and distal polyneuropathy associated with signs of proximal muscular disease /Table 51.1). One patient had involvement of the pyramidal tract with inflammatory changes in the CSF. We did not find any abnormality of muscle enzyme activity, motor nerve conduction velocity or electromyography. These symptoms evolved slowly in spite of strict adherance to a gluten-free diet and of vitamin therapy. Corticosteroid therapy (synthetic ACTH for two months, then oral steroids) was associated with improvement of symptoms in two patients and stabilization in one. The usual aetiologies of such disorders were excluded; in particular, there was no vitamin deficiency, dysglobulinaemia, lupus erythematosus or rheumatoid arthritis. Histological examinations of paraffin-embedded sections from neuromuscular biopsies showed the

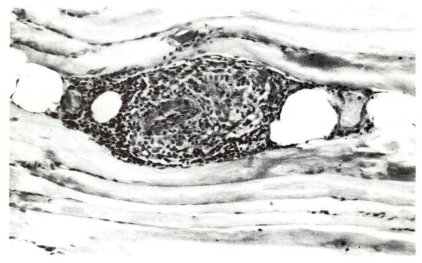

Figure 51.1 Muscle section—P.A.S. × 182. Perivascular inflammatory cuff and occluded lumen

same lesions in nerves and muscles. These lesions (Figure 51.1) consisted of perivascular inflammatory cuffs with mainly lymphocytes and a few histiocytic cells. They involved small diameter arterioles, venules and capillaries. The vascular wall was sometimes affected with little or no fibrinoid necrosis and occasional lumen thrombosis. The lesional pattern was quite focal. These lesions appeared to be of a microvasculitic type, different from periarteritis nodosa. They could be included in the provisional group of 'allergic angeitis' considered to be related to circulating immunocomplexes. Such complexes have been found in coeliac patients on a gluten-free diet[3].

References

1. Cook, W. T. and Smith, W. T. (1966). Neurological disorders associated with adult coeliac disease. *Brain,* **89,** 683
2. Bernier, J. J., Buge, A., Rambaud, J. C., Rancurel, G., Hauw, J. J., Modigliani, R. and Denvil, D. (1976). Polyneuropathies chroniques non carentielles au cours de la maladie coeliaque de l'adulte. *Ann. Med. Int.,* **127,** 721
3. Idris, M., Holborow, E. J., Fry L., Thompson, B., Hoffbrand, A. V. and Stewart, J. S. (1976). Multiple immune complexes and hypocomplementemia in dermatitis herpetiformis and coeliac disease. *Lancet,* **ii,** 487

Discussion of chapter 51

Eggermont	I would suggest caution in concluding that there is a causal relationship between two diseases that happen to occur in the same patient.
Ferguson	I have a patient dying with a neuropathy, but who also has cranial nerve and hypothalamic lesions. Have you, or Dr Cooke, heard of similar patients with central as well as peripheral nervous disease?
L'Hirondel	We have no evidence of central involvement in our patients. With regard to treatment, improvement may be slow and it was eight months before any effect was noted in one patient.
Cooke	Corticosteroids don't help much in the majority of patients, only occasionally.

Poster sessions

1. The incidence of coeliac disease in Newfoundland. S. H. Roberts, Newfoundland and Newcastle-upon-Tyne

2. Screening families for coeliac disease
B. Egan-Mitchell, Fiona M. Stevens, P. F. Fottrell, C. F. McCarthy and B. McNicholl, Galway

3. Histocompatibility antigen involvement in an Irish coeliac disease population
T. J. Murtagh, A. Howe, E. Tempany, D. J. Kelly, J. E. Greally, D. G. Weir, Dublin

4. Schizophrenia and coeliac disease
Fiona M. Stevens, R. S. Lloyd, S. M. J. Geraghty, M. T. G. Reynolds, M. J. Sarsfield, B. McNicholl, P. F. Fottrell, R. Wright and C. F. McCarthy, Galway and Southampton

5. Further evidence of a primary mucosal defect in coeliac disease
H. J. Cornell, C. J. Rolles and C. M. Anderson, Birmingham

6. Chromatographic and electrophoretic properties of gliadin peptides before and after treatment with detoxifying enzymes
W. F. Cleere and J. J. Phelan, Galway

7. *In vitro* digestion of gliadin
H. Carchon and E. Eggermont, Leuven

8. Intestinal peptidases: studies on the specificity of normal and coeliac enzymes
J. J. Phelan, J. Donlon, Fiona M. Stevens, C. F. McCarthy and P. F. Fottrell, Galway

9. The systemic distribution of protein derivatives of gliadin after oral administration
C. Hemmings, W. A. Hemmings and E. W. Williams, Bangor

10. The significance of a high count of intraepithelial lymphocytes in a jejunal biospy
A. Ferguson, J. Gillon and F. Allan, Edinburgh

11. Depression of cell-mediated immunity in coeliac disease
A. W. Bullen, B. B. Scott and M. S. Losowsky, Leeds

12. Splenic atrophy in coeliac disease
A. W. Bullen, R. C. Brown, R. Hall, P. Robinson and M. S. Losowsky, Leeds

13. Coeliac disease 1950–73 at the Birmingham Children's Hospital
M. J. Brueton, C. M. Anderson, A. Regusci, C. J. Rolles, Wai-Kee Sin and T. O. Kyaw-Myint, Birmingham

14. Mucosal recovery in treated childhood coeliac disease
B. McNicholl, B. Egan-Mitchell, Fiona M. Stevens, R. Keane, S. Baker, C. F. McCarthy and P. F. Fottrell, Galway

Index